I0049607

# Health and Wellbeing in Sexual Orientation and Gender Identity

# Health and Wellbeing in Sexual Orientation and Gender Identity

Special Issue Editor

**Catherine Meads**

MDPI • Basel • Beijing • Wuhan • Barcelona • Belgrade • Manchester • Tokyo • Cluj • Tianjin

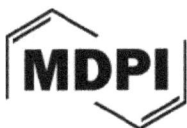

**MDPI**

*Special Issue Editor*
Catherine Meads
Anglia Ruskin University
UK

*Editorial Office*
MDPI
St. Alban-Anlage 66
4052 Basel, Switzerland

This is a reprint of articles from the Special Issue published online in the open access journal *International Journal of Environmental Research and Public Health* (ISSN 1660-4601) (available at: https://www.mdpi.com/journal/ijerph/special_issues/Health_Sexual_Orientation).

For citation purposes, cite each article independently as indicated on the article page online and as indicated below:

LastName, A.A.; LastName, B.B.; LastName, C.C. Article Title. *Journal Name* **Year**, *Article Number, Page Range.*

**ISBN 978-3-03928-368-2 (Pbk)**
**ISBN 978-3-03928-369-9 (PDF)**

© 2020 by the authors. Articles in this book are Open Access and distributed under the Creative Commons Attribution (CC BY) license, which allows users to download, copy and build upon published articles, as long as the author and publisher are properly credited, which ensures maximum dissemination and a wider impact of our publications.

The book as a whole is distributed by MDPI under the terms and conditions of the Creative Commons license CC BY-NC-ND.

# Contents

# About the Special Issue Editor

**Catherine Meads** is a Professor of Health at Anglia Ruskin University and senior systematic reviewer. She has been conducting research into lesbian, gay, bisexual and transgender (LGBT) health since 1992 and has published a number of papers on this topic. Recently she completed a best-evidence review for Public Health England on healthcare experiences and health of UK sexual minority women. She has also delivered numerous public lectures, taught undergraduate medical students, helped develop an e-learning package for GPs and has been on several LGBT conference steering committees. She is currently a member of the UK Government Equalities Office LGBT Advisory Panel.

# Preface to "Health and Wellbeing in Sexual Orientation and Gender Identity"

Improving the health of particular populations is an important objective for public health service planners, policymakers and care delivery staff. This is especially important for disadvantaged minority groups such as people of minority sexual orientation and gender identity populations, where robust evidence to show considerable health inequities is developing. Improving health and wellbeing is an important objective for all who aspire to reduce health inequities (inequalities that are considered preventable). It is important to understand various factors that contribute to lesbian, gay, bisexual, trans and similar (LGBT+) groups' mental and physical health and the mediators and moderators of these relationships. This Special Issue was open to any subject area related to sexual orientation, gender identity, and physical or mental health and wellbeing, and considered systematic reviews as well as primary qualitative or quantitative research. The result is an interesting collection of published papers from around the world. They showed how health inequities in LGBT+ groups of people were found across a wide variety of political environments and health and wellbeing topics. Several focussed on healthcare delivery and its inadequacies regarding the treatment and care of LGBT+ people. The increasing interest in health and wellbeing research for minority sexual orientation and gender identity populations, which have been neglected in the past, shows its growing importance. It is hoped that this collection will contribute to the growing body of evidence around LGBT+ health and wellbeing that can be used by service planners, policymakers and the general public.

**Catherine Meads**
*Special Issue Editor*

International Journal of
*Environmental Research and Public Health*

MDPI

*Article*

# The Power of Recognition: A Qualitative Study of Social Connectedness and Wellbeing through LGBT Sporting, Creative and Social Groups in Ireland

Nerilee Ceatha [1,*], Paula Mayock [2], Jim Campbell [1], Chris Noone [3] and Kath Browne [4]

1   School of Social Policy, Social Work and Social Justice, University College Dublin, Belfield, Dublin 4, Ireland; jim.campbell@ucd.ie
2   School of Social Work and Social Policy, Trinity College, Dublin 2, Ireland; pmayock@tcd.ie
3   School of Psychology, National University of Ireland Galway, Galway, Ireland; chris.noone@nuigalway.ie
4   School of Geography, University College Dublin, Belfield, Dublin 4, Ireland; kath.browne@ucd.ie
*   Correspondence: nerilee.ceatha@ucdconnect.ie

Received: 7 August 2019; Accepted: 24 September 2019; Published: 27 September 2019

**Abstract:** The broad research consensus suggesting substantial vulnerabilities among lesbian, gay, bisexual and transgender (LGBT) communities may fail to recognize the protective factors available to these populations. The sparse literature on mental health promotion highlights the importance of understanding strengths-based community approaches that promote LGBT wellbeing. Informed by the *Ottawa Charter for Health Promotion*, underpinned by Honneth's *Theory of Recognition*, this paper outlines the findings of a qualitative Irish study on LGBT social connectedness through a diverse range of sporting, creative and social interests. Ten in-depth interviews were conducted with 11 people (including one couple) who self-identified as lesbian (5), gay (4), bisexual (1) and transgender (1) aged between 22 and 56 years. A university Research Ethics Committee granted approval. The data were transcribed and coded using thematic analysis, enhanced through a memo-writing approach to reflexivity. The theme of 'connecting' emphasized the shared nature of activities, with like-minded others through groups established by, and for, LGBT communities. Messages from the study reinforce the central role of LGBT communities in the promotion of mental health and social wellbeing, with important policy and practice implications. This requires the contextualization of the contribution of LGBT communities within understandings of social justice, identity and recognition.

**Keywords:** LGBT; wellbeing; Ottawa Charter; recognition; Theory of Recognition; mental health; social inclusion and sense of community; social participation; community participation; social connectedness; community connectedness

## 1. Introduction

According to the World Health Organization (WHO) "wellbeing is fundamental to quality of life, enabling people to experience life as meaningful and to be creative and active citizens" [1]. The WHO makes a further contribution to our understanding of wellbeing through the *Ottawa Charter for Health Promotion*, which defines health promotion as: "the process of enabling people to increase control over, and to improve, their health" [2] The *Charter* emphasizes the need to both change the environment and strengthen the person, acknowledging that:

> *People cannot achieve their fullest health potential unless they are able to take control of those things which determine their health.* [2]

Social connectedness has been identified as a pivotal concept in approaches to mental health promotion and core to wellbeing, as articulated in *Connecting for life: Ireland's national strategy to reduce* suicide 2015–2020 [3]. This strategy seeks to promote a society "where communities and individuals are empowered to improve their mental health and wellbeing" [3]. It highlights protective factors, such as social connectedness, in reducing isolation and promoting help-seeking. The Strategy's second goal is to strengthen community capacity, in recognition that:

> *An empowered community can respond to the needs of its members and protect them in difficult times and can sustain these positive effects over time.* [3]

While *Connecting for Life* adopts a whole population approach, it also identifies specific priority groups, notably those vulnerable to suicide, including lesbian, gay, bisexual and transgender (LGBT) communities. Such policies tend to refer to a broad, albeit contested, notion of heightened LGBT mental health risk, typically contextualized within a minority stress framework [4], describing the consequences of discrimination against, and victimization of, minority groups [3–5]. Thus, it is contended that:

> *LGBT people are at a heightened risk of psychological distress because of the stresses created by stigmatisation, marginalisation and discrimination.* [6]

In this way, *Connecting for Life* aligns with the five-pronged approach outlined in the *Ottawa Charter* [2,6]. As such, the potential of the interconnection of healthy policies and supportive environments, which enable strong connected communities and support individuals' agency in relation to their wellbeing [2], is of particular relevance for LGBT populations [3–6].

The concept of social justice has been identified within the *Ottawa Charter* as one such prerequisite for health [2]. While there are multiple definitions of the concept, distinctions have been drawn between redistributive and recognitive forms of justice. Redistributive justice identifies the political-economic structures as causing social injustice with Fraser expanding the concept to include recognition: "*Cultural injustice is rooted in social patterns of representation, interpretation and communication* [7]. Fraser's notion of "recognitive justice" [7] highlights the importance of revaluing disrespected identities and argues for recognition of the cultural axis of injustice in order to promote cultural diversity through group differentiation [7]. Honneth, drawing on the work of Hegel, Mead and Taylor, further developed these ideas on recognition:

> *The moral quality of social relations cannot be measured only in terms of the fair and just distribution of material goods, rather, our notion of justice is also linked very closely to how, and as what, subjects mutually recognise each other.* (p. 17). [8]

In Honneth's *Theory of Recognition*, such forms of recognition are critical in revaluing disrespected identities [9]. Honneth applies his framework of social justice to emancipation struggles which can promote cultural diversity through group differentiation [10]. In this way, the struggle for recognition provides the impetus for social change [8,9]. Importantly, claims for rightful identity recognition are the motivation for social transformation [9]. This application includes activism by LGBT communities described as:

> *culturally integrated communities with a common history, language and sensibility ... [who] developed a self-understanding ... a transformation of collective self-understanding ... that could lead to the claim for recognition of one's own culture ... The concept of "identity politics" captures this idea.* [10]

The tripartite framework developed by Honneth has three interlinking spheres of recognition: intersubjective recognition; recognition of individual members through community and social networks; and legal recognition of universal rights [9]. This tripartite framework is outlined in Table 1 below:

**Table 1.** Honneth's Theory of Recognition [9].

| Forms of Recognition | Interpersonal Relations | Community Relations | Legal Relations |
|---|---|---|---|
| Mode | Intersubjective | Community contribution | Universal rights and inclusion |
| Potential | Security and resilience | Valuing strengths and competence | Empowerment |
| Impact | Self-confidence | Self-esteem | Self-respect |
| Community impact | Social networks | Social solidarity | Social integrity |

Honneth argued that intersubjective recognition is reciprocal in that there is mutual recognition by others whom one also recognizes. This supports the development of security and resilience: "The certainty about the value of one's own needs can be called "self-confidence" [9]. However, the *Theory of Recognition* both encompasses and surpasses interpersonal relationships to include the recognition of the unique contribution of community members and legal recognition of universal human rights [9]. He identified that recognition is through community relations where: "the individual is recognized as a person whose capabilities are of constitutive value to a concrete community" [9]. This acknowledgment results in self-worth. Honneth identified that recognition necessarily required forms of legal relations involving rights that have "the character of universal human treatment". This, in turn, promotes empowerment whereby "such a type of certainty about the value of one's own judgment can be called self-respect" [9].

In this way, Honneth emphasized the importance of recognition for LGBT people and communities, highlighting the potential of the social environment to enable strong, connected communities that support LGBT wellbeing [2]. This provides a basis for evaluating whether LGBT communities are supported through interpersonal, community and legal recognition in order to gain control over health, which is fundamental to health promotion [2,9]. This is of particular relevance given that policy approaches frequently recognize that LGBT people are at heightened mental health risk [3–5]. On the other hand, a number of researchers have cautioned against such overly negative discourses which tend to offer limited framing of LGBT lived experience, particularly that of LGBT youth [11–15]. It is important, therefore, to acknowledge alternative narratives that explore positive connotations of mental health and social wellbeing, consistent with the *Social Determinants of Health*:

> *As social beings, we need … to feel valued and appreciated … Belonging to a social network of communication and mutual obligation … has a powerful protective effect on health.* [16]

The predominant focus on LGBT mental health risk has tended to obscure alternative approaches that emphasize LGBT strengths-based community approaches to LGBT social connection and wellbeing [17]. It has been argued that "current conceptualizations fail to explain why many LGBT people enjoy good health despite adversity" (p. 5). [17]. Hass et al., while confirming the consensus of health inequalities for LGBT communities, equally acknowledge the limitations of the existing research base, arguing that "(r)elatively little research has been done on factors that protect the large majority of LGB people from suicidal behavior" [3] (pp. 26). They go on to recommend that future research priorities should:

> *Conduct studies of factors that protect against or mitigate the impact of suicide risk factors … and factors that contribute to the development of resiliency … studies should also include potentially protective factors such as … community connectedness.* [3]

In conclusion, the important principles of the *Ottawa Charter*, underpinned by Honneth's *Theory of Recognition* [8–10], offers the the potential for novel approaches to social and community connectedness that highlight more positive aspects of LGBT individual and collective wellbeing. This will now be explored in relation to the following: healthy policies; supportive environments; community action; personal skills; and reorienting health services [2].

## 1.1. Building Health-Promoting Policy

LGBT communities have been at the forefront of long-standing activism in relation to legal recognition in Ireland [18]. While homosexuality was not decriminalized until 1993, there has since been greater recognition of LGBT rights. In 2014, at the *International Day Against Homophobia and Transphobia*, the Irish Government became a signatory to the non-binding *Declaration of Intent*, which asserts that:

> *Human beings are entitled to the full enjoyment of all human rights, regardless of sexual orientation and/or gender identity.* (p. 1) [19]

This commitment informed legislative and policy measures including those seeking to combat discrimination. In 2015, a referendum was passed which amended the Irish Constitution, providing for marriage-equality legislation [20]. That same year, Ireland enacted the Gender Recognition Act [21], with a review making further recommendations for people under 18 years of age [22]. Such initiatives may provide a foundation for a society committed to respecting diversity and empowering LGBT communities, as advocated by Honneth [8–10]. However, it is not clear how well such ideas have been translated into health policies and the promotion of wellbeing, and specifically, in relation to protective factors for LGBT communities. *Connecting for Life* asserted that:

> … *research [is] under-developed in the Irish context, and identified as [a] priority: focus on the protective factors for mental health* … *and how these can be ameliorated within prevention programmes.* [3]

Further, the publication of the *LGBTI+ National Youth Strategy* as part of the Irish programme government acknowledged the "limited availability of Irish-specific data, statistics and … research relating to young LGBTI+ people in Ireland and, more broadly, the general LGBTI+ population" (p. 13) [23]. In response, the Strategy identified three overarching goals, with the third of these prioritizing the development of the research and data environment with a specific objective to "develop research into the factors that support positive mental health for LGBTI+ young people" [23] (p.31).

## 1.2. Creating Supportive Environments

The importance of supportive social environments has been identified as essential in empowering individuals [2,3]. The Irish Department of Justice is currently developing an LGBT inclusion strategy to: "target discrimination, promote inclusion, and improve quality of life and wellbeing for LGBTI people" [24]. While such strategies are welcome, it has been acknowledged that homonegativity and transphobia do not disappear as a result legislative and policy changes [25]. Thus, broader supportive societal environments are recognized as key factors in promoting LGBT wellbeing. Such approaches have been embraced with the development of LGBT inclusion strategies by mainstream sporting bodies, for example [26]. Yet Abichahine and Veenstra found that while lesbian or bisexual women are more likely to involved in sport, the trend is reversed for gay and bisexual men [27]. Denison and Kitchen highlighted the gender-normative and homophobic experiences of LGBT-identified people within mainstream sport [28]. This may, in part, explain the reluctance to engage in sport within LGBT communities, particularly by gay, bisexual and transgender men. Ceatha has suggested that LGBT community involvement in interest sharing provides opportunities to challenge stereotypes, for example, regarding gay men and their interests [29]. Further, Browne, Bakshi and Lim suggest that LGBT community spaces, both formal and informal, may provide a sense of safety, beyond heteronormative and gendered assumptions [25].

Perhaps such experiences account for the global proliferation of groups, established by and for LGBT communities, over the past 45 years [30]. These groups include: Frontrunners, established in 1974, with over 100 LGBT athletics clubs worldwide [31]; *Various Voices*, a biannual LGBT choir festival [32]; the *Bingham Cup*, an annual international rugby competition [28]; a plethora of LGBT film festivals [33]; an International Theatre Festival [34]; and the *Gay Games* [35]. In applying recognition theory to these contexts, it is possible to understand how such social solidarity contributes to the creation of supportive environments established by and maintained for LGBT communities [2,8–10].

### 1.3. Strengthening Community Action

The literature tends to highlight the potential for social connectedness through LGBT communities to impact positively on LGBT identity and wellbeing [36–39]. Formby explored LGBT people's understanding and experience of 'community' and the impact on self-reported wellbeing [36]. She found that most participants expressed a sense of belonging through an LGBT identity with 'like-minded' others, with others identifying collective LGBT identity as formed through shared experiences of discrimination [36]. Further, Detrie and Lease explored a sense of connection within LGBT communities where collective self-esteem tended to contribute to participants' psychological wellbeing [37]. Similarly, DiFulvio found an association between positive self-identification, social support within LGBT communities and greater social and psychological wellbeing [38]. An alternative finding by Kertzner et al. highlighted the potential negative impact of LGBT social and community connections [39]. This, perhaps, may explain Formby's finding that some participants resisted the commonly used term 'LGBT community' as a singular readymade entity which assumes an inevitable sense of belonging [36].

While not all people who identify as LGBT have a social connection to a singular 'LGBT community', Formby suggests a more appropriate usage may be reference to 'LGBT communities', which emphasizes the diversity 'within and between' those who identify as LGBT [36].

### 1.4. Developing Personal Skills

Building individual skills in promoting social, mental and physical health, it has been argued, involves sharing the requisite knowledge to empower, foster mastery and promote self-esteem. The *Ottawa Charter* emphasizes the need to strengthen the person within the context of a changed environment [2], recognising the structural constraints on LGBT agency. Wilkinson and Marmot concur, noting in the *Social Determinants of Health* that exclusion has a social meaning and impacts negatively on health and wellbeing [16]. This is consistent with Meyer's concept of minority stress [4].

Androite highlighted DeVries' emphasis on the importance of LGBT social connections in attenuating the impact of minority stress [40]. Others have argued that community connectedness may ameliorate the effects of stigmatization, prejudice and discrimination [37–41], a position which accords with Honneth's ideas [8–10]. The concept of interpersonal recognition has the potential to develop individual resilience and promote self-confidence [9]. In addition, Heard, Lake and McCluskey suggested that the connection with others and their positive response through affirmation or encouragement, increases creativity and vitality with a subsequent increase in the sense of wellbeing [42]. Spencer and Patrick identify the importance of the concept of mastery and social support, which they suggest could account for differences in self-reported LGBT psychological wellbeing [43]. A similar conclusion was drawn by Ceatha in a project that found that involvement in LGBT community groups facilitated 'mastering wellness' through a broad understanding of wellbeing [29].

### 1.5. Reorienting Health Services

The *Ottawa Charter* provides for a holistic model of service provision premised on three health promotion strategies: advocacy for heath; enabling all to achieve their full health potential; and mediating between different interests [2]. The Institute of Medicine emphasized the challenges in addressing stigma, distinguishing between structural stigma and personally enacted stigma [44]. Formby noted the potential risk of heteronormative institutions and practices to impact negatively on LGBT identity and wellbeing [36]. Further, Haas et al. conceded that the current research focus limits the capacity to monitor and assess the full impact of policies and practices seeking to promote improved LGBT mental health and wellbeing [5]. This stigma, at both the structural and personal levels, may extend to a limited recognition of the cultural and social capital embedded within LGBT networks [45]. This is somewhat surprising given the inverse relationship between mental ill-health and social capital [46]. However, a commissioned report carried out in Ireland claimed that "LGBT people have less access to 'social capital'" [45]. This failure by health services to recognize the individual and collective contribution of LGBT communities may inadvertently create barriers to healthcare access [47]. This suggests that in order to reorient health services, policy development and implementation of practice should be informed by research recognising the contribution of LGBT communities [3,5].

Given the exponential growth of groups, set up by, and for, LGBT communities [30], the lack of research into LGBT social connectedness through involvement in interest groups is surprising. The sparse literature on mental health promotion highlights the importance of understanding strengths-based community approaches that promote LGBT wellbeing. This study is aligned with emerging research trends calling for an exploration of protective factors that promote LGBT wellbeing [3,5,11–15,17,23].

## 2. Materials and Methods

Qualitative methodologies provide a nuanced picture of the meanings, understandings, and experiences of a social group [48]. These factors may remain hidden if quantitative approaches are used [49]. An exploratory qualitative approach sought to illuminate an under-researched topic with a view to "generating results and theories that are understandable and experientially credible both to the people being studied and to others" [49]. The research process was informed by an "iterative design" [50] from the framing of research questions through to describing, analyzing and interpreting the rich data.

### 2.1. Research Aims and Objectives

The research aim was to explore the social meaning and significance of LGBT social and community through their sporting, creative or social pursuits. Giving voice to LGBT people's perspectives and priorities is of paramount importance, with the recognition of mental health inequalities for people from minority sexual orientation and gender identity populations [3–5]. The study prioritized the involvement of LGBT stakeholders and communities in recognition that some LGBT voices may be under-researched [51]. Drawing from Baker and Beagan's emphasis on "learning *with*" LGBT communities [52], the research sought to problematise the assumption that LGBT communities are a universally vulnerable group [11,12]. This approach strengthened the research process, from design to dissemination, enhancing the quality of the study [51]. It also ensured diverse representation across age, sexual orientation, gender and gender identity, nationality and sporting, creative and social interests, informed by Rubin and Rubin's concept of a "conversational partner" [50].

### 2.2. Access, Recruitment and Sampling

A range of LGBT stakeholders, known to the first author, identified potential participants and provided introductions, thus validating researcher credibility and facilitating access to participants who may be considered potentially 'under-researched'. A sampling strategy, comprising a mix of purposive and targeted sampling techniques [50,51], was designed to identify appropriate places and contexts for the recruitment of study participants. LGBT people, aged 18 years or older, who were living in Dublin and were involved in sporting, creative or social groups were recruited. LGBT communities and participants were enthusiastic about the study. Due to the level of interest expressed by LGBT community groups and to ensure inclusion, 11 people participated in 10 interviews, with one joint interview. The sample sought to include a broad age range of LGBT people, with four people in their 20s, three in their 30s, two in their 40s, and two in their 50s. Although all participants resided in Dublin at the time of interview, a number were from rural localities and two were born outside Ireland.

### 2.3. Data Collection

The qualitative interview was the core data collection method informed by Kvale and Brinkmann's description of an *InterView*; an inter-change of views resulting in the co-construction of knowledge [48].

Rubin and Rubin identify four core characteristics of 'responsive interviewing': 1. choosing interviewees who are knowledgeable about the research problem; 2. listening carefully to what they tell you; 3. asking additional questions until their answers are fully understood; and 4. seeking depth, detail and richness derived from interviewees' first-hand experiences [50]. While the interview was largely unstructured, it focused on four broad areas: background, joining groups, wellbeing, and interests. A pilot interview was conducted to ensure shared meanings, clarify understanding of questions and identify any potential gaps in the interview schedule. A reflexive approach, where the researcher is aware of, and openly acknowledged, their role in the study and how they may affect the process, was adopted during the data collection and analysis processes [49].

*2.4. Data Management and Analysis*

Interviews were transcribed verbatim, with all identifying information removed from the transcripts. An open coding technique reduced the data into concepts and categories that were identified on an iterative basis [53]. The identification of themes woven through the interviews and the technique of linking categories aided the identification differences and similarities across participants' accounts. The analysis sought to recognize diversity by accounting for negative instances and incorporating data that contradicted emergent or dominant ideas. The coding categories permitted the presentation of individual stories to give 'voice' to both typical and unique experiences [52]. Due to the exploratory nature of the research, the study did not seek to achieve 'saturation' [49].

*2.5. Ethical Considerations*

According to Maxwell, the four key ethical issues that require consideration in the conduct of research are informed consent; privacy; harm and future research [49]. The voluntary, informed consent of individuals was obtained prior to their participation in the study. Stakeholders disseminated information sheets outlining the purpose of the research and what participation involved. All participants were given between one and three weeks to consider whether they wished to participate, and it was explained that they could withdraw from the study without explanation or negative consequence at any time. Assurances of privacy and confidentiality were also provided. To ensure the anonymity of participants, pseudonyms were used and all potentially identifying information (names of places, people and so on) removed from the transcripts. In order to address potential harm, member checking was achieved through dissemination of the study findings and themes to participants and their feedback sought. Due to the ongoing interest in the study, LGBT stakeholder engagement facilitated dissemination of the research with participants, stakeholders and LGBT communities. Consent was sought throughout this process and specifically in relation to presentations sharing the research within LGBT sporting, creative and social groups. The involvement of LGBT communities from design to dissemination suggested directions for future research. Ethical approval was granted by a Research Ethical Approval Committee in Trinity College Dublin (REAC ref: 521).

## 3. Findings

*3.1. The Sample*

The eleven respondents included five lesbian women, four gay men, one bisexual person and one transgender person who were involved in 15 LGBT groups and 16 non-LGBT groups. Participants' interests included physical activities (athletics, hiking, roller derby, rugby), creative pursuits (theatre, art, choir, creative writing) and social groups (dining, online MeetUp for socialising). The youngest participant was 22 years and the oldest was 56. The majority ($n = 10$) were fully open about their gender identity and sexual orientation, with all describing their annual participation in the Dublin Pride Parade, possibly reflecting their connectedness to LGBT communities. Most participants were in a relationship at the time of interview ($n = 7$), including civil partnerships and marriages; three of the study's participants had children. Nine participants were Irish, while one was born in a European country and one in North America. All lived in the greater Dublin area and a majority (*n* = 10) had completed university education. A large number pursued their primary interest through LGBT groups (*n* = 7), with group membership ranging from between two and 14 years. Others have overlapping interests within and outside LGBT communities (*n* = 4). These four participants have long-standing involvement in their interests (5–28 years), with their involvement in LGBT groups being more recent, but extensive nonetheless (1–11 years). This article will focus on experiences within LGBT sporting, creative and social community groups.

Three key themes—'connecting', 'mastering wellness' and 'making a difference'—were identified following a detailed analysis of the interview data. The following sections examine the theme of 'connecting', highlighting several forms of connecting, including through shared interests or skills; connecting as LGBT; connecting socially; and connecting with LGBT communities.

### 3.1.1. Connecting through Shared Interests

Interests played a pivotal role in the lives of all participants, with activities referred to as "central to nearly everything", a "huge part of my life" and an "integral part of my day and my life as it "holds the key for everything". Enjoyment of these activities was enhanced through these social connections. For some, group membership was "primarily about the people" who are "my type of people". As one participant explained:

> I think it's important . . . as a part of a sense of self . . . to be a fully-rounded person . . . as part of your identity . . . you need to have something more in common than you're just LGBT (MeetUp, 27)

This appears to disrupt Honneth's idea of 'identity politics' and the "claim for recognition of one's own culture" [10]. As such, LGBT community groups may create a space where sexual and gender minority identities are assumed, but which may not be defining, even if recognized by others. However, all respondents (*n* = 11) were involved in shared interests with others within LGBT community groups rather than as solo activities. Participants (*n* = 8) expressed a sense of belonging with like-minded others:

> It's the place to meet like-minded people . . . it was our love of food and wine-matching that was the connection . . . it connects me to the wider community . . . I connected it with being gay (dining, 56)

> I'm part of this community and feel included and involved in it . . . because there's lots of different types of like-minded people there . . . It's a thing that the community really celebrates diversity in that sense . . . I just feel that I am accepted—it's wonderful, it's so validating (roller derby, 27)

> But the main connection for everybody is the love of being outdoors on mountains or hills . . . Sharing my enjoyment of the activity . . . there's an on-par thing now—a shared thing together . . . A coterie of like-minded people can go and do more adventurous things . . . and there's a thrill in that (hiking, 53)

Shared interests appeared to play an important role in creating social networks and community connections. This concurs with Formby's findings which highlighted a sense of belonging to LGBT communities with like-minded others [36] and is reminiscent of Honneth's idea of the importance of interpersonal recognition [8–10]. It appears from these narratives that this recognition was reciprocated, offering a sense of connection, through the shared interests [9]. This has important implications for policy and practice in recognising the importance of such connections. While there is no singular way in which the connections with LGBT community groups are formed, albeit through food or hills, theses narratives suggest that feeling included and 'part of something' was critical.

### 3.1.2. Connecting through Skills

The organic, yet exponential, growth of LGBT community groups in Ireland offer a wide range of activities and pursuits, perhaps reflecting the breadth of diversity 'within and between' LGBT communities [36]. Such groups appear to support the acquisition or development of personal skills [9,42,43]. Study respondents spontaneously mentioned the importance of having peers with a shared interest in understanding the activity and the challenges associated with the acquisition of new skills:

> *It evolved into a support network where we help each other by giving critical feedback on each other's work. So, it's evolved ... and now it's become really quite a solid unit that's a support network for me (art, 23)*

> *The people in the creative writing groups have a very good understanding of what it is I'm trying to do ... It's what I can achieve, what I want to achieve ... It is honouring what somebody does well (creative writing, 44)*

> *Just makes me happy ... Yeah, quite relaxing, calming ... and, from the choir point of view, fulfilling as well ... just being able to achieve something, even small, at the end of a rehearsal (choir, 32)*

In this way, the social networks formed through shared interests appeared to provide encouragement and motivation [42]. Participants frequently mentioned group members who recognized the effort involved in developing competence or mastery of the activity as providing affirmation:

> *The dynamic in the group is very supportive ... If they see improvements, they say: 'That's a good one today.' I'd be the same, I'd say: 'I can see you are really coming on: the speedwork is really helping' (athletics, 46)*

> *Every time I tried something new I was getting better; seeing the recognition on people's faces when they would see me in the rink and me improving as well ... (roller derby, 27)*

These narratives point to a sense of the importance of peer validation of achievements and the support provided in overcoming challenges in acquiring new skills [42]. Honneth also highlights the importance of mutual interpersonal recognition with others who share common interests, which can contribute to self-confidence [9]. In this way, the social networks explored in the study, appeared to provide an important form of recognition, described by Honneth as competence and community contribution [9]. This also reflects Spencer and Patrick's notion of mastery and social support [43] and Ceatha's concept of 'mastering wellness' [29].

For all of the participants ($n = 11$), the importance attributed by them to their shared interests was evident in terms of levels of engagement. This included attending training and workshops, personal investment, in time, equipment and travel; the level of support, both to others and the group; and the extent to which their interests have developed over time. Further, the recognition of the individual contribution of members within these communities appears to positively contribute to self-confidence for the individual and self-esteem for the collective [8–10]. While this has important policy and practice implications, it appears that outside of LGBT communities, such contributions have been largely unrecognized, particularly in the health policy arena.

### 3.1.3. Connecting through LGBT Identity

It was evident from the interviews that, for a number of participants ($n = 9$), having shared interests facilitated entry to a group, established by, and for, LGBT communities. Respondents conveyed a nuanced understanding of the interconnection between their interests and their LGBT identity. Many, for example, identified their sexual orientation or gender identity as an incentive for joining a group established by, and maintained for, LGBT communities:

> *I found myself in a situation where I had no gay friends and it was a connection that I missed ... I figured the only way to really make friends who are also LGBT was to join some sort of a club that had LGBT participants (MeetUp, 27)*

In this way, it appears that it is the interlinking of the interest and LGBT identity that creates the connection; there is a need for both, one without the other would be insufficient. However, this is seemingly contested by those who feel that they do not necessarily connect to LGBT people or need LGBT-specific communities. This may accord Formby's findings that challenged the assumption of the inevitability of a connection to a readymade 'community' [36]. An example of this is outlined below:

> I think I'm defined first and foremost by the fact that I am really passionate about acting and really passionate about theatre and performance. That's my main thing (theatre, 22)

Nonetheless, the presence and visibility of LGBT or gay people in ways that are normalized cannot be underestimated [10]. As such, in spaces where people feel a sense of connection they may not seek out 'like-minded' people around sexual orientation and gender identity, because they are already part of a world where they feel included and supported. While their interest is predominant, this participant expanded on this:

> And plus is the fact that there's always lots of actors who are gay, a lot of theatre makers who are gay; so it's like I fit right in (theatre, 22)

In this way, it appears that while participants' shared interests are to the forefront, these shared interests also provide opportunities for connection with LGBT communities. While there was evidence of "collective self-understanding" [10], other perspectives emerged:

> First I said to myself 'Ok, there is a gay rugby team, I'm not going to play for a gay rugby team just because I'm gay' (rugby, 31)

However, this participant subsequently became involved through a tournament:

> For the first time in my life I was socialising with all gay people ... something just, I don't know if it clicked, or if it felt comfortable ... and I thought 'Actually, this is pretty cool: I feel like I belong here, I feel at ease here, I feel comfortable' (rugby, 31)

While the LGBT group provided a sense of belonging, further elaboration was provided:

> I'd describe myself as ... interested in sports ... yeah, I'm gay ... but I wouldn't want it to be, and I don't think that it should be, one of the first words that I'd choose to describe myself (rugby, 31)

This narrative suggests that while there was no 'need' for a gay team, as sexual orientation is only one form of identity enactment. However, connection with a gay team, through a shared interest in rugby, became a space of connection that moved beyond sexuality. As such, it was both the shared sporting interest and the inclusion through sexual orientation and gender identity that were critical factors. In this way, it appears that self-identification through shared interests provides an opportunity for the salience of these identities to be contextually determined.

While Honneth suggests that the recognition of "rightful identity" [10] provides an impetus for emancipation, it appears that LGBT social networks provide spaces that extend beyond identification solely on the basis of sexual orientation or gender identity. Thus, recognition of the multiplicity of identities is enabled, with the sporting, creative or social interest of increased salience within the group. This finding suggests that it is the shared interests that encompass and expand the concept of a singular LGBT 'community' [36].

### 3.1.4. Connecting Socially

Although Honneth specifically mentioned 'identity politics' in relation to LGBT communities, respondents' accounts strongly suggest that they had a more nuanced understanding of the interconnection between their interests and their LGBT identity [10]. In particular, their social networks offered important forms of interpersonal recognition and a sense of belonging [9,16]. Such groups provided alternatives to the LGBT pub–club scene and, for some, this community connection was an incentive to join the group:

*How do you get to know people?—You share an interest, join a sports team, join a choir … a big group of friends and family, but big and gay and in Dublin. [It] was something you could do that was gay and wasn't just going to a bar... (choir, 36)*

The importance of these groups in facilitating connection to LGBT communities at the time of 'coming out' was mentioned by three participants. The age of 'coming out' ranged from 16 to 44 years, with an average age of 23 years for the sample. Some participants were very clear about their age on 'coming out' while others described a process:

*I loved it, I was going every two weeks, never missed it … it's not a vehicle for 'coming out' and, in a sense, I did use it for 'coming out' … I was very, very nervous going to my first meal and I've met a lot of people who have been very nervous … It has become where I've met my best friends and quite a lot of acquaintances (dining, 56)*

*When I found out there was a gay choir, it seemed obvious thing. People were so welcoming and really, really lovely. It was my first experience of lots of gay people who weren't just the same age as me … I was immersed in it quite quickly—it was everything that I wanted it to be—a great way into the community … it wasn't too much outside my comfort zone (choir, 32)*

While none of the sporting, creative or social groups was depicted by participants as a support group when 'coming out', it may be that sharing interests acted as a conduit for those exploring and questioning their LGBT identity. Further, such supportive environments [2,3] may provide interpersonal recognition through LGBT connection at critical time points, including throughout the 'coming out' process [10].

For others, the social element within the LGBT community groups established by, and for, LGBT communities, provided the motivation to join:

*One of the great things about it is … they meet for coffee and buns afterward and it is a lovely social occasion … even if you're feeling crap you will plan your weekend around [the] Saturday morning run (athletics, 46)*

It appears that the availability of the broad range of interest groups [30] facilitates the recognition of diversity within and between LGBT people [36]. This emphasises the importance of recognition of diversity across LGBT communities as a key aspect of social connectedness. LGBT sporting, creative and social groups seem to be affirmed by members for their promotion of the diversity of LGBT interests. The plethora of LGBT community groups established by, and for, LGBT communities attests to this [26–35].

### 3.1.5. Connecting with LGBT Communities

Most participants felt that they were part of a wider network of LGBT communities, characterized as a "very welcoming and open club" which was "safe and accepting" and fostered feelings of being "included and involved." The importance of safe spaces that were accepting is consistent with Browne, Bakshi and Lim [25]. In the context of perceived societal progress, there was recognition of the potential for present and future policies could impact positively on LGBT wellbeing in Ireland [8–10], particularly given the rapid sense of legislative attitudinal shifts that had occurred during the past decade. This echoes Honneth's appeal for universal legal rights, empowering communities and supporting social integrity [8–10]. Equally, there was an awareness of the limitations of legislative changes [25]. As such, the importance of the empowerment of LGBT communities extended to challenging stereotypes ($n = 6$) and creating visibility ($n = 6$) through involvement in LGBT community groups:

*Some people don't know any gay people, or don't know they know any gay people or it's this 'other' thing and they see it as the stereotypes … We're a choir who mostly happen to be gay (choir, 32)*

*... and a choir singing—especially a relatively traditional choir—is very non-threatening and quite accessible and quite different (choir, 36)*

The discussion above, mentioning that the choir 'mostly happen to be gay' and 'non-threatening', suggests that others' perceptions of LGBT people and social connectedness beyond LGBT communities is also important. However, while visibility matters, it appears to be premised on an expectation that a visible 'non-threatening' LGBT presence will be greeted positively and not result in heteronormative or gendered responses. This perspective was shared by a number of respondents who mentioned the importance of creating visibility (*n* = 6) to counter dominant representations of LGBT lives. Additionally, the importance of a visible presence focused on creating connections within and between LGBT communities [35]:

*It is good to show up and have a presence, a visibility for LGBT people ... If you see somebody representing the lesbian and gay community running at the same event you're running at, that has to allow you to have some sense of belonging or affinity or potential to be ... not so alienated (athletics, 46)*

*A lot of my friends have said to me that they felt like I did pave the way; that me 'coming out' gave them the courage to afterwards ... I think young people now consider to be homophobic ... to be just medieval. My generation doesn't really care anymore what you are and that's pretty good (art, 23)*

This relies on specific understandings of a 'new' Ireland with a younger generation as inherently more open and accepting and who 'doesn't really care' about others' sexual orientation or gender identity. However, reflecting the contested and contradictory nature of these debates, other participants were less certain that societal progress was reflected in LGBT people's lived experience:

*There's still a lazy portrayal of gays in the media ... where being gay is everything about them or just with their mincing characteristics or they speak in one way and they're flamboyantly gay, which ... does exist ... But ... anyone, regardless of their temperament or how they act, can be gay (theatre, 22)*

There were recurring references to homonegativity and the prevalence of the "presumption of heterosexuality":

*It's the same, say for any say teenage boy growing up, when the person asks: 'got a girlfriend?' they never ask ... 'or a boyfriend?' When people assume I'm straight I nearly feel an obligation ... to tell them I'm gay ... It's the way of life to be straight (rugby, 31)*

Perhaps, due to such experiences of homonegativity, heteronormativity and gendered assumptions, some respondents felt it was important for their wellbeing to be involved with an LGBT sporting, creative or social group [26–35]. This is consistent with Browne, Bakshi and Lim's suggestion of such groups providing safe spaces [25]. It may also be that LGBT groups serve an important purpose in providing a sense of belonging [16], promoting wellbeing [3,5,17] and ameliorating the effects of minority stress [38–40]. While it has been suggested that this contributes to the development of personal resilience [9,37,39], this too was questioned by one participant:

*I think to make resilience the focus of the solution is to shift the responsibility from the perpetrator to the person who's been affected by the behaviour ... I'm very resilient. I shouldn't have to be resilient all the time. My life shouldn't be a battle (creative writing, 44)*

Major events, such as 'coming out', forming or ending relationships, parenthood and loss through bereavement, were all cited as examples that participants felt created pressure in negotiating assumptions and stereotypes. It also appeared to provide an impetus for calls for recognition [10]. A considerable number of participants (*n* = 7) specifically mentioned the contribution of LGBT communities to these societal changes:

> *Those challenges and activism have actually led to the changes that we have now ... The challenge is*
> *trying to change society to be more just and more diverse ... whether that's racially ... or sexuality*
> *or gender—a thriving society is one that is diverse economically and creatively and socially generally*
> *(hiking, 53)*

The potential contribution of LGBT community groups in creating formal and informal safe spaces [25] and establishing and maintaining groups that potentially ameliorate the effects of minority stress [39–41] may, in part, explain the longevity and continued demand for such groups [26–35]. This suggests that LGBT communities are pivotal in creating social networks and a sense of connection [9,16,36]. As argued by Honneth, LGBT social networks appear to play an important role in the continued empowerment of LGBT communities, with a positive impact on individual self-confidence and collective self-respect [8–10].

## 4. Discussion

This in-depth exploration of how LGBT people describe the meaning and significance of their shared interests, hobbies and pursuits reveals there is a lot to "learn *with*" LGBT communities [52]. The findings presented suggest that groups, by and for LGBT communities, are pivotal in raising aspects of recognition, both in terms of interpersonal and community contribution as well as right-based activities [8–10]. However, the contribution of LGBT communities in promoting wellbeing appears to have been largely unrecognized. This will now be discussed in light of Honneth's tripartite framework of interpersonal, community and rights-based recognition [8–10].

### 4.1. Interpersonal Recognition

The people in this study actively sought avenues of social networking that facilitated engagement with interests that were personally significant and represented positive contributions to their lives. In many cases, respondents appeared to benefit from experiences of mutual recognition from like-minded others [8–10] because it provided affirmation, validation [41,42] and a sense of belonging [16].

Involvement with an LGBT group also provided safe spaces [25] and, as such, were a mechanism for circumnavigating gendered and heteronormative assumptions [36]. Respondents were acutely aware that social exclusion and societal treatment that is less than equal has the potential to impact negatively on their wellbeing and that of wider LGBT communities [2–6,16]. In this way, LGBT social and community connectedness may provide a buffer against the effects of minority stress [37–41]. These findings are consistent with Formby's, where collective LGBT identity emerged as a bond that developed through a sense of belonging and, for some, through shared experiences of discrimination [36].

Participants' understanding of their experiences, provide considerable insight into the unacknowledged, underlying influences on their wellbeing. The ability to exercise agency is the product of cultural meanings that are both constructed and constrained [54]. While respondents were adept at recognizing constraints on their agency, this recognition, in itself, may lead to a perception of choice. This underscores the emphasis placed throughout the *Ottawa Charter* on changing the environment alongside strengthening the person [2].

### 4.2. Community Recognition

There was a sense that respondents had often exercised agency in relation to self-definition and identity enactment through interest sharing. These provided opportunities for social and community connectedness [37,38,41]. Perhaps, through the creation of spaces where one's LGBT identity is assumed, other forms of identity enactment, in such sporting, creative and social interests, are enhanced. In this way, LGBT groups, by and for LGBT communities, appear to both encompass and extend beyond what Honneth termed 'identity politics' [10]. The formation of these groups around shared interests may have provided opportunities for side-stepping Honneth's suggestion of "collective self-understanding" and "claims for recognition" solely on the basis of sexual orientation or gender identity. Rather, through group membership, participants appeared to move beyond the potential for a limited and limiting monostaticity of identity.

These narratives point to the wealth of cultural and social capital embedded within LGBT networks. Contrary to claims that LGBT communities have less access to social capital [45], it appears such groups play an important role in recognising diversity within and between LGBT communities [36]. It may be that, in these circumstances, LGBT communities in Ireland appear to be at the forefront of mental health promotion [2,3,16]. With strengthened community capacity, LGBT interest groups may provide an example of the second goal of *Connecting for Life* [3] since empowered communities that respond to the needs of members can provide a buffer against the effects of minority stress [3–5,37–41] and help to sustain these benefits over time [42,43].

Through community membership of such groups, participants sought recognition of LGBT human rights through creating visibility and challenging stereotyped assumptions [8–10]. Despite this important contribution by LGBT communities, when viewed through the lens of Honneth's tripartite framework [9], there appears to be a lack of recognition by policy makers of the strengthened LGBT community action in creating these supportive environments, which enhances the development of personal skills [2].

### 4.3. Recognition of LGBT Human Rights

While policy is specifically designed to address identified problems, it is possible that polices, and, therefore, practice, remains trapped in negative connotations of the problem [55,56]. Thus, the broad research consensus of elevated mental health risk [3–6,46,47], as a consequence of stigma and discrimination [3–5], may have inadvertently led to a tendency to focus on resultant deficits. Thus, people who are LGBT may be perceived only as the recipients of healthcare rather than as contributors to their own wellbeing and that of others within LGBT communities. This lack of recognition at interpersonal and community levels, as outlined in Honneth's tripartite framework [9], may inadvertently reinforce structural and personally enacted stigma within health and social care policy and practice [44].

The dearth of literature on mental health promotion within LGBT communities has been acknowledged nationally [3] and internationally [5]. However, in the absence of such research, the direction of policy and practice for health promotion, prevention and intervention with LGBT communities, may be solely informed by the current focus on identifying risk factors for mental health [3,5,6,46,47]. This underscores an anomaly whereby policy makers generally recognize the importance of community connectedness [3–6,46,47], yet fail to recognize such community connectedness within LGBT communities [6,46,47]. This paper highlights the critical importance of recognition of LGBT social networks and calls for shifts in policy and practice frameworks which recognize the strengths embedded within LGBT communities.

### 4.4. Study Limitations

This was a qualitative exploratory study with 11 participants and did not seek to achieve 'saturation'. As such, the findings presented cannot be claimed to be generalizable to other LGBT populations. However, by gathering in-depth accounts, the research provides important insights into LGBT people's understandings of their social and community connectedness and the positive role that LGBT communities could potentially play in health care and health promotions policies. This suggests that further research, particularly mixed-methods research, is clearly needed, in order to identify factors that promote LGBT wellbeing, consistent with current policy [3,23]. Studies of this kind should seek to ensure the inclusion of people from diverse socio-economic and cultural backgrounds, as well as young people, particularly in light of recent research suggesting substantial vulnerabilities among LGBT youth [47].

## 5. Conclusions

This in-depth exploration of how LGBT communities describe the meaning and significance of their shared interests, hobbies and pursuits suggests there is a lot to "learn *with*" LGBT communities [52]. However, within policy, the contribution of LGBT communities in promoting wellbeing appears to have been largely unrecognized. Despite the limitations of the study, the findings provide valuable, alternative views that may contradict policy norms. A health promotion approach, informed by the *Ottawa Charter* and underpinned by Honneth's *Theory of Recognition*, makes it possible to envisage some shifts, from individual health toward service reorientation paradigms. Messages from the study reinforce the central role that LGBT communities can play in the promotion of mental health and social wellbeing, with important policy and practice implications. It would appear that while LGBT communities are in some ways affirmed by members for their role in promoting LGBT wellbeing through social support and mutual reciprocity, this has been largely unrecognized in the health and social policy fields in Ireland. This study exemplifies the social and cultural capital embedded within LGBT networks and the contributory role of interest groups, established by, and maintained for, LGBT communities, in enhancing social connectedness. It may be that future studies in this area can shed more light on these policy-making lacunae, especially given recent trends towards social prescribing to promote community involvement and address social isolation. Finally, the use of alternative theoretical frameworks to enhance debates in this area, in particular, notions of rights-based recognition, where issues of social justice and identify are fore fronted is necessary if health promotion in this area is to be effective.

**Author Contributions:** Conceptualization, N.C. and P.M.; Data curation, N.C.; Formal analysis, N.C.; Investigation, N.C.; Methodology, N.C. and P.M.; Project administration, N.C.; Supervision, P.M.; Visualization, N.C. and P.M.; Writing—original draft, N.C. and P.M.; Writing—review & editing, N.C., P.M., J.C., C.N. and K.B.

**Funding:** This research received no external funding.

**Acknowledgments:** Nerilee Ceatha would like to acknowledge the feedback on an earlier version of this article from Prof. Ivan Perry and Prof. Margaret Barry. The authors would like to acknowledge all within the Dublin LGBT communities for their contributions and continued enthusiasm for this research. Thanks, in particular, to the 11 inspirational participants for sharing their journeys.

**Conflicts of Interest:** Nerilee Ceatha was a member of the Oversight Committee for the Irish *LGBTI+ National Youth Strategy*.

## References

1. WHO. *Mental Health Atlas 2005*; A Report by the Department of Mental Health and Substance Dependence; World Health Organization: Geneva, Switzerland, 2005; p. 1.
2. WHO. *Ottawa Charter for Health Promotion: An International Conference on Health Promotion, the Move Towards a New Public Health*; World Health Organization: Ottawa, ON, Canada, 1986; pp. 1–2.
3. National Office for Suicide Prevention. *Connecting for Life: Ireland's National Strategy to Reduce Suicide 2015–2020*; Health Services Executive: Dublin, Ireland, 2014; pp. 931–3250.
4. Meyer, I.H. Prejudice, social stress, and mental health in lesbian, gay, and bisexual populations: Conceptual issues and research evidence. *Psychol. Bull.* **2003**, *129*, 674–697. [CrossRef] [PubMed]
5. Haas, A.P.; Eliason, M.; Mays, V.M.; Mathy, R.M.; Cochran, S.D.; D'Augelli, A.R. Suicide and suicide risk in lesbian, gay, bisexual, and transgender populations: Review and recommendations. *J. Homosex.* **2010**, *58*, 10–51. [CrossRef] [PubMed]
6. HSE National Social Inclusion Governance Group. *LGBT Health: Towards Meeting the Health Care Needs of Lesbian, Gay, Bisexual and Transgender People*; Health Services Executive: Dublin, Ireland, 2009; p. 24.
7. Fraser, N. *Justice Interruptus: Critical Reflections on the "Postsocialist" Condition*; Routledge: New York, NY, USA, 1997; pp. 12, 14.
8. Honneth, A. Recognition and Social Obligation. *Soc. Res.* **1997**, *64*, 16–35.
9. Honneth, A. *The Struggle for Recognition: The Moral Grammar of Social Conflicts*; The MIT Press: Cambridge, MA, USA, 1995; pp. 26–30.

10. Fraser, N.; Honneth, A. *Redistribution or Recognition: A Political-Philosophical Exchange*; Verso: London, UK; New York, NY, USA, 2003; p. 162.
11. Bryan, A.; Mayock, P. Supporting LGBT lives? Complicating the suicide consensus in LGBT mental health research. *Sexualities* **2017**, *20*, 65–85. [CrossRef]
12. Bryan, A.; Mayock, P. Speaking back to dominant constructions of LGBT Lives: Complexifying 'at riskness' for self-harm and suicidality among lesbian, gay, bisexual and transgender youth. *Ir. J. Anthropol.* **2012**, *15*, 8–15.
13. Marshall, D. Popular culture, the 'victim' trope and queer youth analytics. *Int. J. Qual. Stud. Educ.* **2010**, *23*, 65–85. [CrossRef]
14. Savin-Williams, R.C. *The New Gay Teenager*; Harvard University Press: Cambridge, MA, USA, 2005; Volume 3.
15. Talburt, S.; Rofes, E.; Rasmussen, M.L. Transforming discourses of queer youth and educational practices surrounding gender, sexuality and youth. In *Youth and Sexualities: Pleasure, Subversion, and Insubordination in and out of Schools*; Rasmussen, M.L., Rofes, E., Talburt, S., Eds.; Palgrave Macmillan: New York, NY, USA, 2004.
16. Wilkinson, R.G.; Marmot, M.G. *Social Determinants of Health: The Solid Facts*; World Health Organization: Geneva, Switzerland, 2003; pp. 922.
17. Fredriksen-Goldsen, K.I.; Kim, H.-J.; Lehavot, K.; Walters, K.L.; Yang, J.; Hoy-Ellis, C.P. The Health Equity Promotion Model: Reconceptualization of Lesbian, Gay, Bisexual, and Transgender (LGBT) Health Disparities. *Am. J. Orthopsychiatry* **2014**, *84*, 653–663. [CrossRef]
18. Kuhl, M. Ireland wins LGBT+ activism award at World Pride in New York. In *Gay Community News*; NXF: Dublin, Ireland, 2019.
19. International Day Against Homophobia and Transphobia (IDAHOT). Declaration of Intent, 2014. Available online: http://www.justice.ie/en/JELR/Pages/PR14000118 (accessed on 18 March 2018).
20. Attorney General of Ireland. *Marriage Act 2015. Irish Statute Book*; Oireachtas: Dublin, Ireland, 2015.
21. Attorney General of Ireland. *Gender Recognition Act 2015. Irish Statute Book*; Oireachtas: Dublin, Ireland, 2015.
22. Department of Employment Affairs and Social Protection. Minister Doherty Publishes the Report of the Group Established to Review the Operation of the Gender Recognition Act 2015, Press Office, 18 July 2018. Available online: https://www.welfare.ie/en/pressoffice/pdf/pr180718.pdf (accessed on 9 September 2019).
23. DCYA. *LGBTI+ National Youth Strategy*; Department of Children and Youth Affairs; The Stationery Office: Dublin, Ireland, 2018. Available online: https://www.dcya.gov.ie/documents/20180709LGBTINationalYouthStrategyRev.pdf (accessed on 28 July 2018).
24. DoJ. National LGBTI Inclusion Strategy. Department of Justice, 2018. Available online: https://www.gov.ie/en/consultation/91c3ed-national-lgbti-inclusion-strategy/ (accessed on 16 June 2019).
25. Browne, K.; Bakshi, L.; Lim, J. 'It's Something You Just Have to Ignore': Understanding and Addressing Contemporary Lesbian, Gay, Bisexual and Trans Safety Beyond Hate Crime Paradigms. *J. Soc. Policy* **2011**, *40*, 739–756. [CrossRef]
26. Krane, V. Sport for LGBT athletes. In *Routledge International Handbook of Sport Psychology*; Schinke, R.J., McGannon, K.R., Smith, B., Eds.; Routledge: New York, NY, USA, 2016.
27. Abichahine, H.; Veenstra, G. Inter-categorical intersectionality and leisure-based physical activity in Canada. *Health Promot. Int.* **2017**, *32*, 691–701. [CrossRef]
28. Denison, E.; Kitchen, A. *Out on the Fields: The First International Study on Homophobia in Sport*; Nielsen, Bingham Cup Sydney 2014; Australian Sports Commission, Federation of Gay Games: Sydney, Australia, 2015; Available online: https://www.outonthefields.com (accessed on 28 June 2018).
29. Ceatha, N. Mastering wellness: LGBT people's understanding of wellbeing through interest sharing. *J. Res. Nurs.* **2016**, *21*, 199–209. [CrossRef]
30. GCN. Directory: Dublin & The East. In *Gay Community News*; National Lesbian & Gay Federation Ltd.: Dublin, Ireland, 2019.
31. Cocciolo, A. Community Archives in the Digital Era: A Case from the LGBT Community. *Preserv. Digit. Technol. Cult.* **2017**, *45*, 157–165. [CrossRef]
32. Beale, C. "A Different Kind of Goosebump:" Notes Toward an LGBTQ Choral Pedagogy. In *The Oxford Handbook of Choral Pedagogy*; Abrahams, F., Head, P.D., Eds.; Oxford University Press: Oxford, UK, 2017.
33. Binnie, J.; Klesse, C. The politics of age and generation at the GAZE International LGBT Film Festival in Dublin. *Sociol. Rev.* **2018**, *66*, 191–206. [CrossRef]

34. Loist, S.; Zielinski, G. On the development of queer film festivals and their media activism. *Film Festiv. Yearb.* **2012**, *4*, 49–62.
35. Lee, S.; Kim, S.; Love, A. Coverage of the Gay Games from 1980–2012 in U.S. Newspapers: An Analysis of Newspaper Article Framing. *J. Sport Manag.* **2012**, *28*, 176–188. [CrossRef]
36. Formby, E. *Exploring LGBT Spaces and Communities: Contrasting Identities, Belongings and Wellbeing*; Routledge: London, UK, 2017.
37. Detrie, P.M.; Lease, S.H. The relation of social support, connectedness, and collective self-esteem to the psychological well-being of lesbian, gay, and bisexual youth. *J. Homosex.* **2007**, *53*, 173–199. [CrossRef]
38. DiFulvio, G.T. Sexual minority youth, social connection and resilience: From personal struggle to collective identity. *Soc. Sci. Med.* **2011**, *72*, 1611–1617. [CrossRef]
39. Kertzner, R.M.; Meyer, I.H.; Frost, D.M.; Stirratt, M.J. Social and psychological well-being in lesbians, gay men, and bisexuals: The effects of race, gender, age, and sexual identity. *Am. J. Orthopsychiatry* **2009**, *79*, 500. [CrossRef]
40. Andriote, M. The Power of Choosing Resilience. The Atlantic, 2013. Available online: http://www.theatlantic. com/health/archive/2013/02/the-power-of-choosing-resilience/273245/2/ (accessed on 12 September 2019).
41. Frost, D.M.; Meyer, I.H. Measuring community connectedness among diverse sexual minority populations. *J. Sex Res.* **2012**, *49*, 36–49. [CrossRef]
42. Heard, D.; Lake, B.; McCluskey, U. *Attachment Therapy with Adolescents and Adults: Theory and Practice Post Bowlby*; Karnac Books: London, UK, 2012.
43. Spencer, S.M.; Patrick, J.H. Social support and personal mastery as protective resources during emerging adulthood. *J. Adult Dev.* **2009**, *16*, 191–198. [CrossRef]
44. IOM. *The Health of Lesbian, Gay, Bisexual, and Transgender People: Building a Foundation for Better Understanding*; The National Academies Press: Washington, DC, USA, 2011; Available online: http://iom.nationalacademies.org/Reports/ 2011/The-Health- of-Lesbian-Gay-Bisexual-and-Transgender-People.aspx?_ga=1.39552099.1521693205.1452111936 (accessed on 18 March 2018).
45. Smyth, B. *LGBT Resilience: Building Strong and Inclusive Communities*; A Regional Strategy for Lesbian, Gay, Bisexual and Transgender (LGBT) Inclusion and Support in the South East (Waterford, Wexford, Wicklow, Kildare, Kilkenny and Carlow); Health Services Executive: South East, Ireland, 2012; p. 10.
46. De Silva, M.J.; McKenzie, K.; Harpham, T.; Huttly, S.R. Social capital and mental illness: A systematic review. *J. Epidemiol. Community Health* **2005**, *59*, 619–627. [CrossRef]
47. Higgins, A.; Doyle, L.; Downes, C.; Murphy, R.; Sharek, D.; DeVries, J.; Begley, T.; McCann, E.; Sheerin, F.; Smyth, S. *The LGBTIreland Report: National Study of the Mental Health and Wellbeing of Lesbian, Gay, Bisexual, Transgender and Intersex People in Ireland*; GLEN: Dublin, Ireland; BeLonGTo: Dublin, Ireland, 2016.
48. Kvale, S.; Brinkmann, S. *InterViews: Learning the Craft of Qualitative Research Interviewing*, 2nd ed.; Sage Publications: Los Angeles, CA, USA, 2009.
49. Maxwell, J.A. Designing a qualitative study. In *The SAGE Handbook of Applied Social Research Methods*; Leonard, B., Rog, D.J., Eds.; SAGE Publications Incorporated: Los Angeles, CA, USA, 2009; p. 221.
50. Rubin, H.J.; Rubin, I.S. *Qualitative Interviewing: The Art of Hearing Data*; SAGE Publications Incorporated: Los Angeles, CA, USA, 2005; pp. 14, 30.
51. Ceatha, N. Conducting Insider Ethnography in Under-Researched Communities: The Roles of Researcher and Gatekeepers. SAGE Research Method Cases, 2017. Available online: http://methods.sagepub.com/case/ ethnography-in-under-researched-communities-researcher-and-gatekeepers (accessed on 16 July 2019).
52. Baker, K.; Beagan, B. Making Assumptions, Making Space: An Anthropological Critique of Cultural Competency and Its Relevance to Queer Patients. *Med. Anthropol. Q.* **2014**, *28*, 578–598. [CrossRef] [PubMed]
53. Boeije, H.R. *Analysis in Qualitative Research*; SAGE: London, UK, 2010.
54. Goffman, E. *The Presentation of Self in Everyday Life*; Penguin: London, UK, 1959.
55. Cairney, P.; Jones, M.D. Kingdon's Multiple Streams Approach: What Is the Empirical Impact of this Universal Theory? *Policy Stud. J.* **2016**, *44*, 37–58. [CrossRef]

56. Bacchi, C. Problematizations in health policy: Questioning how "problems" are constituted in policies. *SAGE Open* **2016**, *6*, 2158244016653986. [CrossRef]

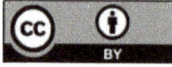

© 2019 by the authors. Licensee MDPI, Basel, Switzerland. This article is an open access article distributed under the terms and conditions of the Creative Commons Attribution (CC BY) license (http://creativecommons.org/licenses/by/4.0/).

International Journal of
*Environmental Research
and Public Health*

MDPI

*Article*

# A Comparative Analysis of Lifetime Medical Conditions and Infectious Diseases by Sexual Identity, Attraction, and Concordance among Women: Results from a National U.S. Survey

Kelly Horn * and James A. Swartz[iD]

Jane Addams College of Social Work, University of Illinois at Chicago, Chicago, IL 60607, USA; jaswartz@uic.edu
* Correspondence: khorn2@uic.edu; Tel.: +1-630-677-9975

Received: 12 March 2019; Accepted: 16 April 2019; Published: 18 April 2019

**Abstract:** There have been limited studies assessing the differences in chronic health conditions between sexual minority (those who identify as lesbian or bisexual) and sexual majority (heterosexual) women. Research has primarily focused on overall physical and mental health or behavioral issues and not on specific health conditions. The addition of sexual orientation and attraction questions to the National Survey on Drug Use and Health (NSDUH) now allows for research regarding health conditions using a national survey that identifies participant sexual orientation and attraction. This study sought to compare the prevalence/odds of having 10 medical conditions/infectious diseases among women, assessing for differences associated with sexual identity, sexual attraction, and the degree of concordance between sexual identity and attraction. Data from 67,648 adult female participants in the 2015–2017 NSDUH survey were analyzed using bivariate and multivariable logistic regression models to assess for differences in prevalence/odds of seven medical conditions. Multivariable models adjusted for demographics, substance abuse/dependence, and mental illness. We found significant differences by sexual identity, but not sexual attraction or concordance. Compared with heterosexually identified women, women who identified as bisexual had significantly higher odds of having three medical conditions and two infectious diseases than heterosexual or lesbian women. The findings generally support those based on studies using more limited geographical samples. There are a number of potential associated and underlying factors that contribute to bisexual women reporting overall poorer health than heterosexual or lesbian women. The factors discussed include stigma, delays in seeking care, lack of insurance and access, and sexual minority women receiving poorer health care generally.

**Keywords:** women's health; sexual identity; chronic health conditions

---

## 1. Introduction

Research on health disparities among sexual minorities–those who identify as gay, lesbian, or bisexual–has focused on general physical well-being and the presence of mental health concerns such as depression and anxiety [1,2]. Other focal areas of health-related research among sexual minorities include behavioral health issues such as smoking, substance use, and binge drinking, as well as other health-related behaviors and social issues that affect health such as obesity, poor diet, inter-partner violence, stigma, and stress [3–6]. Until recently, there has been relatively little direct examination of the distal consequences of these behaviors and issues like the prevalence of specific chronic medical conditions (CMCs) such as heart disease, diabetes, asthma, or cancer in sexual minorities [7–11].

Gaining a complete understanding of the physical health of sexual minority men and women has been challenging due to the historical exclusion of questions on sexual identity from nationally representative health surveys. Consequently, earlier studies on sexual minority health were not nationally representative and restricted to using largely state-based data or data derived from broad-based surveys that nevertheless use state-based sampling such as the Behavioral Risk Factor Surveillance Study (BRFSS) [7–13]. The findings across these studies are difficult to compare, owing to the different sampling frames, instruments, and conditions assessed. However, in general, these studies most consistently found sexual minority participants, with results varying by gender, to be at risk for poorer health overall and at greater risk for poorer health given higher rates of behaviors such as smoking and substance use [3,8,14–18]. Less consistent were the findings for differing rates/odds of specific CMCs by sexual identity, which seem to vary the most from study to study [19].

The inclusion of measures related to sexual orientation, such as sexual identity and attraction, in surveys such as the National Health Interview Survey (NHIS) added in 2013 [20], and the National Survey on Drug Use and Health (NSDUH) added in 2015 [20] now permit broader and more detailed examinations of sexual minority health and specific CMC prevalence using nationally representative samples. For instance, a recent study using NHIS data found male and female sexual minority participants to have higher odds of multiple health risk factors (e.g., smoking, heavy drinking, psychological distress) and multiple CMCs than their heterosexual peers (but did not report on specific CMC prevalence) [10].

An understudied aspect of the association between sexual orientation and health is concordance between sexual identity and attraction, as health disparities could depend on the degree of concordance between the two [21]. Those whose sexual identity and attraction match are considered concordant, whereas those whose sexual identity and attraction do not match are discordant [21]. One might hypothesize that discordance is associated with increased stress and, consequently, individuals whose sexual identity is discordant with sexual attraction could be at higher risk for poor health. To the best of our knowledge, this hypothesis was only tested in a parallel study assessing the same data with exclusively men [22]. Using a nationally representative data set, this study sought to examine the relative health effects of sexual identity, attraction, and concordance comparing sexual minority and majority women on a set of CMCs as well as infectious diseases. The findings of a companion study of men using the same comparisons and parallel statistical analyses was published elsewhere [22]. This current study was done to examine the unique experiences of women.

*Objectives*

The purpose of the current study was to determine the prevalence of chronic health conditions and infectious diseases among women, specifically assessing differences between sexual minority women and heterosexual women. This study examined the prevalence of health conditions and infectious diseases based on three distinct constructs: Sexual identity, sexual attraction, and concordance between sexual identity and attraction.

## 2. Method

This study was a secondary analysis of data collected for the 2015–2017 NSDUH. Details regarding the NSDUH methodology are available at the Substance Abuse and Mental Health Data Archive (https://www.datafiles.samhsa.gov/) [23].

*2.1. Sample*

As those under 18 are not asked questions about sexual identity or attraction, the sample was restricted to the 67,648 female participants aged 18 years or older. Sample size was reduced to 63,495 after removing 4153 (6.2%) participants with missing data on sexual identity and attraction. For the multivariable model with HIV/AIDS status as the dependent variable, sample size was further reduced to 63,346 owing to missing data for this variable ($N = 149$, 0.03%).

## 2.2. Measures

### 2.2.1. Sexual Identity, Attraction, and Concordance

Sexual identity was evaluated using a three-category self-reported variable: Heterosexual, bisexual, or gay/lesbian. Sexual attraction was measured as a self-reported interval-level variable based on a single question that asked respondents to rate sexual attraction using a five-point scale that ranged from "only attracted to the opposite sex" (1) to "only attracted to the same sex" (5). A two-category variable was created to assess sexual concordance/discordance between sexual identity and attraction. Concordance was defined as identifying as heterosexual and reporting sexual attraction only to the opposite sex, identifying as gay or lesbian and reporting sexual attraction to only the same sex, or identifying as bisexual and reporting sexual attraction to either sex. Participants who did not meet these criteria were categorized as discordant, meaning there was some discrepancy between their identified sexual identity and sexual attraction.

### 2.2.2. Demographics

The multivariable models controlled for the following demographics: Race/ethnicity (White, African-American/Black, Hispanic, and Asian/Pacific Islander/Multi-ethnic/Other); age (five categories from 18–25 years through 65 and older); education (four categories from less than high school through college graduate); marital status (married, widowed, separated/divorced, never married); poverty level (living in poverty, income up to twice the poverty level, and income greater than twice the poverty level); population density (living in a core-based statistical area (CBSA) with greater than a million people, living in a CBSA with fewer than a million, and not living in a CBSA). Population density is based on Core Based Statistical Areas (CBSAs), which are used by the U.S. Office of Management and Budget to determine population centers in the United States. Body mass index (BMI) was measured as an interval-level variable calculated from participant weight and height.

### 2.2.3. Past-Year Mental Illness

Past-year mental illness was assessed as a four-category variable (none, mild, moderate, severe). This variable was based on predicted probabilities of having a mental illness and severity level of the mental illness given the participant's age, level of functional disability, suicidal ideation, and major depressive episode based on NSDUH subsample validation studies that compared this measure with the results of clinical interviews using a semi-structured diagnostic instrument [24].

### 2.2.4. Substance Abuse/Dependence

Alcohol and other drug abuse/dependence excluding nicotine were based on self-report and assessed with two binary (no/yes) variables reflecting past-year alcohol abuse/dependence and past-year abuse/dependence on drugs other than alcohol. Criteria for abuse/dependence were based on the Diagnostic and Statistical Manual of Mental Disorders, Fifth Edition (DSM-IV) diagnostic criteria [25]. Past-month nicotine dependence was also assessed as a binary variable based on participant responses to the Nicotine Dependence Syndrome Scale embedded in the NSDUH survey [26].

## 2.3. Dependent Variables

### Medical Conditions and Infectious Diseases

NSDUH participants were asked if they were told by a doctor or other health care professional that they had any of the following eight medical conditions: Asthma, heart condition, hypertension, diabetes, chronic bronchitis or chronic obstructive pulmonary disease (COPD), cirrhosis, kidney disease, or any kind of cancer. Cirrhosis was dropped from the analysis due to the small number of participants who reported ever having that condition ($N = 154$). The survey also asked about the lifetime presence of any of the following infectious diseases: Hepatitis B or C; sexually transmitted infections (STIs) other than HIV/AIDS, such as syphilis, gonorrhea, chlamydia, or herpes; or HIV/AIDs. All medical conditions and infectious diseases included in the analysis were coded as binary (yes/no) variables.

*2.4. Analyses*

Analyses were conducted using Stata 14.2. (StataCorp LLC, College Station, TX, USA) [27]. Data were weighted for selection probability and standard errors were adjusted to reflect NSDUH design characteristics owing to clustering and stratification [24]. Bivariate analyses were first run to obtain the unadjusted prevalence rate for each medical condition or infectious disease by sexual identity. The bivariate prevalence rates for each medical condition were obtained by cross-tabulating the condition with the three-category variables used to represent sexual identity and obtaining the percentage positive for that condition within each sexual identity category. In the multivariable models, the adjusted odds ratios (AORs) of having each medical condition or infectious disease for sexual identity, attraction, and concordance were determined in separate binary logistic models. Interaction effects were also conducted to determine if there were any significant associations between sexual identity and concordance/discordance. Model covariates included: Demographics, mental illness, substance abuse/dependence, and nicotine dependence. All multivariable models also adjusted for HIV/AIDS, except in the model in which HIV/AIDS was the dependent variable.

## 3. Results

*3.1. Demographics*

Table 1 presents sample demographics by sexual identity. There were significant demographic differences by sexual identity for all demographic variables. Individuals between the ages of 18–34 were more likely to report being bisexual than any other age group (70%), whereas those who were 65 and older were much more likely to report being heterosexual (21.9%) than bisexual (2.4%) or lesbian (12.0%; $F_{(5.1, 253.9)} = 131.8$, $p < 0.001$). Bisexual women were more likely to report having some college (38.4%) than a high school degree (26.9%) or a college degree (21.8%) or some high school (13.0%; $F_{(4.8, 238.4)} = 14.0$, $p < 0.001$). Heterosexual participants were more like to report being married (51.5%), whereas those who identified as lesbian/gay (59.4%) or bisexual (58.4%) were more likely to have never been married ($F_{(4.23, 211.6)} = 188.7$, $p < 0.001$). Bisexual women also reported higher rates of poverty (26.4%) than lesbian/gay (18.9%) or heterosexual women (15.7%), with heterosexual women more likely to report incomes greater than twice the federal poverty level (63.4%; $F_{(3.3, 166.9)} = 40.2$, $p < 0.001$).

Table 1. Demographics and Self-reported Sexual Attraction by Sexual Identity.

| Sexual Identity | Heterosexual (N = 62,038) % | [95% CI] | Gay or Lesbian (N = 1321) % | [95% CI] | Bisexual (N = 4289) % | [95% CI] | Totals (N = 67,648) % | [95% CI] | Sig |
|---|---|---|---|---|---|---|---|---|---|
| Race/Ethnicity | | | | | | | | | ** |
| Non-Hispanic white | 64.7 | [63.9, 65.5] | 63.8 | [59.9, 67.8] | 61.3 | [59.4, 63.3] | 64.6 | [63.8, 65.3] | |
| Non-Hispanic black/African-American | 12.4 | [11.9, 13.0] | 15.7 | [13.0, 18.8] | 14.1 | [12.7, 15.7] | 12.5 | [12.0, 13.0] | |
| Hispanic | 15.1 | [14.5, 15.7] | 14.3 | [11.7, 17.4] | 15.7 | [14.2, 17.3] | 15.1 | [14.5, 15.7] | |
| Asian/Pacific Islander/Native American/multi-ethnic | 7.9 | [7.5, 8.2] | 6.2 | [4.6, 8.4] | 8.9 | [7.5, 10.5] | 7.9 | [7.5, 8.2] | |
| Age (in years) | | | | | | | | | *** |
| 18–25 | 12.4 | [12.1, 12.8] | 20.9 | [18.5, 23.5] | 41.5 | [39.5, 43.6] | 13.7 | [13.3, 14.0] | |
| 26–34 | 14.8 | [14.5, 15.2] | 20.6 | [17.6, 24.1] | 28.5 | [26.6, 30.4] | 15.5 | [15.1, 15.8] | |
| 35–49 | 24.6 | [24.0, 25.1] | 23.0 | [20.1, 25.6] | 19.8 | [17.9, 21.9] | 24.4 | [23.9, 24.9] | |
| 50–64 | 26.2 | [25.6, 26.9] | 23.5 | [19.2, 28.4] | 7.8 | [5.9, 10.3] | 25.5 | [24.9, 26.1] | |
| 65+ | 21.9 | [21.2, 22.7] | 12.0 | [8.1, 17.4] | 2.4 | [1.6, 3.6] | 21.0 | [20.4, 21.7] | |
| Education (highest grade) | | | | | | | | | *** |
| Less than high school | 11.9 | [11.3, 12.4] | 10.4 | [8.2, 13.3] | 13.0 | [11.8, 14.3] | 11.9 | [11.4, 12.4] | |
| High school graduate | 23.5 | [23.0, 24.0] | 19.5 | [16.5, 22.9] | 26.9 | [25.5, 28.3] | 23.6 | [23.1, 24.0] | |
| Some college/associate's degree | 32.8 | [32.2, 33.4] | 35.2 | [31.1, 39.5] | 38.4 | [36.5, 40.3] | 33.0 | [32.5, 33.6] | |
| College graduate | 31.9 | [31.1, 32.7] | 35.0 | [30.3, 39.8] | 21.8 | [19.7, 24.0] | 31.6 | [30.8, 32.3] | |
| Marital Status | | | | | | | | | *** |
| Married | 51.5 | [50.8, 52.3] | 25.5 | [20.9, 30.7] | 24.8 | [23.0, 26.6] | 50.1 | [49.3, 50.8] | |
| Widowed | 8.9 | [8.5, 9.3] | 3.2 | [1.7, 5.9] | 1.1 | [0.8, 1.5] | 8.5 | [8.1, 8.9] | |
| Divorced or Separated | 15.9 | [15.3, 16.4] | 11.9 | [9.9, 14.1] | 15.7 | [14.0, 17.7] | 15.8 | [15.3, 16.3] | |
| Never been married | 23.8 | [23.2, 24.3] | 59.4 | [54.3, 64.4] | 58.4 | [56.3, 60.5] | 25.7 | [25.1, 26.2] | |
| Poverty Level | | | | | | | | | *** |
| Living in poverty | 15.7 | [15.2, 16.2] | 18.9 | [15.6, 22.6] | 26.4 | [24.8, 28.1] | 16.2 | [15.6, 16.7] | |
| Income up to twice the federal poverty level | 21.0 | [20.4, 21.4] | 19.5 | [16.3, 23.3] | 24.3 | [22.7, 26.0] | 21.0 | [20.5, 21.5] | |
| Income greater than twice the federal poverty level | 63.4 | [62.7, 64.1] | 61.6 | [56.8, 66.2] | 49.3 | [47.1, 51.5] | 62.8 | [62.1, 63.6] | |
| Population Density [a] | | | | | | | | | ** |
| CBSA > 1 million | 53.5 | [52.7, 54.2] | 54.0 | [49.4, 58.6] | 55.9 | [53.9, 58.0] | 53.6 | [52.9, 54.3] | |
| CBSA < 1 million | 40.7 | [39.9, 41.7] | 42.1 | [37.5, 47.0] | 39.6 | [37.9, 41.4] | 40.7 | [39.9, 41.4] | |
| Not in CBSA | 5.9 | [5.4, 6.4] | 3.8 | [2.5, 5.8] | 4.5 | [3.7, 5.5] | 5.8 | [5.3, 6.3] | |
| Sexual Attraction [b] | | | | | | | | | *** |
| Only attracted to opposite sex | 91.6 | [91.3, 91.8] | 3.7 | [2.1, 6.2] | 5.6 | [4.4, 7.3] | 87.0 | [86.7, 87.3] | |
| Mostly attracted to opposite sex | 6.2 | [6.0, 6.4] | 3.5 | [1.9, 6.3] | 28.6 | [26.7, 30.5] | 7.0 | [6.8, 7.2] | |
| Equally attracted to both sexes | 1.6 | [1.4, 1.7] | 4.5 | [3.0, 6.6] | 59.4 | [57.1, 61.7] | 3.8 | [3.6, 3.9] | |
| Mostly attracted to same sex | 0.1 | [0.1, 0.2] | 32.3 | [28.9, 35.9] | 6.1 | [5.1, 7.2] | 0.9 | [0.8, 0.9] | |
| Only attracted to same sex | 0.5 | [0.5, 0.6] | 56.1 | [52.1, 60.0] | 0.3 | [0.1, 0.6] | 1.4 | [1.3, 1.6] | |
| Sexual Attraction (mean score) | 1.1 | [1.1, 1.1] | 4.3 | [4.2, 4.4] | 2.7 | [2.6, 2.7] | 1.3 | [1.1, 1.13] | |
| Sexual Identity and Attraction | | | | | | | | | *** |
| Concordant | 89.7 | [89.4, 90.0] | 55.0 | [51.0, 58.9] | 94.1 | [92.4, 95.4] | 89.3 | [88.6, 89.9] | |
| Discordant | 10.3 | [100, 10.6] | 45.0 | [48.1, 49.0] | 5.9 | [4.6, 7.6] | 10.7 | [10.1, 11.4] | |

Note: All figures reflect weighted percentages and are based on 67,648 female NSDUH participants 18 years of age and older. Sample N's at the top of each column are unweighted. All figures are percentages unless otherwise indicated. Design-based F-tests based on the weighted data and controlling for stratification and clustering were used to test statistical significance. [a] Population density is based on Core Based Statistical Areas (CBSA), which are used by the U.S. Office of Management and Budget to define population centers in the U.S. [b] Sexual attraction was self-reported using a scale from 1 to 5 with the lowest score indicating exclusive attraction to members of the opposite sex and higher scores indicating increasingly greater attraction to the same sex. 95% CI= 95% Confidence Interval. Sig=significance level. ** $p < 0.01$; *** $p < 0.001$.

There was a strong and positive correlation between sexual identity and sexual attraction ($r = 0.78$, $p < 0.01$). Those who reported being attracted only to those of the opposite sex were also more likely to identify as heterosexual (91.6%), while those who identified as lesbian reported being only attracted to the same sex (56.1%) and mostly attracted to the same sex (32.3%; $F_{(6.3, 313.7)} = 1125.7$, $p < 0.001$). Women who identified as bisexual were the most likely to report concordance in their sexual identity and attraction (94.1%; $F_{(1.92, 96.0)} = 229.9$, $p < 0.001$), followed by heterosexual (89.7%) and lesbian participants (55%). This result demonstrates that self-reported sexual identity may, in some instances, be in conflict with self-reported sexual attraction and may cause discordance.

### 3.2. Medical Conditions, Infectious Diseases, and Behavioral Health Issues

Table 2 shows the results for the bivariate comparisons of the unadjusted lifetime prevalence rates of the seven medical conditions and three infectious diseases by sexual identity. Several of the medical conditions showed significant differences attributable to sexual identity. Bisexual (18%) and gay/lesbian (16.5%) women were more likely than heterosexual (10.8%) women to report having asthma ($F_{(2.0, 99.4)} = 36.4$, $p < 0.001$). Conversely, lifetime prevalence of hypertension was reported more often by heterosexual women (22%) compared with lesbian (15.1%) and bisexual women (9.7%; $F_{(1.92, 96.1)} = 84.9$, $p < 0.001$).

Heterosexual women were also more likely to report having a heart condition (9.6%) than bisexual women (6.5%) or lesbian identified women (7.4%; $F_{(1.9, 98.8)} = 8.6$, $p < 0.01$), and both lesbian women (10.1%) and heterosexual women (10.7%) were more likely than bisexual women (6.1%) to report having diabetes ($F_{(1.74, 87.1)} = 15.5$, $p < 0.01$).

There were significant associations between sexual identity and two of the three infectious diseases. Bisexual women (2%) reported higher rates of hepatitis B/C than gay/lesbian (1.5%) or heterosexual women (0.98%; $F_{(1.9, 99.0)} = 5.6$, $p < 0.01$). Similarly, bisexual women were more likely to report having had an STI in the past 12 months (5.8%) compared to lesbian (2.2%) and heterosexual (2.2%) women ($F_{(1.9, 95.0)} = 46.7$, $p < 0.001$). However, there was no significant difference in the prevalence of HIV/AIDS by sexual identity.

### 3.3. Multivariable Models of Medical Conditions and Infectious Diseases

Table 3 shows the AORs of having any medical condition or infectious disease for sexual identity, attraction, and concordance. The overall significance for each multivariable chronic condition model was assessed using the adjusted Wald F-test to account for any survey design effects [28]. There were significant associations between sexual identity and the odds of having three medical conditions and two of the three infectious diseases. Bisexual women (AOR = 1.5, $p < 0.001$) and lesbian women (AOR = 2.0, $p < 0.05$) had higher odds of ever having asthma than heterosexual women, while both bisexual (AOR = 1.8, $p < 0.01$) and lesbian/gay women (AOR = 3.0, $p < 0.05$) had higher odds of reporting chronic bronchitis/COPD relative to heterosexual women. Bisexual women were also more likely to report lifetime prevalence of any cancer (AOR = 1.9, $p < 0.05$) than heterosexual women. Among the infectious diseases examined, bisexual women had higher odds of reporting hepatitis B/C (AOR = 2.8, $p < 0.05$) and any STIs in the past 12 months (AOR = 2.1, $p < 0.01$) than heterosexual women.

**Table 2.** Bivariate Comparisons of the Lifetime Prevalence of Medical Conditions, Infectious Diseases, and Behavioral Health Issues by Sexual Identity.

| Sexual Identity | Heterosexual (N = 62,038) | | Gay or Lesbian (N = 1321) | | Bisexual (N = 4289) | | Totals (N = 67,648) | | Sig |
|---|---|---|---|---|---|---|---|---|---|
| | % | [95% CI] | % | [95% CI] | % | [95% CI] | % | [95% CI] | |
| Asthma | 10.8 | [10.5, 11.2] | 16.5 | [13.5, 20.0] | 18.0 | [16.1, 20.2] | 11.2 | [10.8, 11.6] | *** |
| Medical Conditions | | | | | | | | | |
| Heart condition | 9.6 | [9.2, 10.0] | 7.4 | [5.3, 10.2] | 6.5 | [5.4, 8.0] | 9.4 | [9.0, 9.8] | ** |
| Hypertension | 22.0 | [21.5, 22.6] | 15.1 | [12.3, 18.4] | 9.7 | [8.4, 11.2] | 21.4 | [20.9, 22.6] | *** |
| Diabetes | 10.7 | [10.3, 11.2] | 10.1 | [7.3, 13.8] | 6.1 | [5.1, 7.3] | 10.5 | [10.1, 11.0] | *** |
| Chronic bronchitis or COPD | 5.4 | [5.1, 5.7] | 6.9 | [4.4, 10.6] | 5.6 | [4.7, 6.6] | 5.5 | [5.2, 5.8] | NS |
| Cirrhosis | 0.2 | [0.1, 0.3] | 0.2 | [0.003, 0.2] | 0.3 | [0.1, 0.9] | 0.2 | [0.2, 0.3] | NS |
| Kidney Disease | 2.2 | [2.0, 2.4] | 1.3 | [0.5, 3.2] | 1.6 | [1.1, 2.3] | 2.1 | [1.9, 2.3] | NS |
| Cancer (any kind) | 7.3 | [6.9, 7.6] | 5.9 | [3.7, 9.2] | 3.9 | [3.0, 5.2] | 7.1 | [6.8, 7.5] | ** |
| Infectious Diseases | | | | | | | | | |
| Hepatitis B or C | 1.0 | [0.9, 1.1] | 1.5 | [0.6, 3.0] | 2.0 | [1.4, 2.8] | 1.0 | [0.9, 1.2] | ** |
| Sexually transmitted infections [a] | 2.2 | [2.0, 2.4] | 2.2 | [1.4, 3.4] | 5.8 | [5.0, 6.8] | 2.3 | [2.2, 2.5] | *** |
| HIV/AIDS | 0.1 | [0.1, 0.1] | 0.2 | [0.1, 0.5] | 0.1 | [0.0, 0.4] | 0.1 | [0.1, 0.1] | NS |
| Behavioral Health Issues | | | | | | | | | |
| Body Mass Index | 28.1 | [28.0, 28.2] | 29.1 | [28.5, 29.6] | 28.8 | [28.4, 29.1] | 28.7 | [28.3, 29.0] | *** |
| Past-year mental illness [b] | | | | | | | | | *** |
| Mild | 10.4 | [10.1, 10.7] | 13.1 | [10.6, 16.0] | 17.1 | [15.6, 18.8] | 10.6 | [10.4, 11.0] | |
| Moderate | 5.6 | [5.3, 5.8] | 6.1 | [4.8, 7.8] | 14.0 | [12.6, 15.5] | 5.9 | [5.7, 6.1] | |
| Serious | 4.9 | [4.6, 5.1] | 12.6 | [10.1, 15.6] | 20.3 | [18.6, 22.1] | 5.6 | [5.3, 5.9] | |
| Past-year substance abuse or dependence | | | | | | | | | |
| Nicotine | 10.0 | [9.6, 10.3] | 16.2 | [13.3, 19.6] | 20.0 | [18.4, 21.7] | 10.5 | [10.1, 10.8] | *** |
| Alcohol | 3.9 | [3.7, 4.1] | 7.7 | [6.0, 9.9] | 12.5 | [11.2, 13.8] | 4.3 | [4.0, 4.7] | *** |
| Other drugs | 1.6 | [1.5, 1.7] | 4.3 | [3.3, 5.7] | 8.5 | [7.4, 9.8] | 1.9 | [1.8, 2.0] | *** |

Note. All figures reflect weighted percentages and are based on 67,648 female NSDUH participants 18 years of age and older. Subgroup N's at the top of each column are unweighted. All figures are percentages unless otherwise indicated. Design-based F-tests based on the weighted data and controlling for stratification and clustering were used to assess statistical significance. [a] Sexually transmitted infections includes gonorrhea, chlamydia, syphilis, or herpes. [b] Past-year mental illness category is based on thresholds derived from a logistic regression model of mental illness as predicted by age, functional disability, thoughts of suicide, and major depressive episode. 95% CI = 95% Confidence Interval. Sig = significance level. NS = non-significant; ** $p < 0.01$; *** $p < 0.001$.

**Table 3.** Bivariate Logistic Regression Results for Medical Conditions and Infectious Diseases.

| Medical Condition/Infectious Disease | Asthma AOR | 95% CI | Heart Condition AOR | 95% CI | Hypertension AOR | 95% CI | Diabetes AOR | 95% CI | Chronic Bronchitis/COPD AOR | 95% CI |
|---|---|---|---|---|---|---|---|---|---|---|
| Sexual Identity (Heterosexual = reference) | | | | | | | | | | |
| Bisexual | 1.5 | [1.2, 2.0] | 1.2 | [0.8, 1.7] | 1.0 | [0.7, 1.4] | 1.4 | [1.0, 2.0] | 1.8 | [1.2, 2.7] ** |
| Gay | 2.0 *** | [1.1, 3.5] | 0.7 * | [0.3, 1.7] | 0.8 | [0.4, 1.6] | 1.8 | [0.4, 4.6] | 3.0 | [1.2, 7.7] * |
| Sexual attraction [b] | 0.9 | [0.8, 1.0] | 1.1 | [0.9, 1.3] | 1.0 | [0.9, 1.1] | 0.8 | [0.7, 1.0] | 1.0 | [0.8, 1.1] |
| Discordant sexual identity and attraction (Concordant = reference) | 1.2 | [1.0, 1.5] | 1.1 | [0.8, 1.4] | 1.0 | [0.7, 1.3] | 1.3 | [0.9, 1.8] | 1.0 | [0.7, 1.5] |
| Sexual Identity and Concordance Interaction (concordant + bisexual discordant + gay discordant = reference) | | | | | | | | | | |
| Bisexual and Discordant | 0.5 * | [0.2, 1.0] | 1.0 | [0.4, 2.7] | 0.6 | [0.3, 1.5] | 0.6 | [0.2, 2.0] | 1.3 | [0.4, 4.5] |
| Gay and Discordant | 0.8 | [0.5, 1.3] | 1.1 | [0.5, 2.3] | 1.0 | [0.4, 2.3] | 1.0 | [0.3, 2.6] | 0.4 | [0.1, 1.2] |
| Race/ethnicity (White = reference) | | | | | | | | | | |
| Non-Hispanic black/African-American | 0.9 | [0.8, 1.0] | 0.6 | [0.5, 0.7] | 1.8 *** | [1.6, 2.0] | 1.6 *** | [1.4, 1.8] | 0.6 | [0.4, 0.7] |
| Hispanic | 0.8 *** | [0.7, 0.9] | 0.6 | [0.4, 0.7] | 0.8 ** | [0.7, 0.9] | 1.6 *** | [1.4, 1.9] | 0.5 | [0.4, 0.7] |
| Asian/Pacific Islander/Native American/multi-ethnic | 1.0 | [0.8, 1.2] | 0.7 ** | [0.5, 0.9] | 1.2 * | [1.1, 1.5] | 1.8 *** | [1.4, 2.3] | 0.9 | [0.7, 1.2] |
| Age in years (18–25 = reference) | | | | | | | | | | |
| 26–34 | 0.8 *** | [0.7, 0.9] | 1.0 | [0.8, 1.4] | 2.3 *** | [2.0, 2.7] | 1.9 *** | [1.6, 2.3] | 1.4 ** | [1.1, 1.8] |
| 35–49 | 0.7 *** | [0.6, 0.8] | 1.8 | [1.5, 2.0] | 5.8 | [5.1, 6.7] | 3.9 *** | [3.2, 4.7] | 2.6 *** | [2.1, 3.2] |
| 50–64 | 0.7 *** | [0.6, 0.7] | 3.6 | [3.0, 4.2] | 16.7 | [14.5, 19.3] | 8.4 *** | [6.9, 10.2] | 6.7 *** | [5.4, 8.3] |
| 65+ | 0.7 | [0.6, 0.8] | 9.6 | [8.2, 11.2] | 37.6 | [32.6, 43.5] | 14.2 *** | [11.6, 17.4] | 12.9 *** | [10.3, 16.3] |
| Education level (Less than high school = reference) | | | | | | | | | | |
| High school graduate | 1.0 | [0.9, 1.2] | 0.9 | [0.8, 1.1] | 1.3 | [1.2, 1.5] | 0.9 | [0.7, 1.1] | 1.0 | [0.8, 1.3] |
| Some college/associate's degree | 1.2 ** | [1.0, 1.4] | 0.9 | [0.7, 1.0] | 1.4 | [1.2, 1.6] | 0.8 *** | [0.7, 0.9] | 0.9 | [0.8, 1.1] |
| College graduate | 1.4 *** | [1.1, 1.6] | 0.9 | [0.7, 1.1] | 1.2 | [1.1, 1.5] | 0.6 | [0.5, 0.7] | 0.7 | [0.5, 0.9] |
| Marital Status (Married = reference) | | | | | | | | | | |
| Widowed | 0.8 | [0.7, 1.0] | 1.5 | [1.3, 1.8] | 1.2 * | [1.0, 1.4] | 1.1 | [0.9, 1.3] | 1.3 * | [1.0, 1.6] |
| Divorced or separated | 1.3 *** | [1.2, 1.4] | 1.2 | [1.0, 1.4] | 1.0 | [0.9, 1.1] | 1.0 | [0.9, 1.1] | 1.4 ** | [1.1, 1.7] |
| Never been married | 1.1 | [1.0, 1.2] | 1.0 | [0.9, 1.03] | 0.9 | [0.8, 1.0] | 0.9 * | [0.8, 1.0] | 1.0 | [0.8, 1.3] |
| Poverty Level (Living in poverty = reference) | | | | | | | | | | |
| Income up to twice the federal poverty level | 1.2 | [1.1, 1.3] | 1.3 | [1.1, 1.6] | 1.0 | [0.9, 1.1] | 1.1 | [1.0, 1.3] | 1.5 | [1.3, 1.9] |
| Income greater than twice the federal poverty level | 1.0 ** | [0.9, 1.1] | 1.2 | [1.0, 1.4] | 1.1 | [1.0, 1.2] | 1.3 | [1.2, 1.5] | 1.3 *** | [1.1, 1.5] |
| Population Density [c] (Not in CBSA = reference) | | | | | | | | | | |
| CBSA > 1 million | 1.1 | [0.9, 1.3] | 0.8 | [0.7, 0.9] | 0.9 | [0.8, 1.1] | 0.9 | [0.8, 1.1] | 0.9 | [0.8, 1.1] |
| CBSA < 1 million | 1.1 | [1.0, 1.3] | 0.9 | [0.7, 1.1] | 1.0 | [0.9, 1.1] | 1.0 | [0.9, 1.2] | 0.9 | [0.8, 1.1] |
| HIV/AIDS ever (Never/unknown = reference) | 0.8 | [0.3, 2.1] | 2.6 | [0.7, 9.9] | 1.8 | [0.6, 5.4] | 1.9 | [0.7, 5.6] | 1.1 | [0.3, 5.0] |
| Body Mass Index | 1.0 *** | [1.0, 1.04] | 1.0 | [1.0, 1.03] | 1.1 | [1.1, 1.1] | 1.1 | [1.1, 1.1] | 1.0 | [1.0, 1.04] |
| Past-year mental illness [d] (None = reference) | | | | | | | | | | |
| Mild | 1.3 | [1.2, 1.5] | 1.6 | [1.4, 1.9] | 1.0 | [0.8, 1.1] | 1.4 *** | [1.2, 1.6] | 1.9 | [1.6, 2.3] |
| Moderate | 1.7 | [1.5, 2.0] | 1.8 | [1.5, 2.1] | 1.1 | [0.9, 1.1] | 1.4 *** | [1.2, 1.7] | 2.3 | [1.8, 2.9] |
| Serious | 2.1 | [1.9, 2.4] | 2.1 | [1.8, 2.5] | 1.1 | [1.0, 1.2] | 1.7 | [1.4, 2.1] | 2.1 | [1.6, 3.8] |
| Past-month nicotine dependence (Not dependent = reference) | 0.9 | [0.8, 1.1] | 0.9 | [0.7, 1.1] | 0.9 | [0.8, 1.1] | 1.2 | [1.0, 1.4] | 2.8 | [2.4, 3.1] |
| Past-year alcohol dependence/abuse (Not dependent/abusing = reference) | 1.0 | [0.8, 1.2] | 0.9 | [0.7, 1.1] | 1.0 | [0.9, 1.2] | 0.7 * | [0.5, 1.0] | 0.7 * | [0.6, 1.0] |
| Past-year other drug dependence/abuse (Not dependent/abusing = reference) | 1.3 | [1.0, 1.5] | 1.6 * | [1.2, 2.1] | 1.4 | [1.1, 1.8] | 1.0 | [0.7, 1.4] | 1.5 | [1.1, 2.0] |
| **Model Statistics and Diagnostics** | | | | | | | | | | |
| $F_{(31, 20)}$ [e] | 50.4 *** | | 59.9 *** | | 145.5 *** | | *** | | 50.9 *** | |
| Squared Residuals [f] | −4.20 | NS | −0.80 | NS | −6.20 | NS | NS | | 0.06 | NS |
| Coefficient of Discrimination [g] | −47.0 *** | | −110.0 *** | | −160.0 *** | | NS | | −90.1 *** | |

| Medical Condition/Infectious Disease | Kidney Disease AOR | 95% CI | Cancer AOR | 95% CI | Hepatitis B or C AOR | 95% CI | Sexually Transmitted Infections [a] AOR | 95% CI | HIV/AIDS AOR | 95% CI |
|---|---|---|---|---|---|---|---|---|---|---|
| Sexual Orientation (Heterosexual = reference) | | | | | | | | | | |
| Bisexual | 1.2 | [0.6, 2.5] | 1.9 | [1.0, 3.3] | 2.8 | [1.1, 7.5] | 2.1 ** | [1.3, 3.6] | 0.5 | [0.1, 5.1] |
| Gay | 0.5 | [0.1, 4.0] | 1.5 | [0.5, 4.6] | 2.2 | [0.3, 16.0] | 1.9 | [0.5, 7.1] | 0.3 | [0.004, 14.6] |
| Sexual attraction [b] | 1.0 | [0.7, 1.3] | 0.9 | [0.7, 1.7] | 0.9 | [0.6, 1.4] | 0.8 | [0.6, 1.1] | 1.7 | [0.7, 4.2] |
| Discordant sexual identity and attraction (Concordant = reference) | 1.3 | [0.7, 2.4] | 1.1 | [0.7, 1.7] | 1.1 | [0.6, 2.3] | 2.2 *** | [1.5, 3.1] | 0.7 | [0.1, 6.4] |
| Sexual Identity and Concordance Interaction (concordant + bisexual discordant + gay discordant = reference) | | | | | | | | | | |
| Bisexual and Discordant | 2.1 | [0.4, 11.7] | 0.5 | [0.1, 2.4] | 1.7 | [0.3, 9.5] | 0.2 ** | [0.1, 0.5] | 1.0 | [0.01, 97.7] |
| Gay and Discordant | 1.7 | [0.2, 15.2] | 0.8 | [0.3, 1.9] | 0.8 | [0.2, 4.6] | 0.2 * | [0.1, 0.8] | NE | [0.01, 97.7] |

**Table 3.** *Cont.*

| | Kidney Disease | | | Cancer | | | Hepatitis B or C | | | Sexually Transmitted Infections [a] | | | HIV/AIDS | | |
|---|---|---|---|---|---|---|---|---|---|---|---|---|---|---|---|
| | AOR | 95% CI | | AOR | 95% CI | | AOR | 95% CI | | AOR | 95% CI | | AOR | 95% CI | |
| **Race/ethnicity (White = reference)** | | | | | | | | | | | | | | | |
| Non-Hispanic black/African-American | 1.2 | [0.8, 1.6] | | 0.4 | [0.3, 0.5] | *** | 0.7 | [0.5, 1.1] | | 1.5 | [1.2, 1.8] | ** | 3.2 | [1.3, 7.9] | * |
| Hispanic | 1.1 | [0.7, 1.4] | | 0.5 | [0.4, 0.6] | *** | 1.1 | [0.8, 1.6] | | 0.9 | [0.7, 1.2] | | 1.3 | [0.2, 6.6] | |
| Asian/Pacific Islander/Native American/multi-ethnic | 0.9 | [0.6, 1.4] | | 0.6 | [0.4, 0.7] | *** | 1.6 | [1.1, 2.3] | * | 0.7 | [0.6, 0.9] | * | 1.8 | [0.4, 8.2] | |
| **Age in years (18–25 = reference)** | | | | | | | | | | | | | | | |
| 26–34 | 1.5 | [1.1, 2.1] | | 2.7 | [2.0, 3.7] | *** | 2.3 | [1.3, 3.8] | ** | 0.8 | [0.7, 1.0] | * | 0.9 | [0.3, 3.3] | |
| 35–49 | 2.7 | [1.9, 3.8] | ** | 6.1 | [4.6, 8.0] | | 4.0 | [2.3, 6.9] | *** | 0.6 | [0.5, 0.8] | *** | 3.6 | [1.2, 11.4] | * |
| 50–64 | 4.3 | [3.0, 6.2] | *** | 15.1 | [11.1, 20.6] | | 7.9 | [4.4, 14.3] | *** | 0.5 | [0.4, 0.7] | *** | 5.6 | [1.8, 17.6] | ** |
| 65+ | 11.1 | [7.8, 15.8] | *** | 31.8 | [23.4, 43.3] | *** | 8.9 | [4.6, 17.5] | *** | 0.4 | [0.3, 0.5] | *** | 1.3 | [0.3, 5.2] | |
| **Education level (Less than high school = reference)** | | | | | | | | | | | | | | | |
| High school graduate | 0.9 | [0.7, 1.2] | | 1.3 | [1.1, 1.7] | * | 0.9 | [0.6, 1.3] | | 1.3 | [1.0, 1.7] | * | 0.3 | [0.1, 0.7] | ** |
| Some college/associate's degree | 1.1 | [0.8, 1.5] | | 1.6 | [1.2, 2.0] | ** | 0.8 | [0.6, 1.2] | | 1.2 | [1.0, 1.5] | | 0.2 | [0.1, 0.7] | ** |
| College graduate | 0.8 | [0.6, 1.1] | | 1.7 | [1.3, 2.2] | *** | 0.9 | [0.6, 1.3] | | 1.4 | [1.1, 1.9] | ** | 0.0 | [0.0, 0.2] | *** |
| **Marital Status (Married = reference)** | | | | | | | | | | | | | | | |
| Widowed | 1.2 | [0.9, 1.6] | | 1.1 | [0.9, 1.2] | | 1.3 | [0.9, 2.1] | | 0.8 | [0.5, 1.3] | | 3.4 | [1.0, 12.4] | * |
| Divorced or separated | 1.1 | [0.9, 1.5] | | 1.1 | [1.0, 1.3] | | 1.1 | [0.9, 1.5] | | 2.0 | [1.6, 2.6] | *** | 3.9 | [1.3, 11.6] | * |
| Never been married | 1.0 | [0.8, 1.4] | | 1.1 | [0.9, 1.4] | *** | 1.2 | [0.8, 1.8] | | 1.5 | [1.3, 1.8] | *** | 3.4 | [1.1, 10.5] | * |
| **Poverty Level (Living in poverty = reference)** | | | | | | | | | | | | | | | |
| Income up to twice the federal poverty level | 1.5 | [1.1, 2.0] | * | 0.8 | [0.7, 1.0] | * | 2.3 | [1.5, 3.4] | *** | 1.1 | [0.9, 1.3] | | 1.3 | [0.5, 3.1] | |
| Income greater than twice the federal poverty level | 1.4 | [1.2, 1.7] | ** | 1.0 | [0.8, 1.1] | | 1.2 | [0.8, 1.7] | | 1.1 | [0.9, 1.3] | | 2.0 | [0.9, 4.6] | |
| **Population Density [c] (Not in CBSA = reference)** | | | | | | | | | | | | | | | |
| CBSA > 1 million | 0.8 | [0.6, 1.3] | | 1.2 | [1.0, 1.4] | * | 1.3 | [0.8, 2.1] | | 1.0 | [0.8, 1.4] | | 3.9 | [1.1, 13.9] | * |
| CBSA < 1 million | 0.9 | [0.7, 1.3] | | 1.2 | [1.0, 1.4] | * | 1.4 | [0.9, 2.3] | | 1.1 | [0.8, 1.4] | | 2.1 | [0.6, 8.0] | |
| HIV/AIDS ever (Never/unknown = reference) | 6.0 | [1.0, 35.1] | | 1.7 | [0.4, 7.5] | | 10 | [2.6, 38.1] | *** | 4.2 | [1.5, 12.0] | ** | NE | | |
| Body Mass Index | 1.0 | [1.0, 1.04] | * | 1.00 | [1.0, 1.0] | | 1.0 | [1.0, 1.0] | * | 1.0 | [1.0, 1.0] | | 1.0 | [0.9, 1.0] | |
| **Past-year mental illness [d] (None = reference)** | | | | | | | | | | | | | | | |
| Mild | 1.9 | [1.4, 2.4] | | 1.2 | [1.0, 1.4] | * | 2.0 | [1.5, 2.7] | *** | 1.7 | [1.4, 2.1] | *** | 2.4 | [0.7, 8.8] | |
| Moderate | 2.0 | [1.4, 3.0] | | 1.3 | [1.0, 1.6] | | 1.9 | [1.2, 2.9] | * | 1.6 | [1.3, 2.9] | *** | 4.5 | [1.9, 10.9] | *** |
| Serious | 2.9 | [2.0, 4.2] | *** | 1.8 | [1.5, 2.2] | *** | 1.8 | [1.1, 2.7] | * | 1.9 | [1.6, 2.3] | *** | 1.4 | [0.5, 4.3] | |
| Past-month nicotine dependence (Not dependent = reference) | 0.8 | [0.6, 1.0] | | 1.0 | [0.8, 1.1] | | 1.6 | [1.2, 2.2] | *** | 1.3 | [1.1, 1.5] | * | 1.2 | [0.4, 4.2] | |
| Past-year alcohol dependence/abuse (Not dependent/abusing = reference) | 0.3 | [0.2, 0.6] | ** | 0.9 | [0.7, 1.3] | | 1.3 | [0.8, 2.0] | | 1.8 | [1.5, 2.2] | | 2.2 | [0.9, 5.3] | |
| Past-year other drug dependence/abuse (Not dependent/abusing = reference) | 1.0 | [0.6, 1.8] | | 1.1 | [0.8, 1.6] | | 4.0 | [2.6, 6.2] | | 1.8 | [1.5, 2.1] | *** | 1.2 | [0.3, 4.5] | |
| **Model Statistics and Diagnostics** | | | | | | | | | | | | | | | |
| $F_{(29, 22)}$ [e] | 27.3 | *** | | 34.9 | *** | | 18.2 | | | 14.2 | *** | | 47.2 | *** | |
| Squared Residuals [f] | 1.00 | NS | | 0.25 | NS | | 1.07 | NS | | -1.83 | NS | | 0.60 | NS | |
| Coefficient of Discrimination [g] | -44.9 | *** | | -96.1 | *** | | -50.0 | *** | | -46.7 | *** | | -24.4 | *** | |

Note. Bivariate logistic regression models are based on analysis NSDUH 2015–2017 data obtained from 67,648 female respondents 18 years of age and older. Owing to missing data on covariates, the unweighted N for HIV/AIDS was 63,346 and 63,495 for all other medical conditions. Data were weighted to adjust for variation in sampling probabilities. Standard error estimates and significance levels account for design effects owing to stratification and clustering. [a] Sexually transmitted infections includes gonorrhea, chlamydia, syphilis, or herpes. [b] Sexual attraction was self-reported using a scale from 1 to 5 with the lowest score indicating exclusive attraction to members of the opposite sex and higher scores indicating increasingly greater attraction to the same sex. [c] Population density is based on Core Based Statistical Areas (CBSA), which are used by the U.S. Office of Management and Budget to define population centers in the U.S. [d] Past-year mental illness category is based thresholds as derived from a logistic regression model of mental illness as predicted by age, functional disability, thoughts of suicide, and major depressive episode. [e] Reflects an F statistic testing improvement in model fit with included parameters versus a model with only the constant term. Significance indicates a statistically reliable improvement in model fit with inclusion of the parameter estimates. [f] Reflects a t-test of the squared residuals term after fitting the main effects model. Significance indicates unexplained residual variance for the main effects only model and potential model misspecification. [g] Based on the mean difference between the predicted probabilities of having a condition for observed cases and non-cases. Significance was assessed using a t-test. NS = Not significant; NE = Not estimated; * $p < 0.05$, ** $p < 0.01$; *** $p < 0.001$.

To assess whether the effects of sexual identity varied by concordance/discordance status in influencing the prevalence of each chronic condition, the authors included terms representing the interaction between these two primary predictors in each multivariable model. The decision to retain the interaction as having additional influence was based on the significance level of the term, as well as comparison of standard model fit statistics, such as BIC and change in the log-likelihood ratio between the main effects only model and the model containing the interaction term. There was only a single significant difference for identity/attraction concordance: Women who were discordant regardless of sexual identity had higher odds of having STIs (AOR = 2.2, $p < 0.001$) than women whose sexual identity and attraction were concordant. There were no significant associations for any of the assessed conditions or infectious diseases and sexual attraction, although there was one significant interaction effect for sexual identity and concordance. Women who reported being bisexual and discordant (AOR = 0.2, $p < 0.01$) and gay and discordant (AOR = 0.2, $p > 0.05$) had higher odds of reporting STIs than those who had concordance between sexual identity and sexual attraction.

## 4. Discussion

### 4.1. Main Findings

Similar to other studies that examined health disparities related to sexual identity [3,9,10,14–19], our analyses demonstrate differences in the prevalence and odds of a number of CMCs for sexual minority and majority women. Our results augment the findings of earlier studies by supporting their generalizability to a national sample. Most of the significant differences were among women identifying as bisexual in comparison to self-identified heterosexual women [29]. There were fewer significant differences among women identifying as lesbian/gay and no differences in health conditions based on sexual attraction. Although there was one significant difference between sexual minority women and sexual majority women based on concordance between sexual identity and sexual attraction, the overall pattern of results suggests that a person's sexual identity has a greater bearing on health than attraction or the degree of concordance between identity and attraction.

There are likely a number of structural and psychosocial disparities that underlie the cross-study findings of poorer health among sexual minorities, particularly women, that are present in our results: Greater unaffordability of medical care due to health care insurance coverage, poorer quality of care, delays seeking medical care, and greater stress specifically due to identifying as a sexual minority. In this regard, our results could be viewed as supporting intersectionality theory whereby social and economic inequalities owing to race, gender, and sexual identity are related and have larger health effects than would be predicted if considered independently [30].

In our study as well as in previous research, bisexual women were more likely to be socioeconomically disadvantaged and living in impoverished conditions relative to other women [29]. Although the multivariable models in this analysis adjusted for poverty level, other poverty-related factors, such as poorer diet, could have increased the odds of having certain health conditions among bisexual participants and contributed to an inability to afford medical care. Blosnich et al. [31] found that bisexual and lesbian women had much lower odds of seeking medical care owing to cost compared to heterosexual women.

Sexual minority women reported receiving lower quality of medical care received even when they are able to afford care, leading to delays seeing a general practitioner or gynecologist [32]. Hesitation seeking medical care due to stigma and increased stress levels is particularly relevant for bisexual women who had the highest prevalence/odds for multiple health conditions. Research demonstrated that bisexual women report greater stigmatization and social exclusion within lesbian and gay communities as well as from heterosexual communities, resulting in less social support [33]. Greater social isolation could also account for bisexual women seeking more sexual partners in order to develop a sense of belonging, putting them at greater risk for STIs including infection with the human papilloma virus (HPV).

Stress among sexual minority women related to external prejudice, internalized homophobia, and environmental stress at work, school, or home have also been shown to affect health [34,35]. For instance, perceived prejudice related to sexual identity is associated with increased odds of experiencing physical health problems among LGB women even after adjusting for general stressful life events [34]. Additionally, the cumulative effects of persistently increased levels of stress in the lives of sexual minority women could contribute to deterioration in physical health over time. Our findings demonstrated that bisexual women, in particular, had increased odds of reporting any past-year mental illness, which could account for increased stress that may affect health and the development of chronic health conditions.

The findings of higher odds of CMCs and infectious diseases among sexual minority women stands in contrast to our parallel study of sexual minority men [22]. We found no significant associations between the same set of CMCs and infectious diseases and sexual identity, attraction, or concordance, with the exception of HIV/AIDS. The reasons for this gender-based discrepancy is unclear given that gay and bisexual men likely experience some of the same issues (e.g., stigma, medical care affordability) as sexual minority women warranting further study of these gender discrepancies.

## 4.2. Limitations

The NSDUH is cross-sectional and does not allow for assessment of health over the course of life. It is possible health disparities and the effects of sexual identity, attraction, and concordance change over time. Younger participants, especially those with a co-occurring mental illness or substance abuse issues, might not manifest adverse health consequences until later life. Additionally, self-report could generate under- or over-reporting of the CMCs or discrepancies in other measures like mental health, substance use, poverty level, or education. Individuals may have a condition of which they are unaware, particularly if it is asymptomatic or may report a condition that does not meet clinical diagnostic criteria. Furthermore, self-reporting can result in under- or over-reporting due to social desirability bias or recall bias [36]. Although this is a limitation, a review of the literature on the validity of self-reported health data found that self-reported health information is generally valid and reliable [37].

Another limitation is the absence of sexual behavior measures in the NSDUH. Although sexual identity and attraction are important, sexual behavior is another potentially important health-related dimension of sexuality [20]. For example, women who identify as bisexual may be attracted to both men and women but could be exclusively homosexual or heterosexual in their relationships. Questions on sexual behavior would be important additions to national surveys to gain a fuller picture of health related to different aspects of sexuality. Finally, only a limited number of CMCs were assessed with different results possible for excluded conditions.

## 4.3. Implications for Practice

Because both lesbian and bisexual women may not seek medical care to the extent that heterosexual women do, greater education should be given to physicians about sexual minorities and how best to care for them. Disclosing sexual identity to a physician can be seen as challenging as coming out to others for sexual minority patients [38]. Physicians should be mindful of creating a space that allows for disclosure of sexual identity and regularly asking individuals about their sexual preference in order to reduce stigma among sexual minorities and create a safe place for lesbian and bisexual women to share their health concerns. If sexual minority women feel more comfortable to seek care from a primary care physician or gynecologist, this may reduce the risk of developing health problems over time. Physicians who are working with bisexual women should be educated on the various implications and risks of having sexual partners of both sexes. Physicians who create a strong therapeutic relationship with sexual minority patients can enable those patients to discuss health issues more openly and disclose their sexual identity, leading to an increased comfort in seeking medical care as needed [38].

In addition, other professionals working with sexual minority women, such as social workers or counselors, should be aware of the potential increase of chronic health conditions and how that may impact treatment in therapeutic settings or settings that provide resources to sexual minority women. Providing resources for these women could have an impact for future health and providing a safe space for sexual minority women to share their concerns may help encourage women to seek medical help more regularly. If sexual minority women have greater odds of having chronic health conditions or infectious diseases, one potential way of reducing those odds is by creating spaces in which these women feel comfortable seeking medical or other care.

Future research should continue to explore the experiences of sexual minority women and health care. Studies that explore a larger number of CMCs, such as specific cancers, and which use longitudinal data to assess temporal changes would be especially valuable. Qualitative studies to assess the experiences of bisexual women seeking medical care to understand hindrances would allow development of strategies to foster higher engagement in medical care. Understanding health-related differences among sexual minority women related to poverty, racism, and stigma and how these intersect to produce poorer health is also critically important.

## 5. Conclusions

Using a nationally representative sample, we found significant differences in CMCs and infectious diseases for sexual minority in comparison to sexual majority women, especially those who identified as bisexual. Greater understanding and acceptance of bisexuality by both the heterosexual and gay communities could be beneficial in encouraging bisexual women to seek medical care or explore their sexuality in safe ways, which could help to prevent STIs or other CMCs from developing. Bisexual-specific organizations are on the rise [33] and future research could assess the extent to which these environments impact bisexual women's health, tendency to seek medical care, and attitudes about sexuality.

**Author Contributions:** Conceptualization, J.A.S. and K.H. Writing-original draft preparation, K.H. and J.A.S. Writing-review and editing, K.H. and J.A.S. Formal analysis, J.A.S. and K.H.

**Funding:** This research received no external funding.

**Acknowledgments:** The authors have no further acknowledgments.

**Conflicts of Interest:** The authors declare no conflict of interest.

## References

1. Lehavot, K.; Simoni, J.M. The impact of minority stress on mental health and substance use among sexual minority women. *J. Consult. Clin. Psychol.* **2011**, *79*, 159–170. [CrossRef] [PubMed]
2. Lick, D.J.; Durso, L.E.; Johnson, K.L. Minority Stress and Physical Health Among Sexual Minorities. *Perspect. Psychol. Sci.* **2013**, *8*, 521–548. [CrossRef] [PubMed]
3. Boehmer, U.; Maio, X.; Linkletter, C.; Clark, M.A. Adult health behaviors over the life course by sexual orientation. *Am. J. Public Health* **2012**, *102*, 292–300. [CrossRef]
4. Hequembourg, A.L.; Dearing, R.L. Exploring shame, guilt, and risky substance use among sexual minority men and women. *J. Homosex.* **2013**, *60*, 615–638. [CrossRef]
5. Matthews, A.K.; Cho, Y.; Hughes, T.; Wilsnack, S.C.; Johnson, T.; Martin, K. The relationships of sexual identity, hazardous drinking, and drinking expectancies with risky sexual behaviors in a community sample of lesbian and bisexual women. *J. Am. Psychiatr. Nurses Assoc.* **2013**, *19*, 259–270. [CrossRef] [PubMed]
6. Persson, T.J.; Pfaus, J.G.; Ryder, A.G. Explaining mental health disparities for non-monosexual women: Abuse history and risky sex, or the burdens of non-disclosure? *Soc. Sci. Med.* **2015**, *128*, 366–373. [CrossRef] [PubMed]
7. Beach, L.B.; Elasy, T.A.; Gonzales, G. Prevalence of self-reported diabetes by sexual orientation: Results from the 2014 behavioral risk factor surveillance system. *Lgbt Health* **2018**, *5*, 121–130. [CrossRef] [PubMed]

8. Garland-Forshee, R.Y.; Fiala, S.C.; Ngo, D.L.; Moseley, K. Sexual orientation and sex differences in adult chronic conditions, health risk factors, and protective health practices, Oregon 2005–2008. *Previous Chronic Dis.* **2014**, *11*, E136. [CrossRef] [PubMed]
9. Gonzales, G.; Henning-Smith, C. Health disparities by sexual orientation: Results and implications from the Behavioral Risk Factor Surveillance System. *J. Community Health* **2017**, *42*, 1163–1172. [CrossRef]
10. Gonzales, G.; Przedworski, J.; Henning-Smith, C. Comparison of health and health risk factors between lesbian, gay, and bisexual adults and heterosexual adults in the United States: Results from the National Health Interview Survey. *Jama Intern. Med.* **2016**, *176*, 1344–1351. [CrossRef] [PubMed]
11. Boehmer, U.; Maio, X.; Linkletter, C.; Clark, M.A. Health conditions in younger, middle, and older ages: Are there differences by sexual orientation? *Lgbt Health* **2014**, *1*, 168–176. [CrossRef] [PubMed]
12. Swartz, J.A. The relative odds of lifetime health conditions and infectious diseases among men who have sex with men compared with a matched general population sample. *Am. J. Men's Health* **2015**, *9*, 150–162. [CrossRef] [PubMed]
13. Swartz, J.A. Multi-Group latent class analysis of chronic medical conditions among men who have sex with men. *Aids Behav.* **2016**, *20*, 2418–2432. [CrossRef] [PubMed]
14. Cochran, S.D.; Mays, V.M. Physical health complaints among lesbians, gay men, and bisexual and homosexually experienced heterosexual individuals: Results from the california quality of life survey. *Am. J. Public Health* **2007**, *97*, 2048–2055. [CrossRef] [PubMed]
15. Conron, K.J.; Mimiaga, M.J.; Landers, S.J. A population-based study of sexual orientation identity and gender differences in adult health. *Am. J. Public Health* **2010**, *100*, 1953–1960. [CrossRef] [PubMed]
16. Fredriksen-Goldsen, K.I. Disparities in health-related quality of life: A comparison of lesbians and bisexual women. *Am. J. Public Health* **2010**, *100*, 2255–2261. [CrossRef]
17. Landers, S.J.; Mimiaga, M.J.; Conron, K.J. Sexual orientation differences in asthma correlates in a population-based sample of adults. *Am. J. Public Health* **2011**, *101*, 2238–2241. [CrossRef] [PubMed]
18. McNair, R.; Szalacha, L.A.; Hughes, T.L. Health status, health service use, and satisfaction according to sexual identity of young australian women. *Women's Health Issues* **2011**, *21*, 40–47. [CrossRef]
19. Caceres, B.A.; Brody, A.; Luscombe, R.E.; Primiano, J.E.; Marusca, P.; Sitts, E.M.; Chyun, D. A systematic review of cardiovascular disease in sexual minorities. *Am. J. Public Health* **2017**, *107*, e13–e21. [CrossRef]
20. Patterson, J.G.; Jabson, J.M.; Bowen, D.J. Measuring sexual and gender minority populations in health surveillance. *Lgbt Health* **2017**, *4*, 82–105. [CrossRef]
21. Wolff, M.; Wells, B.; Ventura-DiPersia, C.; Renson, A.; Grov, C. Measuring sexual orientation: A review and critique of U.S. data collection efforts and Implications for health policy. *J. Sex. Res.* **2017**, *54*, 507–531. [CrossRef] [PubMed]
22. Swartz, J.A.; Horn, K. A Comparative Analysis of Lifetime Medical Conditions and Infectious Diseases by Sexual Identity, Attraction, and Concordance: Results from a National U.S. Survey. Available online: https://journals.ke-i.org/index.php/mra/article/view/1452/1130 (accessed on 17 April 2019).
23. United States Department of Health and Human Services; Substance Abuse and Mental Health Service Administration; Center for Behavioral Health Statistics and Quality. National Survey on Drug Use and Health, 2015–2017. Available online: https://www.datafiles.samhsa.gov/ (accessed on 18 April 2019).
24. Center for Behavioral Health Statistics and Quality. *2015 National Survey on Drug Use and Health Public Use File*; Substance Abuse and Mental Health Services Administration: Rockville, MD, USA, 2016.
25. American Psychiatric Association (Ed.) *Diagnostic and Statistical Manual of Mental Disorders, Text.-Revision*; American Psychiatric Association: Washington, DC, USA, 2002.
26. Shiffman, S.; Waters, A.; Hickox, M. The nicotine dependence syndrome scale: A multidimensional measure of nicotine dependence. *Nicotine Tob Res.* **2004**, *6*, 327–348. [CrossRef] [PubMed]
27. StataCorp. *Stata 14.2 for PC.*; StataCorp: College Station, TX, USA, 2017.
28. Korn, E.; Graubard, B. Simultaneous testing of regression coefficients with complex survey data: Use of Bonferroni t statistics. *Am. Stat.* **1990**, *4*, 270–276. [CrossRef]
29. Gorman, B.K.; Denney, J.T.; Dowdy, H.; Medeiros, R.A. A new piece of the puzzle: Sexual orientation, gender, and physical health status. *Demography* **2015**, *52*, 1357–1382. [CrossRef] [PubMed]
30. Veenstra, G. Race, gender, class, and sexual orientation: Intersecting axes of inequality and self-rated health in Canada. *Int. J. Equity Health* **2011**, *10*, 1–11. [CrossRef] [PubMed]

31.  Blosnich, J.R.; Farmer, G.W.; Lee, J.G.L.; Silenzio, V.M.B.; Bowen, D.J. Health inequalities among sexual minority adults: Evidence from ten U.S. states. *Am. J. Prev. Med.* **2014**, *46*, 337–349. [CrossRef] [PubMed]

32.  Smith, E.M.; Johnson, S.R.; Guenther, S.M. Health care attitudes and experiences during gynecologic care among lesbians and bisexuals. *Am. J. Public Health* **1985**, *75*, 1085–1087. [CrossRef] [PubMed]

33.  Balsam, K.F.; Mohr, J.J. Adaptation to sexual orientation stigma: A comparison of bisexual and lesbian/gay adults. *J. Couns. Psychol.* **2007**, *54*, 306–319. [CrossRef]

34.  Frost, D.M.; Lehavot, K.; Meyer, I.H. Minority stress and physical health among sexual minority individuals. *J. Behav. Med.* **2015**, *38*, 1–8. [CrossRef]

35.  Sherry, A. Internalized homophobia and adult attachment: Implications for clinical practice. *Psychother. Theory Res. Pract. Train.* **2007**, *44*, 219. [CrossRef]

36.  Chapman Institute. *How Valid is Self-Reported Health Data?* Chapman Institute: Seattle, WA, USA, May 2012.

37.  Althubaiti, A. Information bias in health research: Definition, pitfalls, and adjustment methods. *J. Multidiscip. Healthc.* **2016**, *9*, 211–217. [CrossRef] [PubMed]

38.  Law, M.; Mathai, A.; Webster, F.; Mylopoulos, M. Exploring lesbian, gay, bisexual, and queer (LGBQ) people's experiences with disclosure of sexual identity to primary care physicians: A qualitative study. *BMC Fam. Pract.* **2015**, *16*, 175. [CrossRef] [PubMed]

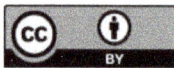

© 2019 by the authors. Licensee MDPI, Basel, Switzerland. This article is an open access article distributed under the terms and conditions of the Creative Commons Attribution (CC BY) license (http://creativecommons.org/licenses/by/4.0/).

International Journal of
*Environmental Research and Public Health*

MDPI

*Article*

# Inferring Opinions and Behavioral Characteristics of Gay Men with Large Scale Multilingual Text from Blued

Ge Huang [1], Mengsi Cai [1] and Xin Lu [1,2,3,*]

[1]  College of Systems Engineering, National University of Defense Technology, Changsha 410073, China; gehuang_nudt@hotmail.com (G.H.); caimengsi18@nudt.edu.cn (M.C.)
[2]  School of Software Engineering, Shenzhen Institute of Information Technology, Shenzhen 518172, China
[3]  School of Business, Central South University, Changsha 410083, China
*  Correspondence: xin.lu@flowminder.org

Received: 5 September 2019; Accepted: 24 September 2019; Published: 26 September 2019

**Abstract:** Gay men in many countries are increasingly using geosocial networking applications (GSN apps), thus offering new opportunities for understanding them. This paper provides a comprehensive content analysis of posts and opinions on Blued, the world's largest gay social networking dating app, to infer and compare opinions and behavioral characteristics of gay men in different countries. Machine learning and linguistic programming approaches were used to extract themes and analyze sentiments of posts. The results show that the majority of posts are related to daily life activities, and less are related to sensitive topics. While most posts are positive or neutral, negative emotions, including anxiety, anger, and sadness, are mainly distributed in posts related to self-identification and sexual behaviors in China and to relationships in other countries. Voting items indicate that only 50.52% of the participants will take regular HIV tests while 50.2% would have casual sex when they are single. Additionally, 35.8% of the participants may try drugs when invited by friends. Our findings suggest an opportunity and necessity for researchers and public health practitioners to use open source data on GSN apps and other social medias to inform HIV interventions and to promote social inclusion for sexual minorities.

**Keywords:** gay men; content analysis; behavioral characteristics; GSN apps; Blued

## 1. Introduction

Social media provide an important platform for people to communicate and interact online. As new technologies are developed, geosocial networking applications (GSN apps) on mobile phones are gradually replacing traditional social media in people's lives. GSN apps are diverse with regard to their customer bases, points of interest, and operator interfaces. Studying the usage patterns of social media or applications for specific populations allows us to better understand their behavior and inform interventions [1,2]. In sexual minorities, GSN apps, such as Blued, Grindr, and HER, have been commonly used since 2009, helping individuals from these groups to socialize, seek partners, and obtain support. For example, the world's largest GSN APP, Blued, originating from China, is now a very popular social media worldwide, especially in the Asia-Pacific region. However, recent data from The Joint United Nations Programme on HIV/AIDS (UNAIDS) show that, since 2016, the rate of new human immunodeficiency virus (HIV) infections in the Asia-Pacific region has stopped decreasing. According to the analysis, about 30% of new infections in the Asia-Pacific region occur in men who have sex with men (MSM). HIV prevalence and infection rates have risen sharply among young men who have sex with men (MSM) in countries, such as China and Indonesia [3].

GSN apps provide an effective social platform for sexual minorities, as well as a potential tool for studying their high-risk behaviors [4]. Recent research has examined the sociodemographic characteristics [5], app usage [6], sexual behaviors [7], HIV testing and detection [8,9], drug and alcohol use [10], and efficiency of recruiting MSM using apps [11,12]. It is easily understood why researchers link app usage to high-risk behavior, but the viewpoints and emotions of gay men shown in the discourses have largely been ignored [13]. GSN apps contain a large amount of textual information, which plays a vital role in understanding the behavior and psychological conditions of their users. However, few researchers have paid attention to the text content generated on GSN apps [14,15]. Thus, in this paper, we utilized the textual content generated on a popular GSN app to infer opinions and behavioral characteristics of gay men.

To analyze the discourses generated on social networks, such as tweets and posts, two representations have been widely used. First, theme extraction is commonly employed to characterize the topics being discussed on social media [16–18]. The theme extraction methods are diverse due to the differences in the lengths of texts, the amount of data, and the granularity needed. Second, sentiment values and linguistic styles have been found to be helpful in understanding users' viewpoints [1,19], which generally include lexicon-based and machine learning-based approaches. These two representations enable us to document what users are interested in and how they discuss their interests, providing insights into their life quality and mental status.

In this work, we used a large-scale multi-language text dataset on a popular GSN app for gay men named Blued, which included 1186 topics and all voting items. We focused on three major aspects: (1) What is the thematic content of the posts? (2) what is the sentiment of the posts in each category? and (3) what are the users' views on sensitive issues? Statistical, machine learning, and linguistic programs were used in the analysis.

A key contribution of this paper is to provide a comprehensive view of a GSN app through topic classification as well as sentiment and linguistic analysis. Another contribution is to document the opinion and behavior characteristics of a large number of gay men who use GSN apps. This study demonstrates the potential of GSN apps as a new channel for gay behavior monitoring. Our findings provide data support for research and suggest the potential of machine learning classification and psychoanalysis techniques in the textual content analysis for sexual minorities.

## 2. Data and Methods

### 2.1. Data Collection and Filtering

Blued is a GSN app for gay men that allows users to post and interact through short messages. It was first created for Chinese gay men in 2012 but has since become the largest GSN app for gay men worldwide, with over 40 million users, especially in the Asia–Pacific region. According to the users' locations, the Blued app is divided into Blued (only for gay men in mainland China) and Blued international (for gay men in other parts of China and other countries). The topic data in the Chinese language and all voting data were collected from Blued, while the topic data in non-Chinese languages were collected from Blued international from 1 January 2015 to 28 February 2019.

The topic data were collected by searching posts with specific hashtags in the "Topic List" module in Blued. A hashtag is a type of metadata tag that is widely used on many social networking sites and apps. With Blued, users can create and use hashtags in different languages by placing the pound sign (#) in front of a word or unspaced phrase in a non-Chinese post (e.g., #love) or by placing the pound sign both before and after words in a Chinese post (e.g., #爱自己#). Figure 1 shows the flow of topic collection, filtering, and classification used in this study. We divided hashtags into official-released, user-defined, and domain-specific hashtags. For official-released hashtags, we collected Chinese and English hashtags displayed in the "discovery" interface in Blued and hashtags released by official accounts. For user-defined hashtags, we first collected the 800 most commonly used words in Chinese. Then, we collected the 500 most popular hashtags on Instagram from a website that lists the most popular hashtags on various social networks (Top-Hashtags.com). For domain-specific hashtags, we collected sensitive topics by searching sensitive words related to gay men using the topic search interface in the app, based on our prior knowledge. Then, we used these words and unspaced phrases with the topic search interface on Blued and recorded the hashtags with a large amount of discussion or participation. After the hashtags were identified, we collected all the posts containing them. Non-English hashtags were not considered because trying to find keywords to use to search in 97 languages was not feasible. Up to March 2019, a total of 1186 topics were collected, including 551 Chinese topics and 635 English topics.

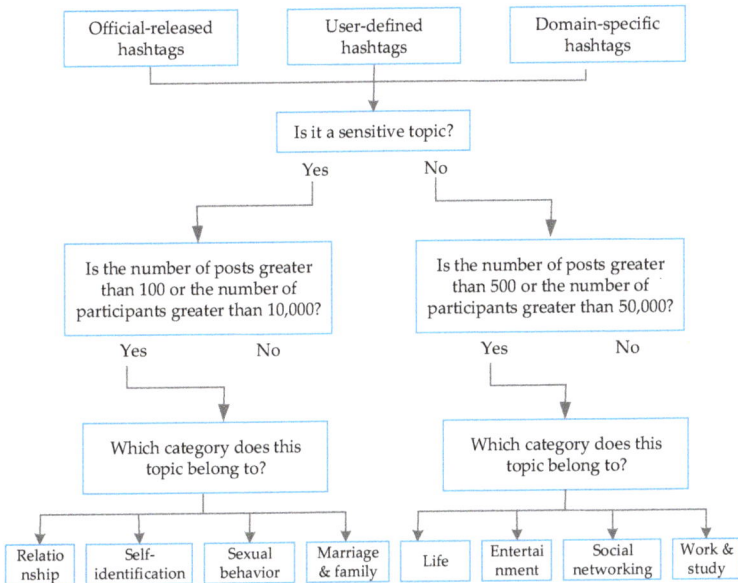

**Figure 1.** Flow of topic collection, filtering, and classification.

For further screening, we divided the topics into sensitive topics-related to love, self-identification, high-risk behaviors, marriage, and family; and non-sensitive topics-related to life, entertainment, friendship, work, and study. Since most of the daily discussions of the users involved non-sensitive topics, we removed non-sensitive ones with less than 500 posts or with less than 50,000 participants (users' behaviors include creating posts, upvoting, or replying to posts) as well as sensitive topics with less than 100 posts or with less than 10,000 participants for subsequent analysis. After removing the unimportant topics, we were left with 1132 topics, including 511 Chinese topics and 621 English topics. The Chinese topic data included 1,100,324 posts while the English topic data included 1,994,167 posts. It must be noted that the topic interface in Blued is a Twitter-style interface that most Chinese users used to release a post with or without a hashtag. While the topic interface in Blued international is an Instagram-style interface, most non-Chinese users tend to incorporate multiple hashtags in a post to increase the exposure of themselves, and then to make more friends. Consequently, there were many duplicate posts in the topic data, especially in non-Chinese posts. After we removed duplicates, 931,109 Chinese posts and 738,203 non-Chinese posts remained for further analysis.

Voting is an important function that reflects the common viewpoints and attitudes of people using social networks. It generally consists of a question with two or more options, and some user comments. "Viewpoint" is a sub-module in an earlier version of the Blued app (the direct entry has now been removed), and the voting questions posted in the module are usually related to sensitive topics. In this work, we collected all the voting data from the "Viewpoint" module in Blued, including 114 voting items, 5,042,240 votes, and 407,453 comments (see Table A1).

### 2.2. Classification

Three of the authors examined the topic dataset independently then discussed and summarized the classification framework. The final categories and selected topic data examples are listed in Table 1, in which all topics are classified into the following eight categories: Life, entertainment, social networking, relationship, self-identification, high-risk behavior, work and study, and marriage and family.

### 2.3. Sentiment and Psychological Analysis

As most Chinese posts included only one hashtag, we classified them manually based on the subject of the hashtag. For the English topic data, we translated all non-English posts to English and used a semi-automatic method to extract themes from the posts. Then, we used psycholinguistic programs to calculate the total number of words each theme used that fell into each affection category and classified the affections expressed in each post. Figure 2 shows the analysis process for the topic data. For voting items, we classified them and identified the main points from the text manually.

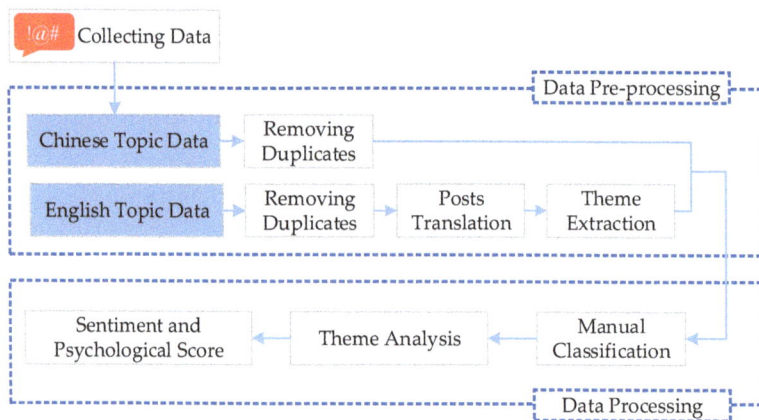

**Figure 2.** Architecture of the analysis process of the topic data.

### 2.3.1. Manual Classification of Chinese Topic Data

Due to differences between Chinese and other languages, the design and use of hashtags in the Chinese language are very different from the design and use of hashtags in other languages. Each Chinese hashtag has a specific meaning (e.g., #ideal lover#, #my future#, #mom, #I want to tell you#) while most English hashtags have no specific meaning (e.g., #gay, #beach, #city). In addition, when publishing a post, Chinese users generally include only one topic hashtag, but most non-Chinese users tend to incorporate multiple hashtags in a post. As a result, the contents of posts in Chinese are more relevant to the hashtags that they are tagged with. Thus, we manually categorized all Chinese topic hashtags according to the classification frame.

Two of the authors independently examined 25% of the hashtags. If a single hashtag contained multiple themes, the hashtag was classified according to the predominant theme of the post to which it was attached. Next, the authors established a classification framework together to avoid ambiguities in category definitions. Finally, the two authors re-examined all the hashtags separately and resolved any differences on classification through discussion.

**Table 1.** Descriptions and examples of topic hashtag categories.

| Category | Description | Hashtag Examples | Example of Voting Items | | Poll Options |
| --- | --- | --- | --- | --- | --- |
| | | | Question | | |
| Life | Talking about health, greetings, pets, memories, festival, photos or videos, tourism, dress up, habit, cooking, travel, plan and wish, bachelor life, etc. | #今日自拍打卡# (selfie of today) #一个人的生活# (single life) | Which do you prefer: comfort or freedom? | | (1) Small city, full of happiness. (2) Big city, just be yourself. |
| Entertainment | Discussing male stars, movies, music, award, constellation, game, sports meeting, etc. | #型男速递# (handsome men) #奥斯卡# (Oscar) | n/a | | n/a |
| Social networking | Searching for new friends, talking about friends, etc. | #最佳损友# (best friend) #漂流瓶# (whispering Sailing) | Do you think it's offensive to call friends sisters? | | (1) Yes. (2) No. |
| Relationship | Expressing preference of boyfriend, confessing to his boyfriend, trying to find a boyfriend, talking about ex-boyfriends, etc. | #我和X先生# (Mr. X and me) #最浪漫的事# (the most romantic thing) | Can you accept a long-distance relationship? | | (1) Yes, true love stands the test of distance. (2) No, lack of safety. |
| Self-identification | Expressing a sense of pride in their identities, talking about sexual orientation, coming out, social support, etc. | #爱自己# (love yourself) #同志骄傲日# (Gay Pride day) | Will you argue with each other when you encounter anti-gay speech? | | (1) Yes. (2) No. |
| Sexual behavior | Talking about HIV detection and precaution measures, drug abuse, etc. | #为艾发声# (speak for AIDS) #青春零艾滋# (no AIDS in youth) | Will you interact with HIV-infected people? | | (1) Yes, he can live normally if he takes medicine regularly. (2) No, I don't want to risk myself no matter how I like him. |
| Work & studies | Sharing experience in school, university or workplace, etc. | #我的校园生活# (my school life) #职场潜规则# (hidden rules in workplace) | Will you hide your sexual orientation at work? | | (1) Yes, for protecting my privacy. (2) No, just be myself. |
| Marriage & family | Expressing emotion about parents, brothers and sisters, sharing opinions about marriage and child, etc. | #父母老了# (parents getting old) #我们结婚吧# (let's get married) | Will you adopt a child in the future? | | (1) Yes. (2) No. |

2.3.2. Semi-Automatic Classification of English Topic Data

When we searched posts by English hashtags, the results contained a large number of posts written in a total of 97 different non-English languages, especially languages from Southeast Asia (see Table 2). Therefore, we developed a post-flow translation code program based on Google Translate and translated all non-English topic posts into English. As mentioned above, the hashtags attached to each non-Chinese post were numerous and had low relevance to the subject of the post, so it was not possible to categorize the posts according to the content of the hashtags directly. Therefore, we used machine-learning methods to cluster the non-Chinese posts.

**Table 2.** Top 20 languages analyzed in the posts data.

| Language Name | Native Name | Number of Posts | Language Name | Native Name | Number of Posts |
|---|---|---|---|---|---|
| Chinese | 中文 | 935,745 | German | Deutsch | 8807 |
| English | English | 482,110 | Malay | Bahasa, Melayu, بهاس ملايو | 8337 |
| Portuguese | Português | 65,107 | Dutch, Flemish | Nederlands, Vlaams | 4117 |
| Spanish, Castilian | Español | 29,775 | Galician | Galego | 3148 |
| Vietnamese | Tiếng Việt | 27,943 | Latin | latine, lingua latina | 3085 |
| Thai | ไทย | 27,904 | Javanese | ꦧꦱꦗꦮ, Basa Jawa | 2949 |
| Indonesian | Bahasa Indonesia | 24,280 | Polish | język polski, polszczyzna | 2926 |
| Tagalog | Wikang Tagalog | 13,073 | Japanese | 日本 (にほんご) | 2618 |
| Italian | Italiano | 10,263 | Finnish | suomi, suomen kieli | 2599 |
| French | français | 9720 | Danish | dansk | 2201 |

We examined the non-Chinese posts and found that, despite having attached hashtags, most of the posts were short, and single posts tended to be about a single theme. Since the standard latent dirichlet allocation (LDA) method generally does not work well with short texts, we applied a modified author-topic model named Twitter-LDA [20], which assumes a single subject assignment for each post. We removed posts that only contained hashtags (more than three) and those from users with fewer than three posts. Then, we used the Twitter-LDA model to automatically extract 110 topic clusters (based on preliminary experiments) across 500 iterations from all the posts. After the noisy topics were removed, we obtained a set of 104 topic clusters, which we manually assigned to one of the eight topic categories mentioned above.

2.3.3. Automatic Sentiment and Psychological Analysis

To measure the sentiment and psychological status of each topic category, we used a computational linguistics program called Linguistic Inquiry and Word Count (LIWC) [21] to analyze non-Chinese posts and a modified Chinese LIWC program called TextMind [22] to analyze Chinese posts. Both programs calculate the percentages of words in a given text that fall into one or more of over 80 linguistic, psychological, and topical categories indicating various cognitive, social, psychological, and affective processes. These programs, for example, help users to determine the degree to which a text uses pronoun or verb, or positive or negative emotions. In this work, we focused on categories related to affections. It must be noted that the core of the programs are dictionaries containing words that belong to predefined categories and the different LIWC indicators are not statistically independent of each other. For example, the word "afraid" is classified into *Anx* (represented for anxiety) category, the *Anx* is a subcategory of *NegEmo* (representing negative emotion), and the *Negative Emotion* is a subcategory of *Affect* (representing affection). The output features related to affective processes are as follows: *Affect*,

*PosEmo, NegEmo, Anx, Anger*, and *Sad*. We counted and compared the output measures of the eight categories of topics separately for the Chinese and English topic data.

### 2.3.4. Classification of Voting Data

We used the same method described in Section 2.3.1 to manually categorize all voting items according to our classification frame. As there were no voting items related to entertainment, we classified all voting items into seven categories. We examined the number of voting items and users involved, the number of comments in each category, and then summarized the main points of each category.

### 2.4. Ethics Approval and Consent to Participate

The study and Liu (2018) [13] were both supported by the Natural Science Foundation of China (91546203, 71771213) and approved by the Medical Ethical Committee of the Institutional Review Board (IRB) at Peking University (IRB00001052–16016). The study did not involve any physical, social, or legal risks to the participants; the data is anonymous; and the confidentiality of the participants' information was strictly protected.

### 2.5. Data Availability

All data analyzed in this study are publicly available; all posts in the datasets can be collected by searching hashtags in the "topic" interface on Blued. Other data that support the findings in this study are available from the corresponding author on reasonable request.

## 3. Results

### 3.1. Topic Data Analysis

#### 3.1.1. Basic Statistical Results

Chinese topic data: There were 511 topics published in Chinese, involving 931,109 posts. There was no significant difference between the distribution characteristics of Chinese topics and those of Chinese posts. As illustrated in Table 3, more than half of the posts were related to daily life, such as publishing photos or videos. The second popular theme was relationships, accounting for 19.2% of the posts, followed by self-identification and entertainment topics, accounting for 7.7% and 6%, respectively. Social networking topics accounted for 3%, and the proportion of the other three topics was less than 2%. Because Blued is a GSN app for gay men, most users are keen to discuss topics closely related to life and love. Due to the particularity of their sexual identity, they also discuss self-identity and sexual behavior. However, only 9.1% of posts shared information about gay identity, and very few posts involved sexual behavior in gay men (<1%). On the one hand, the results revealed the users' motives of "making friends" and "attracting attention". They hoped to increase connection between each other by sharing information about daily lives, and then meet more gay friends. On the other hand, the users tended to be reserved in relating private information, such as high-risk behavior and HIV status, likely because disclosure of this information might have a negative impact on their socialization.

Table 3. The statistical results of topic categories.

| Category | Number of Topics | | Posts Released | | Users Involved | |
|---|---|---|---|---|---|---|
| | CHN | ENG | CHN | ENG | CHN | ENG |
| Life (Life) | 272 | 76 | 567,062(60.9%) | 398,480(74.9%) | 402,257 | 31,009 |
| Entertainment (Ent) | 50 | 6 | 55,998(6.0%) | 17,697(3.3%) | 38,853 | 7245 |
| Social networking (SN) | 15 | 8 | 28,102(3.0%) | 39,350(7.4%) | 20,478 | 10,130 |
| Relationship (Rls) | 107 | 6 | 178,461(19.2%) | 38,144(7.2%) | 143,629 | 11,736 |
| Self-identification(SI) | 41 | 2 | 71,743(7.7%) | 10,652(2.0%) | 61,719 | 4559 |
| Sexual behavior (SB) | 9 | 1 | 12,799(1.4%) | 2822(0.5%) | 9280 | 1574 |
| Work and study (W and S) | 8 | 3 | 9833(1.1%) | 12,506(2.4%) | 8048 | 5643 |
| Marriage and family (M and F) | 9 | 2 | 7111(0.8%) | 12,530(2.4%) | 6345 | 5109 |
| Summary | 511 | 104 | 931,109 | 532,181 | 690,609 | 77,005 |

English topic data: After removing noisy topics, 104 English topics remained, involving 532,181 posts. As illustrated in Table 3, the distribution characteristics of English topics were not significantly different from those of the Chinese topics. The majority of non-Chinese posts were about life, accounting for 74.9% of the posts, followed by social networking and relationship topics, accounting for 7.4% and 7.2%, respectively. An additional 2% of posts reflected self-identification. A smaller number of posts reflected sexual behavior (1.4%) and work and study (1.1%) topics. Very few posts involved marriage and family (<1%). Interestingly, sensitive topics accounted for a lower proportion of total posts in non-Chinese posts than in Chinese posts. The results show that non-Chinese users are more likely to use the software for making friends, and their countries are more open to sexual identity, so these users are less likely to discuss sexual identity and sexual behaviors.

### 3.1.2. Theme Analysis

The common words in each category from the Chinese and English topic data are shown as word clouds in Figure 3. Background statistics are shown as a stacked bar in the center, from which we can see that the proportion distribution of each Chinese topic category was more uniform than that of English topics. The most common words within each category are shown to the left and right. The size of a word correlates with the frequency of the word used in that category. As can be seen from Figure 3, words, such as "love" and "life", appeared frequently in all Chinese and English topics.

Life. Chinese users posted their own photos and discussed single or weekend life, while there were many greeting posts in the English topic. The words "appearance", "wear", and "hair", representing people's physical appearance, can be seen in both Chinese and English topics, indicating the close attention to appearance in the gay community.

Entertainment. Within the entertainment topic, Chinese users focused more attention on anime, comics, and games (ACG), such as Anime Park. There were also many discussions about various horoscopes and male stars in Chinese posts. The most commonly mentioned star was Leslie Cheung, a famous bisexual singer and actor in China in the 1980s. Non-Chinese users paid more attention to photos and videos on Instagram and YouTube.

Social networking. Chinese users shared numerous stories about gay friends and experiences of meeting new gay friends. There were also many posts introducing themselves to make new friends. Non-Chinese users tended to create super groups and invite gay friends to join. There were also many posts inviting friends to follow them in the app or other social networks, such as Instagram, Facebook, and Twitter.

Relationship. High-frequency words in Chinese posts, such as "Valentine's Day" and "Double Seventh Festival", indicate that the Chinese users attached great importance to Valentine's Day. The most discussed related items included the ideal boyfriend type, confessions to a boyfriend, and ending the single life. The high-frequency words in Chinese topics, such as "find" and "boyfriend", and those in non-Chinese posts, "true" and "waiting", reflected their desire for stable relationships.

Self-identification. Chinese users used words like "gay", "1" (top), and "0" (bottom) to talk about their sexual identity and sexual roles. Similarly, Chinese users often used words like "not easy", "thirty" (representing the age of a person), and "monster", indicating that Chinese gay man have problems regarding social identity and may suffer from social discrimination. However, there were still many mutually encouraging posts represented by the word "proud." Non-Chinese users used words like "people", "human", and "rights", indicating that non-Chinese users are more active in fighting for equal rights for gay men.

Sexual behavior. Chinese users posted frequently about "AIDS" and "condom", reflecting the effectiveness of the promotion of acquired immunodeficiency syndrome (AIDS) prevention in China. Meanwhile, Chinese users had many discussions on "hookup", "no hookup", and "419 (for one night)". The words "discrimination" and "solidarity" appeared frequently in the Chinese topics while they were less common in the English topic data. Non-Chinese users talked more about HIV status, testing, and safe sex behavior.

Work and study. The word "busy" was mentioned frequently in the Chinese posts, indicating the current fast-paced lifestyle of Chinese people. In terms of study, there was considerable discussion about the college entrance examination and the graduation season. The discussion on work revolved around what they were doing and unspoken rules for the workplace. Non-Chinese users discussed recreation, taking pictures, and making money more frequently.

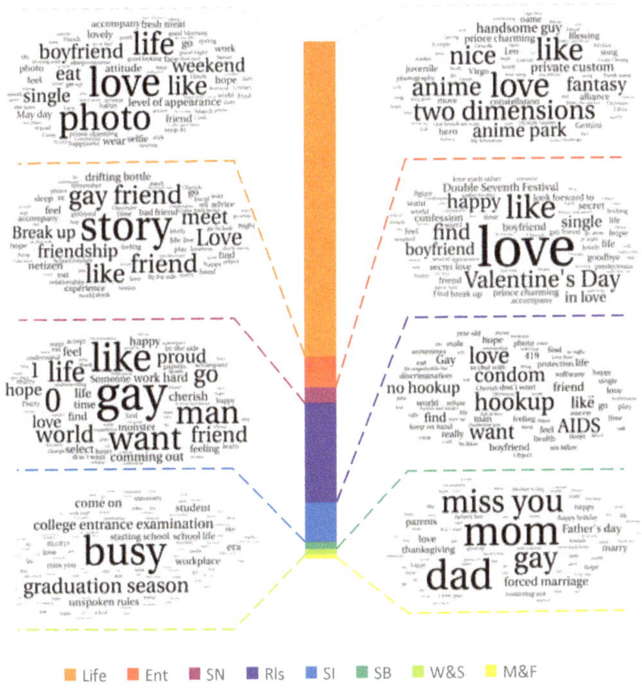

(a)

**Figure 3.** *Cont.*

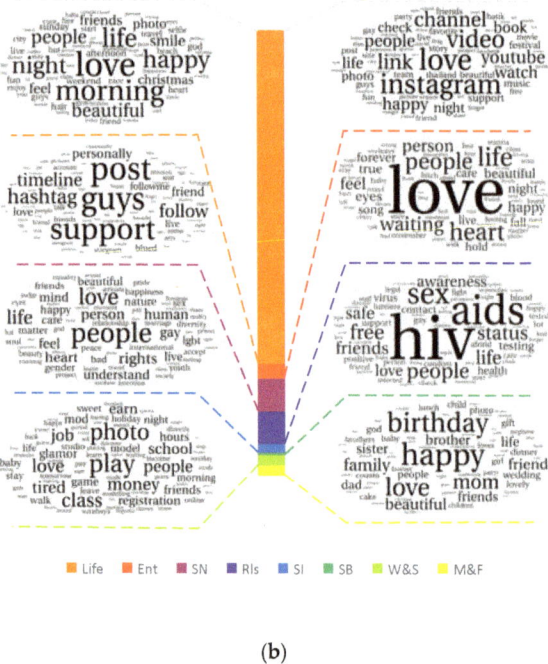

**(b)**

**Figure 3.** Word cloud of the eight categories of (**a**) Chinese and (**b**) English topic data.

Marriage and family. Within the Chinese posts, the Chinese users used words like "mom", "dad", "thanksgiving", "gay", and "hope" to express their mental conflicts between fulfilling filial piety and their sexual identities. The forced marriage phenomenon was also discussed. There were fewer discussions about other brothers and sisters and children. In the non-Chinese posts, many users not only posted about their parents but also shared experiences regarding their brothers and sisters. Others shared more birthday and wedding wishes. The word "happy" was frequently used in the English posts, indicating that the non-Chinese users were generally more positive than the Chinese users.

### 3.1.3. Sentimental and Psychological Analysis

The LIWC and Textmind score represents the ratio of the words in each category relative to the total word count of the queried text file. Table 4 shows the scores of the *Affect*, *PosEmo*, and *NegEmo* categories calculated by the LIWC and Textmind programs, in which bold letters represent relatively higher scores in each column. It is obvious that the proportion of emotional words contained in the Chinese topics was higher than that in the English topics. In the Chinese topics, sensitive topics contained a higher proportion of emotional words than non-sensitive topics, whereas this difference was not obvious in the English topics. From the perspective of positive emotions, Chinese users were more positive about relationships, while non-Chinese users were more positive in the relationship and marriage and family topics. From the perspective of negative emotions, Chinese users were negative about self-identification and sexual behaviors, while non-Chinese users were negative about relationships.

**Table 4.** Affection scores of each category calculated by LIWC programs.

| Category | Affection (%) | | Positive Emotion (%) | | Negative Emotion (%) | |
|---|---|---|---|---|---|---|
| | CHI | ENG | CHI | ENG | CHI | ENG |
| Life | 5.8 | 1.9 | 3.4 | 1.6 | 1.3 | 0.2 |
| Entertainment | 6.3 | 1.6 | 3.8 | 1.4 | 1.4 | 0.1 |
| Social networking | 5.9 | 1.7 | 3.1 | 1.5 | 1.4 | 0.2 |
| Relationship | **7.9** | **2.6** | **4.7** | 2.2 | 1.6 | **0.4** |
| Self-identification | 7.4 | 2.1 | 4.0 | 1.7 | **1.8** | 0.3 |
| Sexual behavior | **8.0** | 1.7 | 3.9 | 1.4 | **1.8** | 0.3 |
| Work and study | 5.2 | 1.8 | 3.0 | 1.5 | 1.3 | 0.2 |
| Marriage and family | 7.8 | 2.5 | 4.0 | **2.3** | 1.5 | 0.2 |

Figure 4 shows the sentiment distribution of the topic data. All posts in each category were classified into positive (POS), negative (NEG), and neutral (NEU). In general, positive emotions were significantly more commonly expressed than negative emotions, especially in Chinese posts. The Chinese and English topics showed the largest difference with regard to social networking while Chinese posts contained more emotions. This is because most Chinese posts were related to gay friend stories, whereas non-Chinese posts were mostly about supergroups. The proportion of affective posts in the life topic was smallest in both the Chinese and English topics, and more than 50% of the posts were neutral. The biggest differences between positive and negative emotions were found in the relationship and marriage and family topics, both in the Chinese and non-Chinese posts. The results indicate that they have positive expectations regarding their future relationships. In terms of the marriage and family topic, the positive sentiments found in the Chinese posts were related to giving thanks to parents while the positive emotions of non-Chinese posts were reflected in family celebrations.

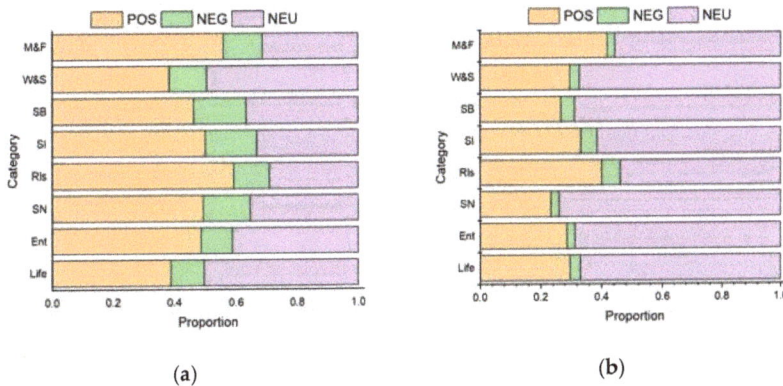

**Figure 4.** Sentiment distribution of (a) Chinese and (b) English topic data.

In LIWC and Textmind, the negative emotion is divided into three categories: *Anx, Anger*, and *Sad*. Table 5 shows the scores of these negative emotions of each category calculated using the LIWC and Textmind programs, in which bold letters represent the highest score in each column. With regard to anxiety, Chinese users tend to be more anxious about self-identification while non-Chinese users were extremely anxious about sexual behaviors. In terms of anger, while it most frequently appeared in the sexual behaviors topic under Chinese posts, it commonly featured in the relationship topic under non-Chinese posts. From the perspective of sadness, the sadness of Chinese users is mainly reflected in their gay identity, since they suffered from more pressure on homosexuality in a conservative society compared to western countries. Compared to Chinese users, non-Chinese users feel sadder when dealing with relationship issues. Therefore, self-identification and sexual behaviors were main triggers of negative feelings of Chinese users, while relationships and sexual behaviors were major causes of negative feelings of non-Chinese users.

**Table 5.** Scores of negative emotions of each category calculated by the LIWC programs.

| Category | Anxiety (‰) | | Anger (‰) | | Sadness (‰) | |
|---|---|---|---|---|---|---|
| | CHI | ENG | CHI | ENG | CHI | ENG |
| Life | 2.1 | 0.2 | 2.0 | 0.3 | 3.8 | 1.1 |
| Entertainment | 2.3 | 0.1 | 2.3 | 0.2 | 3.2 | 0.7 |
| Social networking | 2.3 | 0.1 | 2.6 | 0.2 | 3.4 | 1.2 |
| Relationship | 2.1 | 0.3 | 2.8 | **0.8** | 4.7 | **2.1** |
| Self-identification | **3.6** | 0.2 | 2.9 | 0.6 | **5.9** | 1.5 |
| Sexual behavior | 2.3 | **0.7** | **6.6** | 0.5 | 3.0 | 1.7 |
| Work and study | 1.8 | 0.1 | 2.4 | 0.5 | 3.9 | 0.7 |
| Marriage and family | 2.7 | 0.1 | 2.4 | 0.2 | 3.9 | 1.2 |

Figure 5 shows the distribution of negative emotions in the topic data. Sadness was the most common negative emotion in both the Chinese and non-Chinese posts, and the Chinese posts were more negative than the non-Chinese posts. The proportional differences between the three negative emotions in the Chinese topics were smaller than in the English topics. Except for the sexual behavior topic, the Chinese users tend to be more anxious than the non-Chinese users. Similarly, except for the self-identification and work and study topics, the Chinese posts contain more anger than the non-Chinese posts. The proportion of sadness in the non-Chinese posts was significantly higher than in the Chinese posts. Moreover, the Chinese users expressed anxiety and anger more often than the non-Chinese users. In particular, the Chinese users expressed strong anger in the sexual behavior topic while the non-Chinese users expressed more sadness in this topic.

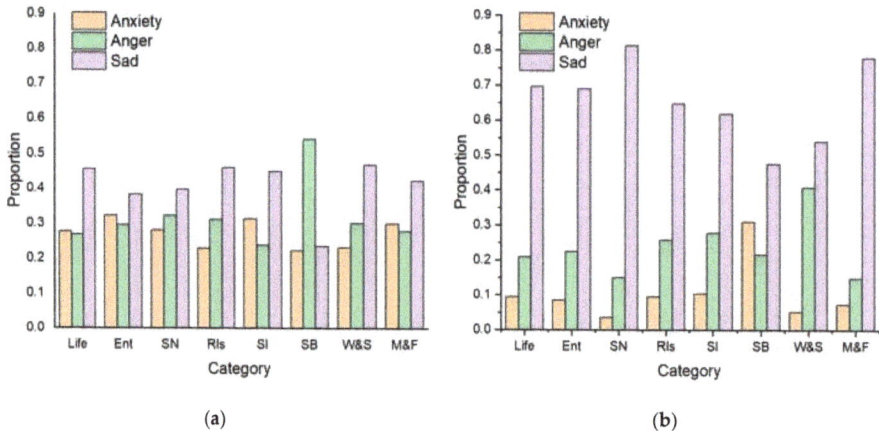

**Figure 5.** Negative emotion distribution of (**a**) Chinese and (**b**) English topic data.

*3.2. Voting Data Analysis*

3.2.1. Basic Statistical Results

Until the collection of data, a total of 114 viewpoints were published in Blued, and the statistical results of the viewpoints for the seven studied categories are presented in Table 6.

**Table 6.** The statistical results of the voting categories.

| Category | Number of Viewpoints | Number of Votes | Number of Comments |
|---|---|---|---|
| Life | 18(15.8%) | 576,839 | 49,615 |
| Social networking | 15(13.2%) | 726,010 | 52,143 |
| Relationship | 57(50.0%) | 2,529,860 | 204,600 |
| Self-identification | 7(6.1%) | 405,017 | 36,819 |
| Sexual behavior | 5(4.4%) | 198,168 | 17,040 |
| Work & study | 5(4.4%) | 261,642 | 20,205 |
| Marriage & family | 7(6.1%) | 344,704 | 27,031 |
| Summary | 114 | 5,042,240 | 407,453 |

### 3.2.2. Main Points by Category

*Life.* Socially, gay men focused more attention on the faces (54.4%) of their partners rather than on their physical shape, and 72% of the participants were willing to accept cosmetic surgery. More than 57% of the participants said they would go to the offline counter to buy skincare products, and nearly half of the participants said they could accept gays who define themselves as "tops" wearing makeup. A total of 77.5% of the participants said that they would continue to maintain their fitness after consummating a stable relationship. According to the comments on this voting item, 66.6% of the participants indicated that they work out for their own health or looks, and the workouts have nothing to do with making friends or maintaining relationships. Meanwhile, 28.8% of the participants said they believe that maintaining a good physical shape is important when participating in a relationship or making friends in a gay group. In terms of physical shape, 61.7% of the participants focused more attention on their partners' hips than on their chests. While there were differences between gay and straight man, they did have some commonalities in their lifestyles: 79.7% of the participants indicated they like to sleep naked, 75.3% said they feel anxious when they are away from their mobile phones, and 51% were uncomfortable with people looking at an embarrassing picture of them.

Social networking. In terms of meeting new friends, 76.9% of the participants said they would respond to greetings from strangers. More than half of the participants said that they would respond to greetings even if the other person did not have an avatar. In order to protect their privacy, 64.7% of the participants said they supported using alternative accounts to make friends online. Additionally, 62% of the participants said they focused heavily on others' appearance in daily interactions, and 73.4% thought that two people with different worldviews could not be compatible with each other. In terms of gender preference, 62% of the participants indicated that they did not mind others' sex role, 64.4% believed that there could be a pure friendship between a "top" and a "bottom", and 57.7% disliked being called "sister" in gay groups.

Relationship. Items related to relationships accounted for half of all voting items. We divided the voting items into dating, in a relationship, and after a breakup. In terms of dating, 64.6% of the participants said that they have no clear standard for a boyfriend, mainly basing their decisions on first appearances. A total of 67.9% of the participants said they did not oppose single people having affairs with multiple partners. When in a relationship, 62.1% of the participants said that they should show conjugal love in social networks, but 74.4% of the participants said they would not display affection in public. Further, 74.9% of the participants thought that there should be privacy between couples. More than half (53.6%) of the participants said they could not accept long-distance relationships because of the lack of safety, but in another voting item, 69.6% of the participants said they would go to where their boyfriend was located. About half (50.8%) of the participants said that they should be away from the gay group when they were in a committed relationship, and 56.8% said they could not accept an open relationship. However, 55.2% of the participants believed that they could keep "back-burner" men while they were in relationships. A total of 65.3% of the participants said that they would not trust their boyfriends to go to a gay bar alone, 61.6% said they are unable to forgive cheaters, and 67% stated that cheaters could no longer be believed. There were also many discussions about money issues in a relationship. A significant majority (73.3%) of the participants said that they ask about their potential partner's income before committing to a relationship while more than half would mind that the other was part of "the moonlight clan" (people who expend their entire salary before the end of each month). Further, 63.5% of the participants would not put their wages together while 65% would share date expenses with their boyfriends. After a breakup, 54.7% of participants said they would not start a new relationship right away.

Self-identification. In terms of self-identification, 65.2% of the participants said that if they had another chance, they would not choose to be gay again. A total of 59.3% of the participants said that they have not kissed girls, 61.7% would not argue with each other when they encountered anti-gay speech, and 62.9% believed that homosexuals are born with their sexual preference. Effeminacy is a feature of some gay men, and 53.1% of the participants believed that gays show a feminine inclination. Moreover, 40% of the participants said they wanted to try wearing women's clothing. In terms of sexual preference, 62% of the participants felt that one's sexual role is unimportant, and 62.5% said they do not believe that there is a pure top in gay relationships.

Sexual behavior. A little more than half (54.3%) of the participants said that they would not interact with HIV-infected people, but more than half of the participants said that they would not give up having sex with others after they end a relationship. The large majority (88.6%) of the participants said that they would get an HIV test routinely when AIDS is curable, but only 50.52% will take regular HIV tests. Additionally, 64.2% of the participants indicated that they would reject an invitation for substance use, while 35.8% of the participants said they would like to try drugs.

Work and study. Disclosing sexual orientation in the workplace will undoubtedly affect a gay individual's work. Thus, 86.3% of the participants said they would hide their sexual orientation at work, although it is still possible to find gay men among their colleagues through the GSN app. A total of 56.5% of the participants said that they would meet other gay men and take care of each other, while 50.9% thought that the benefits of office love outweigh the risks. In the student group, 63.3% of the participants said they would not break up with their partners after graduation.

Marriage and family. Same-sex marriage is not currently recognized by law in China. Unsurprisingly, 68.2% of the participants said that they had not discussed homosexuality with their parents. Further, 65% of the participants said they would resist forced marriage, 53.4% said they would marry lesbians, and 72.4% said that they would break up with their boyfriend once he got married. A significant majority (78.1%) of the participants said they wanted to have a child, and 64.4% indicated that they would adopt a child. Some participants supported giving birth to a child through surrogacy, but they were afraid that their child would have psychological problems or suffer discrimination in the future.

## 4. Discussion and Conclusions

We examined posts and voting projects on the world's largest GSN app for gay men, Blued, to study the publicly textual content of the online gay community in depth, with a focus on investigating the daily behavioral patterns and opinions of members of the gay population. On the one hand, based on the huge number of participants in Blued—181,308,061 participants (the number of posts, comments and likes) to the topic page and 5,449,693 participants (the number of votes and comments) to the voting page—it is easy to see how popular GSN apps are in the gay community. Our analysis of the data indicated that the posts contained more positive than negative emotions. Therefore, GSN app seem to have the potential to inspire gay men to live a more active life. On the other hand, our analysis also found some potential disadvantages.

Our first research focus was theme extraction from all the posts. We divided the posts into eight categories, four of which included sensitive topics. More than 60% of the posts were related to life, especially in the English topics, followed by topics related to relationships and social networking. In fact, nearly one-fifth of the Chinese posts were related to relationships. The results reflect the social needs of users, who hope to extend the connection between each other by sharing details of their daily lives, which is very important for gay men, who cannot expose their sexual orientation on ordinary social platforms. Based on the content of the posts, it is clear that gay men are very concerned about their own appearance, body shape, and clothing. In the Chinese life topic, nearly half of the hashtags were related to selfies. When making friends, gays focus more attention on the other person's face and body shape, whereas there is little mention of the other person's conduct. Although face and body shape are also important in heterosexual interactions, it seems to be a greater focus in the gay community [23]. Related studies have shown that more gay men than heterosexual men feel pressure to be in good physical shape [24]. This leads to a gym culture among gay men. However, the over-emphasis of external appearance and body size within the gay community weakens the role of other factors in making friends, which may lead to unhealthy standards of spouse selection and may cause those who do not have the ideal appearance and body shape to feel inferior. In addition, relatively few posts were related to entertainment and work and study, and the content of these topics in the Chinese and non-Chinese posts varied considerably due to differences in regional cultures.

Among the sensitive topics, less than 8% of the posts were related to gay identity, and there were even fewer such posts in the English topics. From the perspective of the theme, the Chinese users expressed self-awareness, self-encouragement, and a desire for social identity while the non-Chinese users expressed a desire for human rights and equality. Currently, same-sex marriage has been legalized in more than 20 countries; however, it is not recognized by law in China. Even posting videos related to homosexuality in mainstream media and social networks is regarded as a violation. The enormous social pressure caused by this negative attitude has led many sexual minorities to give up their self-identification in order to follow social norms. Relevant research shows that there are 16 million "tongqi" (straight woman married to gay man) in China [25]. Posts related to sexual behaviors accounted for 1.37% of the total Chinese posts, and there were even fewer in the non-Chinese posts. From the perspective of theme, most of the non-Chinese posts were related to HIV testing and safe sex, with less information related to hookups. This may be because the word "hookup" is expressed in different languages, which is difficult to understand using a translation program. Nearly 60% of the Chinese posts were related to "hookup", and one quarter of them were asking for hookups. In fact, the number of posts asking for hookups was more than the number of posts against hooking up. A related study proved the correlation between hookups or casual sex and HIV infection [26]. However, users rarely disclose their HIV status, which further exacerbates the risk of HIV infection among gay men. At the same time, based on the high frequency of the words "AIDS" and "condom", it may reflect the promotion of AIDS prevention in China over the past few years. However, the lack of adolescent sex education and loopholes in the age limits for minors using apps may aggravate the HIV situation.

The second research focus was on identifying emotions in each category of posts. The results suggest that most of the posts were positive. The relationship and marriage and family topics contained the most emotions, especially positive emotions. The proportion of emotional words in the Chinese posts was higher than in the non-Chinese posts in all categories. With regard to distribution patterns, the Chinese and non-Chinese posts were most similar in the life topic and most different in the social networking topic. With regard to negative emotions, both the self-identification and sexual behavior topics contained many negative emotions, but there was a greater difference in the distribution of negative emotions between the Chinese and non-Chinese posts. The results show that the Chinese posts revealed considerable anxiety in the self-identification topic, and words related to death commonly appeared in this topic. The non-Chinese posts revealed more anxiety in sexual behavior, and words related to death appeared more frequently in this topic. Other studies have shown that the incidence of mood and anxiety disorders, the main risk factors for suicidal behavior, are more strongly related to homosexuality, lesbian, or bisexuality identities rather than sexual behavior or attractiveness [27].

The third research focus was on the Chinese users' views on sensitive issues. The voting data show that more than half of the participants would not accept open or long-distance relationships, although 55.2% supported having "back-burner" men when in a relationship. It seems that, when in a relationship, gay men are not only insecure about their partners but also fail to fully focus upon them. With regard to sexual behavior, 54.3% of participants said they would not interact with HIV-infected people, but more than half said they would not give up having sex with others after they end a relationship, and only half of the participants said they would participate in regular HIV testing. It can thus be inferred that the risk of HIV infection in this group is likely to be high. In terms of drug abuse, 64.2% of the participants said that they would reject their friends' drug invitations. The comments on this voting item indicated that most popular drug is "Rush", a club drug used to enhance sexual pleasure. Although "Rush" is not currently defined legally as a drug in China, its sale has recently been banned in the country. Regarding the sexual orientation of homosexuality, more than 60% of the participants said that if they had another chance, they would not want to be gay again, and more than 80% said they would hide their sexual orientation at work because they feared ridicule and discrimination. Nearly 70% of the participants said they have not discussed homosexuality with their parents. In order to maintain their reputations and avoid moral distress and social discrimination [28], more than half of the participants said they would marry a lesbian. The results show that self-identification, family acceptance, and social inclusion tend to be low for Chinese gay men.

Although GSN apps are widely used by the general population, public health practitioners and educators are just beginning to use this resource as a tool for research, education, and sharing information [29]. Our findings suggest that GSN apps can be used to reflect the behavior characteristics of gay men and identify individuals at risk of casual sex and HIV. In addition, although the social inclusion of homosexuality is presently occurring slowly in China, in the context of traditional Chinese culture, gay individuals still face tremendous discrimination and psychological pressure, especially those infected with HIV. Public information about HIV should be promoted more strongly, and sexual education should be popularized for adolescents in China.

Limitations should be considered when interpreting our findings. Our hashtag list did not cover all popular or sensitive topics. Similarly, many popular topics in minority languages were not covered in our research because of the language limitations of the researchers. In addition, we only included posts by searching hashtags in the topic interface, but private messages sent between accounts and posts without hashtags might generate different content. It is also notable that when dealing with English topics, we translated all non-English posts into English posts. As most posts were very short and contained an internet abbreviation spectrum, the machine translation results might not have been accurate and could have negatively affected our analysis. Additionally, as the gay men using the GSN apps were relatively young, the findings of this work may not represent the actual situation among more diverse gay communities.

Despite these limitations, we believe that this study supports the literature on behavior and opinion analyses of sexual minorities through a comparative analysis of themes and sentiments of posts in China and other countries, presenting the main viewpoints of gay individuals toward sensitive issues in Chinese gay communities. Our findings stress the need for continuous research in this area, especially to better understand whether and how this type of content can be used to help those who need interventions. In addition, it would be beneficial for this work to be replicated with other social apps or social networks to identify gay men in mainstream media through the topics they care about and to investigate behaviors and opinions in sexual minorities.

**Author Contributions:** Conceptualization, X.L.; Data curation, G.H. and M.C.; Funding acquisition, X.L.; Investigation, M.C.; Methodology, G.H.; Writing—original draft, G.H.; Writing—review and editing, X.L.

**Funding:** Xin Lu acknowledges the National Natural Science Foundation of China (71771213, 71790615 and 91846301) and the Hunan Science and Technology Plan Project (2017RS3040, 2018JJ1034). Ge Huang and Mengsi Cai is partially supported by the National Natural Science Foundation of China (71690233, 91546203, 71774168).

**Conflicts of Interest:** The authors declare no conflict of interest.

# Appendix A

**Table A1.** A comprehensive list of voting questionnaires on Blued.

| ID | Question | Option 1 | Option 2 |
|----|----------|----------|----------|
| | **Life** | | |
| 1 | Which do you prefer: comfort or freedom? | Small city, full of happiness. | Big city, just be yourself. |
| 2 | Will you continue to work out after consummating a stable relationship? | Yes, I will be attractive if I look handsome. | No, I will indulge myself. |
| 3 | Can you accept 1 wearing makeup? | Yes. | No. |
| 4 | Can you accept massages by strangers in bathhouse? | Yes, it's good social manners. | No, it's embarrassing. |
| 5 | Which would you choose: artificial beauty and natural ugliness? | Artificial beauty. | Natural ugliness. |
| 6 | Which one do you like: nice ass or muscular chests? | Yes. | No. |
| 7 | Have you ever had a wet dream staying with a male star? | Yes. | No. |
| 8 | Which do you value more: body shape or face value? | Body shape. | Face value. |
| 9 | Do you like to sleep naked? | Yes. | No. |
| 10 | Have you ever thought about wearing women's clothing? | Yes. | No. |
| 11 | Are you suffering from mobile phone separation anxiety? | Yes. | No. |
| 12 | Do you mind if others see your previous embarrassing pictures? | Yes. | No. |
| 13 | Will you spend ahead of time to celebrate the upcoming Chinese New Year? | Yes. | No. |
| 14 | Will you give the elders a red envelope in Chinese New Year after having job? | Yes. | No. |
| 15 | Will you go to the offline counter to buy skincare products? | Yes, just be myself. | No, that's embarrassing. |
| 16 | Will you take photos with friends who looks better than yourself? | Yes, I will smile. | No, I will refuse. |
| 17 | Is it your style to be different? | Yes. | No. |
| 18 | Which do you prefer: masturbation cup or vibrator? | Masturbation cup. | Vibrator. |
| | **Making Friends** | | |
| 19 | Is the sexual role 1 (top) and 0 (bottom) important when making friends? | Yes, I will blacklist him if we are in the same sexual role. | No, I just want to meet someone interesting. |
| 20 | Do you care about the other person's face value? | Yes, friends should be handsome. | No, true heart is more important. |
| 21 | Will you respond to greetings if the other person did not have an avatar? | Yes. | No. |
| 22 | Should I tell my fiend if his boyfriend cheated on him? | Yes, it's our duty. | No, I don't want to bother myself about others. |
| 23 | If your idol become a WeChat salesmen, will you still love him? | Yes. | No. |
| 24 | Will you respond to strangers who greeting like "Are you online"? | Yes, I will response politely. | No, I just want to talk to those who is sincere. |
| 25 | Will you tell your friend if he bought a fake item? | Yes, I will kindly remind him to pay attention to being deceived. | No, it's embarrassing. |
| 26 | Will you accept friend requests from the person who unfriend you? | Yes. | No. |
| 27 | Do you think it's offensive to call friends sisters? | Yes. | No. |
| 28 | Do you think two people with different worldviews can be compatible with each other? | Yes. | No. |
| 29 | When making friends, will you consider where they come from? | Yes. | No. |
| 30 | Is there a pure friendship between 1 and 0? | Yes. | No. |
| 31 | Will you choose a private place when you meet gay friend for the first time? | Yes. | No. |
| 32 | Is that all right to use alternative accounts to make friends online? | Yes. | No. |
| 33 | Can you accept the lubricant is not effective? | Yes. | No. |
| | **Relationship** | | |
| 34 | Can you stay friends after a breakup? | Yes, friendship remains even if we break up. | No, I'll blacklist him. |
| 35 | Should single men blame themselves on having affairs with multiple partners? | Yes, I can't stand that. | No, it's none of your business. |
| 36 | "Tiancai" boyfriend (a man who is totally your type) is a playboy, can you accept? | Yes. | No. |

**Table A1.** *Cont.*

| ID | Question | Option 1 | Option 2 |
|----|----------|----------|----------|
| 37 | Can you forgive your boyfriend if he cheated on you? | Yes, but don't do it next time. | No, old habits die hard. |
| 38 | Can you accept a long-distance relationship? | Yes, true love stands the test of distance. | No, lack of safety. |
| 39 | Should you check your boyfriends' phone? | Yes, secret is a time bomb. | No, there should be free space between couples. |
| 40 | Do you trust your boyfriend to go to Gay bar alone? | Yes, he is not dare. | No, I know he can't control himself. |
| 41 | Do you accept sharing date expenses with your boyfriends? | Yes, I support separate finances. | No. |
| 42 | Will you confess to the men who you have secret crushes on? | Yes, don't leave any regrets behind. | No, I'll keep him in my heart. |
| 43 | Are straight men an aphrodisiac or poison to you? | Aphrodisiac. | Poison. |
| 44 | Do you mind if your boyfriend share photos of his body shape on the Internet? | Yes. | No. |
| 45 | Do you want to get away from gay communities after going steady with someone? | Yes, for safety. | No, true love stands the test of interference. |
| 46 | Should gay men show conjugal love in social networks? | Yes, love should be seen by someone. | No. |
| 47 | Do you mind if your boyfriend is in contact with ex-boyfriend? | Yes. | No. |
| 48 | Do you mind if your boyfriend is "the moonlight clan" (people who expend their entire salary before the end of each month)? | Yes. | No. |
| 49 | After the quarrel, should 1 compromise first? | Yes. | No. |
| 50 | Will you pay attention to the status of your ex-boyfriend? | Yes. | No. |
| 51 | Will you get mad when your boyfriend pays more attention to their phone than you? | Yes. | No. |
| 52 | Do you accept open relationships? | Yes. | No. |
| 53 | Should there be any "back-burner" men while you are in a relationship? | Yes, to avoid risk. | No, one life, one love. |
| 54 | If a man you like is boyfriend of your good friend, will you chase him? | Yes, just be myself. | No, bless for my friend. |
| 55 | If you find your boyfriend and you have a common friend in gay group, will you gossip about it? | Yes, I'm curious about sensitive relationship. | No, I don't care. |
| 56 | Do you want to start a new relationship quickly after a breakup? | Yes. | No, I need time to calm down. |
| 57 | Will you lower your standard for a boyfriend if you are single for a long time? | Yes, every man has his fault. | No, there will always be someone worth waiting for. |
| 58 | Should I respond to my ex-boyfriend who want to get back together? | Yes. | No. |
| 59 | Will you share a house with people who like bring people home? | Yes. | No. |
| 60 | Will you contact your first love if he becomes less handsome after grew up? | Yes. | No. |
| 61 | How to do if your boyfriend shows bad sexual skills at date night? | I need to be calm, I am desperate. | It's not a big deal, I will help you with my passion. |
| 62 | Will you confess to your boyfriend the history of your love? | Yes. | No. |
| 63 | Will you go out with your boyfriend if he looks not handsome? | Yes. | No. |
| 64 | Do you have virginity obsession? | Yes. | No. |
| 65 | Will you display affection in public? | Yes. | No. |
| 66 | Can you accept platonic love? | Yes, ideal love is what I pursue. | No, we are human. |
| 67 | Do you dare to test your boyfriend's loyalty? | Yes. | No. |
| 68 | Will you masturbate without your boyfriend knowing? | Yes. | No. |
| 69 | Have you ever been confessed by girl? | Yes. | No. |
| 70 | Do you like to warm up before having sex? | Yes. | No. |
| 71 | Is male masculinism good or bad? | Good. | Bad. |
| 72 | Have you ever kissed a girl? | Yes. | No. |
| 73 | Should you return valuable gifts to your partner after a breakup? | Yes. | No. |
| 74 | Will you go to work where your boyfriend located? | Yes. | No. |
| 75 | Will you ask about your partner's income before committing to a relationship? | Yes. | No. |
| 76 | Are you obsessed with sports boys? | Yes. | No. |

**Table A1.** *Cont.*

| ID | Question | Option 1 | Option 2 |
|---|---|---|---|
| 77 | Will you break up because of disharmony in sexual intercourse? | Yes. | No. |
| 78 | Should there be privacy between couples? | Yes. | No. |
| 79 | Should older virgins be self-confident or inferior? | Self-confident. | Inferior. |
| 80 | Which do you prefer: men from the South or men from the North? | The men in the South. | The men in the North. |
| 81 | Should people be thankful spending money on his boyfriend? | Yes. | No. |
| 82 | Will you put your boyfriends' and your wages together after going steady? | Yes. | No. |
| 83 | Can you believe those who cheated before? | Yes. | No. |
| 84 | Do you think it's necessary to divide household chores clearly in husband & husband life? | Yes. | No. |
| 85 | Would you choose to confess on Valentine's Day? | Yes. | No. |
| 86 | Is it important to have a clear standard when looking for a boyfriend? | Yes, standard is important. | No, mainly basing on first appearances. |
| 87 | Will you love someone because he is good to you? | Yes. | No. |
| 88 | Will you share your passport number with your boyfriend if he asks? | Yes. | No. |
| 89 | Will you have sex with someone when you have prostatitis? | Yes. | No. |
| 90 | Will you blame your boyfriend's inability during of intercourse because of tiredness of journey? | Yes. | No. |
| **Self-Identification** | | | |
| 91 | Do you believe in pure 1? | Yes, there should be pure 1. | No, pure 1 is just a legend. |
| 92 | If you have another chance, will you be a gay again? | Yes, I'm not regret. | No, I just want simple life. |
| 93 | Can you accept that 0 is taller than 1? | Yes. | No. |
| 94 | Do you believe that straight men can be turned into gay men? | Yes. | No. |
| 95 | Will you argue with each other when you encounter anti-gay speech? | Yes. | No. |
| 96 | Do you agree that all gays show feminine inclinations? | Yes. | No. |
| 97 | Do you think homosexuals are born with their sexual preference? | Yes. | No. |
| **Sexual Behavior** | | | |
| 98 | Will you interact with HIV-infected people? | Yes, he can live normally if he takes medicine regularly. | No, I don't want to risk myself no matter how I like him. |
| 99 | Will you give up having sex with others after end a relationship? | Yes, I'll wait for Mr. right. | No. |
| 100 | Do you take regular HIV tests? | Yes. | No. |
| 101 | will you take HIV tests routinely when AIDS is curable? | Yes. | No. |
| 102 | Will you reject their friends' drug invitations? | Yes. | No. |
| **Work & Study** | | | |
| 103 | Will you recognize each other when you meet gay friends in your work? | Yes, take care with each other. | No, just do my own part. |
| 104 | Will you hide your sexual orientation at work? | Yes, for protecting my privacy. | No, just be my self. |
| 105 | Will you share a bed with a straight male colleague? | Yes. | No. |
| 106 | Is office love good or bad? | Good. | Bad. |
| 107 | Will you break up with your boyfriend because of graduating from university? | Yes. | No. |
| **Marriage & Family** | | | |
| 108 | If you your encounter a relative in Blued, will you blacklist him? | Yes, it's embarrassing. | No, we'll take care of each other. |
| 109 | As a gay, do you want to have a child? | Yes, I want to be a father. | No, just two of us. |
| 110 | If your boyfriend gets married with another person, will you break up with him? | Yes, I will break up with him. | No, true heart is more important. |
| 111 | Have you ever discussed homosexuality with your parents? | Yes, proper guidance makes parents more open-minded. | No, that's a sensitive topic. |
| 112 | Will you adopt a child in the future? | Yes. | No. |
| 113 | Will you choose to marry a lesbian? | Yes. | No. |
| 114 | In terms of forced marriage, will you obedient or rebellious? | Obedient. | Rebellious. |

## References

1. Nguyen, T.; Phung, D.; Dao, B.; Venkatesh, S.; Berk, M. Affective and content analysis of online depression communities. *IEEE Trans. Affect. Comput.* **2014**, *5*, 217–226. [CrossRef]
2. Sowles, S.J.; McLeary, M.; Optican, A.; Cahn, E.; Krauss, M.J.; Fitzsimmons-Craft, E.E.; Wilfley, D.E.; Cavazos-Rehg, P.A. A content analysis of an online pro-eating disorder community on Reddit. *Body Image* **2018**, *24*, 137–144. [CrossRef] [PubMed]
3. UNAIDS. Global AIDS Update 2019—Communities at the Centre. Available online: https://www.unaids.org/en/resources/documents/2019/2019-global-AIDS-update (accessed on 12 July 2019).
4. Zou, H.; Fan, S. Characteristics of men who have sex with men who use smartphone geosocial networking applications and implications for HIV interventions: A systematic review and meta-analysis. *Arch. Sex. Behav.* **2017**, *46*, 885–894. [CrossRef]
5. Phillips, G.; Grov, C.; Mustanski, B. Engagement in group sex among geosocial networking mobile application-using men who have sex with men. *Sex. Health* **2015**, *12*, 495–500. [CrossRef] [PubMed]
6. Grosskopf, N.A.; LeVasseur, M.T.; Glaser, D.B. Use of the internet and mobile-based "apps" for sex-seeking among men who have sex with men in New York City. *Am. J. Men's Health* **2014**, *8*, 510–520. [CrossRef] [PubMed]
7. Landovitz, R.J.; Tseng, C.-H.; Weissman, M.; Haymer, M.; Mendenhall, B.; Rogers, K.; Veniegas, R.; Gorbach, P.M.; Reback, C.J.; Shoptaw, S. Epidemiology, sexual risk behavior, and HIV prevention practices of men who have sex with men using GRINDR in Los Angeles, California. *J. Urban Health* **2013**, *90*, 729–739. [CrossRef] [PubMed]
8. Wei, L.; Chen, L.; Zhang, H.; Yang, Z.; Zou, H.; Yuan, T.; Xiao, Y.; Liu, S.; Tan, W.; Xie, W. Use of gay app and the associated HIV/syphilis risk among non-commercial men who have sex with men in Shenzhen, China: A serial cross-sectional study. *Sex. Transm. Infect.* **2019**. [CrossRef]
9. Bien, C.H.; Best, J.M.; Muessig, K.E.; Wei, C.; Han, L.; Tucker, J.D. Gay apps for seeking sex partners in China: Implications for MSM sexual health. *AIDS Behav.* **2015**, *19*, 941–946. [CrossRef]
10. Holloway, I.W. Substance use homophily among geosocial networking application using gay, bisexual, and other men who have sex with men. *Arch. Sex. Behav.* **2015**, *44*, 1799–1811. [CrossRef]
11. Burrell, E.R.; Pines, H.A.; Robbie, E.; Coleman, L.; Murphy, R.D.; Hess, K.L.; Anton, P.; Gorbach, P.M. Use of the location-based social networking application GRINDR as a recruitment tool in rectal microbicide development research. *AIDS Behav.* **2012**, *16*, 1816–1820. [CrossRef]
12. Fields, E.L.; Long, A.; Dangerfield, D.T.; Morgan, A.; Uzzi, M.; Arrington-Sanders, R.; Jennings, J.M. There's an App for That: Using Geosocial Networking Apps to Access Young Black Gay, Bisexual, and other MSM at Risk for HIV. *Am. J. Health Promot.* **2019**. [CrossRef] [PubMed]
13. Liu, C.; Lu, X. Analyzing hidden populations online: Topic, emotion, and social network of HIV-related users in the largest Chinese online community. *BMC Med Inform. Decis. Mak.* **2018**, *18*, 2. [CrossRef] [PubMed]
14. Mo, P.K.; Coulson, N.S. Exploring the communication of social support within virtual communities: A content analysis of messages posted to an online HIV/AIDS support group. *Cyberpsychol. Behav.* **2008**, *11*, 371–374. [CrossRef] [PubMed]
15. Miller, B. "Dude, where's your face?" Self-presentation, self-description, and partner preferences on a social networking application for men who have sex with men: A content analysis. *Sex. Cult.* **2015**, *19*, 637–658. [CrossRef]
16. Bun, K.K.; Ishizuka, M. Topic extraction from news archive using TF* PDF algorithm. In Proceedings of the Third International Conference on Web Information Systems Engineering, WISE 2002, Singapore, 14 December 2002; pp. 73–82.
17. Chen, K.-Y.; Luesukprasert, L.; Seng-cho, T.C. Hot topic extraction based on timeline analysis and multidimensional sentence modeling. *IEEE Trans. Knowl. Data Eng.* **2007**, *19*, 1016–1025. [CrossRef]
18. Wang, X.; Wei, F.; Liu, X.; Zhou, M.; Zhang, M. Topic sentiment analysis in twitter: A graph-based hashtag sentiment classification approach. In Proceedings of the 20th ACM International Conference on Information and Knowledge Management, Glasgow, Scotland, 24–28 October 2011; pp. 1031–1040.
19. Bollen, J.; Mao, H.; Pepe, A. Modeling public mood and emotion: Twitter sentiment and socio-economic phenomena. In Proceedings of the Fifth International AAAI Conference on Weblogs and Social Media, Barcelona, Spain, 17–21 July 2011.

20. Zhao, W.X.; Jiang, J.; Weng, J.; He, J.; Lim, E.-P.; Yan, H.; Li, X. Comparing twitter and traditional media using topic models. In *European Conference on Information Retrieval, Proceedings of the 33rd European Conference on IR Research ECIR 2011, Dublin, Ireland, 18–21 April 2011*; Springer: Berlin/Heidelberg, Germany, 2011; pp. 338–349.

21. Pennebaker, J.W.; Booth, R.J.; Francis, M.E. *Linguistic Inquiry and Word Count: LIWC [Computer Software]*; Liwc. Net: Austin, TX, USA, 2007; Volume 135.

22. Gao, R.; Hao, B.; Li, H.; Gao, Y.; Zhu, T. Developing simplified Chinese psychological linguistic analysis dictionary for microblog. In *Brain and Health Informatics, Proceedings of International Conference on Brain and Health Informatics, BHI 2013, Maebashi, Japan, 29–31 October 2013*; Springer Nature: Basel, Switzerland, 2013; pp. 359–368.

23. Jankowski, G.S.; Diedrichs, P.C.; Halliwell, E. Can appearance conversations explain differences between gay and heterosexual men's body dissatisfaction? *Psychol. Men Masc.* **2014**, *15*, 68. [CrossRef]

24. Yelland, C.; Tiggemann, M. Muscularity and the gay ideal: Body dissatisfaction and disordered eating in homosexual men. *Eat. Behav.* **2003**, *4*, 107–116. [CrossRef]

25. Juan, S. Millions of Wives Wed to Gay Men: Expert. Available online: http://www.chinadaily.com.cn/china/2012-02/03/content_14528838.htm (accessed on 8 June 2019).

26. Garofalo, R.; Kuhns, L.M.; Hidalgo, M.; Gayles, T.; Kwon, S.; Muldoon, A.L.; Mustanski, B. Impact of religiosity on the sexual risk behaviors of young men who have sex with men. *J. Sex Res.* **2015**, *52*, 590–598. [CrossRef]

27. Bostwick, W.B.; Boyd, C.J.; Hughes, T.L.; McCabe, S.E. Dimensions of sexual orientation and the prevalence of mood and anxiety disorders in the United States. *Am. J. Public Health* **2010**, *100*, 468–475. [CrossRef]

28. Ren, Z.; Howe, C.Q.; Zhang, W. Maintaining "mianzi" and "lizi": Understanding the reasons for formality marriages between gay men and lesbians in China. *Transcult. Psychiatry* **2019**, *56*, 213–232. [CrossRef]

29. McHugh, M.C.; Saperstein, S.L.; Gold, R.S. OMG U# Cyberbully! An exploration of public discourse about cyberbullying on twitter. *Health Educ. Behav.* **2019**, *46*, 97–105. [PubMed]

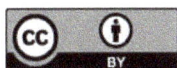

© 2019 by the authors. Licensee MDPI, Basel, Switzerland. This article is an open access article distributed under the terms and conditions of the Creative Commons Attribution (CC BY) license (http://creativecommons.org/licenses/by/4.0/).

International Journal of
*Environmental Research
and Public Health*

MDPI

*Article*

# A Systematic Review of UK Educational and Training Materials Aimed at Health and Social Care Staff about Providing Appropriate Services for LGBT+ People

Ros Hunt, Christopher Bates, Susan Walker, Jeffrey Grierson[ID], Sarah Redsell and Catherine Meads *

Faculty of Health, Education, Medicine and Social Care, Anglia Ruskin University, East Road, Cambridge CB1 1PT, UK; ros.hunt@virgin.net (R.H.); Chrisbates1809@gmail.com (C.B.); susan.walker@anglia.ac.uk (S.W.); jeffrey.grierson@anglia.ac.uk (J.G.); sarah.redsell@anglia.ac.uk (S.R.)
* Correspondence: catherine.meads@anglia.ac.uk; Tel.: +07850-864327

Received: 29 October 2019; Accepted: 1 December 2019; Published: 7 December 2019

**Abstract:** Background: There is greater dissatisfaction with health services by LGBT people compared to heterosexual and cisgender people and some of this is from lack of equality and diversity training for health professionals. Core training standards in sexual orientation for health professionals have been available since 2006. The purpose of this project is to systematically review educational materials for health and social care professionals in lesbian, gay, bisexual, and transgender (LGBT) issues. Methods: A protocol was developed and searches conducted in six databases. Selection criteria: any studies reporting delivery or evaluation of UK education of health and/or social care professionals in LGBT issues, with no language or setting restrictions. Inclusions and data extraction were conducted in duplicate. Narrative synthesis of educational evaluations was used. Educational materials were assessed using thematic synthesis. Results: From the searches, 165 full papers were evaluated and 19 studies were included in the narrative synthesis. Three were successful action-research projects in cancer services and in residential care. Sixteen sets of educational/training materials have been available since 2010. These varied in length, scope, target audience, and extent of development as classroom-ready materials. Conclusions: Despite the availability of appropriate training programmes for post-qualifying staff, recommendations to undertake training, best practice examples, and statements of good intent, LGBT people continue to report that they are experiencing discrimination or direct prejudice from health and/or social care services. Better training strategies using behaviour change techniques are needed.

**Keywords:** lesbian; bisexual; gay; transgender; education; systematic review

## 1. Introduction

The recent survey of 108,100 lesbian, gay, bisexual, and transgender (LGBT) people's experiences of everyday life in the UK, published by the UK Government Equalities Office [1] found that in the preceding 12 months 40% of transgender respondents had had at least one negative experience of healthcare because of their gender identity and that 13% of cisgender respondents had had at least one negative experience of healthcare because of their sexual orientation. This finding echoes that of a recent review of the literature in inequality among LGBT groups in the UK [2] which found greater dissatisfaction with health services by LGBT people compared to heterosexual and cisgender people. They report instances of overt discrimination and inappropriate behaviour by health professionals from a number of different studies included in the review.

A recent grey literature survey of 3000 UK health and social care staff (called the Unhealthy Attitudes Survey) [3] found that 25% of patient-or client-facing staff had heard colleagues make negative remarks about sexual orientation and 20% make negative remarks about gender identity. Five percent of patient-or client-facing staff had witnessed colleagues discriminate against or provide poorer treatment because of their sexual orientation and 7% of health and social care staff said they would not feel comfortable working alongside a trans colleague. Numerous quotes are provided, such as "A colleague who is gay made a remark about his partner and another colleague said 'Oh my god seriously are you gay, gross'. The irony of this was that the remark was made during equality and diversity training." and "A transgender nurse [was] often referred to as 'he-she-it' by other staff and service users" [3]. Staff remarks to other staff have the potential to more clearly indicate their attitudes, whereas staff may be more guarded when talking to patients or service users. It was found that 10% of staff had witnessed a colleague expressing the belief that someone could be 'cured' of their minority sexual orientation [3] despite the fact that conversion therapy has been condemned as ineffective [4] and that the UK government is bringing forward proposals to end the practice of 'conversion therapy' in the UK [5]. High proportions of health and care staff stated that they did not consider sexual orientation relevant to a person's health needs, for example 72% of care workers, 62% of nurses, and 55% of social workers [3]. There is good evidence from the English General Practice Patient Survey [6] that sexual minorities have worse health care experiences than heterosexual people, which probably result in inequalities in family practitioner use [7]. From these results it is clear that health and social care staff need more effective equality and diversity training.

In 2006, Core Training Standards for Sexual Orientation was published with the aim to make national services inclusive for LGB people [8]. In 2010 the UK Parliament introduced the Equality Act (2010) which legally protects LGBT people from discrimination in the workplace and in wider society. The Unhealthy Attitudes Survey [3] found that only 50% of health and care staff reported that they had received equality and diversity training in the previous 12 months, and the majority of this did not address LGBT issues. Therefore, in spite of core training standards being available for 10 years, there continues to be a considerable need to increase the quality and effectiveness of equality and diversity training in the UK.

This systematic review evaluates all relevant materials about the delivery and evaluation of UK education of health and social care professionals in lesbian, gay, bisexual, and transgender (LGBT) issues, in order to obtain a starting point from which to improve training.

## 2. Materials and Methods

### 2.1. Inclusion Criteria

This systematic review was conducted according to a prospective protocol for a student project. Any qualitative or quantitative studies (published or grey literature) with information of interest in any setting and made available between 2010 and 2018 were eligible if they:

- Described evaluations of teaching to UK-based health and/or social care staff around LGBT issues; of
- Described curricula or educational materials for use with UK-based health and/or social care staff around LGBT issues.

LGBT was defined as sexual orientation and gender identity minorities. Sexual orientation could be defined by identity (lesbian, bisexual, gay) or behaviour (women who described themselves as having sex with women, or having sex with women and men; men who described themselves as having sex with men, or having sex with women and men; or by same sex cohabitation status). Gender identity minorities were transgender men and women however defined. The 2010 cut off was chosen because of the UK Equality Act (2010).

Excluded were reports or studies calling for education to be improved, without giving any specific educational materials. Also excluded were reviews and systematic reviews of educational materials, organisational policy documents and materials from outside the UK.

## 2.2. Search Strategy, Study Selection, and Data Extraction

Database searches up to November 2019 were conducted by two reviewers (CB, CM) and checked by another (CM, RH). Databases (on platforms) searched included Applied Social Science Index and Abstracts (ProQuest), Embase (Ovid), Inform Adults (Community Care), Medline (EBSCO), PsychInfo (Ovid), Psychology and Behavioural Sciences Collection (EBSCO), Social Care Online (SCIE), Science and Social Science Citation Indices (Web of Science).

Search terms and appropriate synonyms (as MeSH terms and text words) were developed based on populations and exposures and included 'sexual orientation', 'gender identity' 'gay', 'lesbian', 'bisexual', 'transgender', 'queer', 'questioning', 'cisgender' 'asexual', 'gender dysphoria', 'heteronormativity', 'men who have sex with men' (MSM), 'men who have sex with men and women (MSMW), 'women who have sex with women' (WSW), 'women who have sex with men and women' (WSWM), and 'LGBT' plus services and professionals involved such as 'healthcare', 'social care', 'professionals', and 'practitioners' plus terms around relevant LGBT issues such as 'education' 'knowledge', 'understanding', and 'awareness'. The same search terms were used for each database but adapted where necessary. Database searches were supplemented with searches on Google, Google Scholar, and specific websites—the Stonewall charity, LGBT Partnership, LGBT Consortium, LGBT Foundation, Birmingham LGBT, ACCESSCare, LGBT Health and Wellbeing Scotland, MindOut, and London Friend. References of relevant reviews were sifted and the archives on LGBT health used in other projects by one of the authors (CM) was searched for relevant studies.

All titles found by the above search were assessed for inclusion and abstracts, where available, were read. If any titles and abstracts had relevant information or there was uncertainty, the full study was read and either accepted for the systematic review or rejected based on the above inclusion and exclusion criteria. Full-text assessment to determine inclusion in the systematic review was carried out by both reviewers (RH, CM). Any disagreements were resolved by discussion. Data was extracted by one reviewer (RH) and checked by another (CM). No authors were contacted about data discrepancies.

## 2.3. Data Analysis

Results are discussed narratively, with main themes developed through synthesis of qualitative results, and tabulation where appropriate. One researcher (RH) extracted relevant information from included studies, coded them, and organised them into descriptive themes. These were checked and amended by a second researcher (CM). None of the systematic review authors have been involved in any of the included studies.

## 3. Results

From the database searches 165 full papers were read. From these papers, 19 studies were included in the narrative synthesis, 3 in Group 1 and 16 in Group 2, see Figure 1 (PRISMA flow chart).

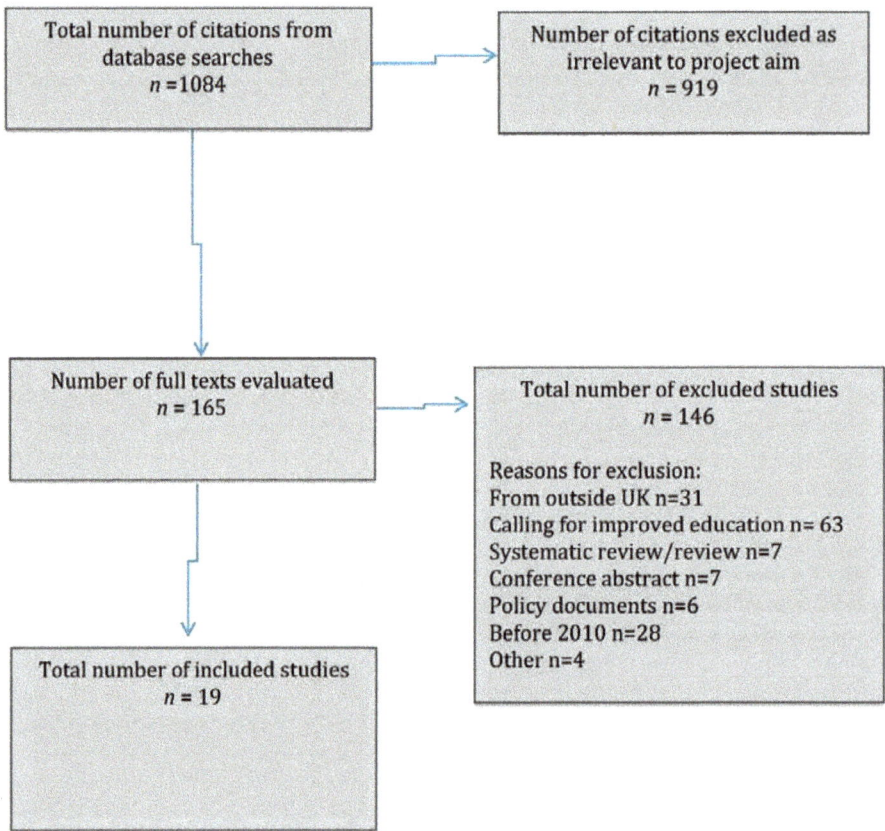

**Figure 1.** Prisma flow diagram.

*3.1. Study Characteristics*

For Group 1 we found three action research projects evaluating teaching around LGBT issues to UK-based health and/or social care staff, one based in six residential care homes for older people [9,10], one with cancer nurses and other health professionals [11] and one with a local branch of a cervical screening programme in NHS Bradford and Airedale [12]. These are detailed in Table 1. There were no evaluations found for other NHS or social care staff training initiatives.

**Table 1.** Characteristics of included teaching project evaluations—Group 1.

| | Service | Project Type | Number of Staff Involved | Number of Community Activists Involved | Actions | Findings | Follow Up | Grant Funding |
|---|---|---|---|---|---|---|---|---|
| Carter 2012 | Cervical screening programme in Bradford and Airedale | Service improvement project for NHS | Not reported (?all staff in the cervical screening programme) | Not reported but some were in the project steering group | Materials for SMW developed with staff (leaflet) and circulated through GP practices, sexual health clinics, LGB venues, and Bradford's gay pride event. | Being involved in update staff training was key to sustaining and widening impact | Evaluation of cervical screening rates in 2012 planned* | Department of Health Pacesetters initiative |
| Fish 2016 | Cancer care | Knowledge exchange project | Approximately 9: Staff from a breast cancer charity, another cancer charity, a cancer research charity, NHS, 2 academics, and 5 cancer service users and carers | Staff from two LGBT community groups. | Funding applications, developing research questions and conducting research, contribution to National Cancer Equalities Initiative, staff seminars, good practice resources for staff, policy briefings, website material. | Wide ranging and successful project, resulted in lesbians and bisexual women being mentioned in policy statements | Not described specifically | National Cancer Action Team, ESRC Knowledge Exchange programme |
| Hafford-Letchfield 2017 and Willis 2018 | Six residential care homes for older people in a large city in England | Service standard improvement for private care home provider | 35 interviews (?all staff in each of the care homes) | 8 (training was given to them) | Community activists co-facilitated staff advisory sessions then started dialogues with staff, with some difficult and important conversations. | Staff perceived sessions as enlightening, educational, and informative | Post-intervention interviews at 7 months | Comic Relief |

* post intervention evaluation never occurred due to lack of funds (personal communication Lesley Hedges 2017).

Action research involves research where the researchers and clients collaborate in the identification and definition of an issue to be addressed and in the development of solutions. All three action-research projects were successfully completed and reported important gains in understanding and attitudes in participants. For example, the residential care home project found at the 7-month-post-intervention interviews that there were small but important shifts in attitudes and gains in awareness. This then translated in more appropriate behaviour at key points. For the breast cancer project, it resulted in increased staff understanding of the distinctive needs of LGBT cancer service users, influencing of their attitudes and assumptions, the provision of tailored information and support from the two cancer charities involved, and wider dissemination through organisation staff members. For the cervical smear project open discussion of issues in training sessions led to successful countering of inaccurate views that might have hindered progress in the project.

For Group 2, we found 16 different sets of training materials around LGBT issues specifically for UK health and social care staff. These are listed in date order:

- Moving forward: working with and for older lesbians, gay men, bisexuals and transgendered people. Training and resource pack. Written by Steve Pugh, Willie McCartney, and Julia Ryan. (2010) [13]
- Working with older lesbian, gay, and bisexual people, a guide for care and support services. Written by James Taylor at Stonewall (2011) [14]
- Supporting older lesbian, gay, bisexual and transgender people, a checklist for social care providers. Written by Opening Doors London and Camden AgeUK (2011) [15]
- Implications for lesbian, gay, bisexual, and transgender (LGBT) people. www.scie.org.uk, written Social Care Institute for Excellence (SCIE) (2011) [16]
- Sexual Orientation: A guide for the NHS. Written by Alice Ashworth for Stonewall (undated but produced in 2012) [17]
- Working with lesbian, gay, bisexual, and transgender older people, by Trish Hafford-Letchfield (2014) [18]
- How to be LGBT+ friendly: Guide for care homes. Written by PrideCymru (2015) [19]
- LGB&T People & Mental Health: Guidance for Services and Practitioners. Written for the LGB&T Partnership by Barker MJ, et al., (2015) [20]
- Lesbian, gay, bisexual, trans and queer good practice guide. Mind and Mind Out (2016) [21]
- Dementia Care and LGBT communities: A good practice paper. Written by National LGBT Partnership and Colleagues (2016) [22]
- Out loud, LGBT voices in health and social care, a narrative account of LGBT needs. Written by LGBT Partnership (2016) [23]
- Best Practice in providing healthcare to lesbian, bisexual and other women who have sex with women. Written by LGBT Partnership (2016) [24]
- Lesbian, gay, bisexual & trans health priorities, building an LGB&T voice into planning systems. Written by LGBT Partnership (2017) [25]
- A whole systems approach to tackling inequalities in health for lesbian, gay, bisexual and trans (LGBT) people, a toolkit. Written by LGBT Partnership (2018) [26]
- Health4LGBTI Trainer's Manual and 4 slide packs-Reducing Health Inequalities experienced by LGBTI People: What is Your Role as a Professional? Written by Zeeman and colleagues for the European Commission (2018) [27]
- Safe to be me. Meeting the needs of older lesbian, gay, bisexual and transgender people using health and social care services. A resource pack for professionals. Written by Sally Knocker and Anthony Smith for Age UK (undated but produced in 2018) [28]

## 3.2. Description of Documents for Group 2

For a brief description of the sixteen sets of training materials please see Table 2.

**Table 2.** Characteristics of training materials—Group 2.

| | Author or Organisation | Target Group | Care Group Age | Target Provider | Length |
|---|---|---|---|---|---|
| 1 | Pugh 2010 | LGBT | Older people | Health and social care | 142 pages |
| 2 | Taylor 2011 | LGB | Older people | Care and support services | 28 pages |
| 3 | Opening Doors London 2011 | LGBT | Older people | Social care providers | 10 pages |
| 4 | SCIE 2011 | LGBT | Personalisation | Social care providers | 6 pages |
| 5 | Ashworth (2012) | LGB | All | Healthcare | 23 pages |
| 6 | Hafford-Letchfield 2014 | LGBT | Older people | Social care providers | 30 pages |
| 7 | PrideCymru 2015 | LGBT+ | People in care homes | Care home providers | 3 pages |
| 8 | Barker 2015 | LGBT | All | Health services and practitioners | 12 pages |
| 9 | Mind 2016 | LGBTQ | All | Mental health service providers | 23 pages |
| 10 | LGBT Partnership 2016a | LGBT | Dementia care | Dementia services | 16 pages |
| 11 | LGBT Partnership 2016b | LGBT | All | Health and social care | 24 pages |
| 12 | LGBT Partnership 2016c | SMW | All | Healthcare | 22 pages |
| 13 | LGBT Partnership 2017 | LGBT | All | Health and social care | 14 pages |
| 14 | LGBT Partnership 2018 | LGBT | All | Health systems | 43 pages |
| 15 | European Commission (2018) | LGBT | All | Healthcare | Trainer's manual 151 pages. Module 1–41 pages Module 2–61 pages Module 3–31 pages Module 4-41 pages |
| 16 | Knocker 2016-8 | LGBT | Older people | Health and social care | 40 pages |

### 3.2.1. Material Recipients

Eleven of the documents were aimed at service managers, planners and/or commissioners. Of these, two [17,19] could have been easily accessed by individual staff to increase their knowledge and awareness. Two documents [14,27] were aimed at trainers and provided the tools to undertake the training of others. Four of the documents [16,18,20,21] were aimed primarily at front line staff and two were aimed at mental health practitioners and two were aimed at social care staff. In many cases, these documents outlined recommendations as to what should be covered in training for various groups of staff and the rationale for providing such training. Some documents were addressed to "anyone working or volunteering" in health and social care. Five documents were specifically aimed at health services only [17,20,21,25,26], six were for those providing health and social care [14,22–24,27,28], and five specifically at those providing social care [13,15,16,18,19]. Social care here is used in its widest sense including residential care and housing providers.

### 3.2.2. Material Format

Only one of the documents contained 'ready to use' training materials [27]. Another provided all that might be required to design appropriate training [13]. Others provided plans of what materials to use dependent on the planned trainees and the level of contact—for example what would be appropriate for use with hospital porters and what would be appropriate in training those responsible for assessing a person's care or health needs (for example SCIE 2011 [16]). Without exception the training materials or plans were for half day or whole day training events.

### 3.2.3. Aims of Training Materials

In some instances, the aims of the training materials were stated directly, for example ensuring that the recipients knew what to do and what policies to implement in order to comply with the law (e.g., complying with Cree 2006 [8]). Others sought to "promote equality" or reduce health inequalities (for example LGB&T Partnership 2017 [25] and European Commission 2018 [27]). Some aimed to offer practical advice to improve services (for example Taylor 2011 [14], Pride Cymru 2015 [19] Barker 2015 [20] and Mind 2016 [21]) or provided checklists for evaluating current service provision (for example Opening Doors (London) 2011 [15] and Knocker and Smith 2018 [28]). Two documents (both of these were written for the NHS) also addressed the needs of LGBT staff and how they should be employed and supported [17,28].

### 3.2.4. Specific Content

All the documents sought to give information in some manner, the aim being to influence recipients of the training to change behaviour. In some instances, this was directed towards those who worked directly with LGBT people as service users/patients as to how they should make services accessible inclusive and/or appropriate to the service user group. Others sought to influence managers in providing and evaluating training for their staff. Content included:

- Use of language—Many items included glossaries, meanings of terms, what words to use and not use, how to avoid being exclusive (for example, by assuming heterosexuality) and offered specific examples of how to ask open questions in a non-exclusive manner. For example: "which people are important in your life?" [14] or "are you in a relationship?" [23] rather than assuming a heterosexual partner. Being seen to be prepared to challenge any homophobic remarks was also essential [28].
- Visual communication—Advice was given on how to promote an LGBT friendly ambience, including the use of pictures of same sex couples in health settings (for example Ashworth 2012 [17]) and in marketing, the use of rainbow images as a sort of kite mark (for example LGBT Partnership 2016a [22]), and the provision of LGBT specific magazines in waiting areas and residential facilities (for example Pride Cymru 2015 [19]) and the prominent display of policies on discrimination [14]. One gave examples of flags used in the community [21].
- Legal and policy position—That required by law was outlined (for example the Equalities Act, 2010; the Gender Recognition Act, 2004). Additionally, the expectations of professionals such as medical professionals (the NHS charter) and social workers (the Knowledge and Skills Framework) were explained and attempts were made to show how these might translate into practice for patients/service users. The organisation's own policy statement was often explored with indications as to what should be done in order to comply.
- LGBT history—Some documents, particularly those aimed at individuals and organisations working with older people, explained what LGBT people's life experience was likely to have been. The aim here was information giving but also so that training recipients could gain some insight

into older LGBT people's life history and expectations of discrimination when receiving health or care services.

- Checklists against which organisations and individuals could assess themselves were provided, together with examples of good practice: for example, Opening Doors (London) 2011 [15] and Knocker and Smith 2018 [28]. One provided an example of a monitoring form for sexual orientation and gender identity [21].
- Intersectionality was a common feature of the documents (for example Knocker and Smith 2018 [28]). It was frequently highlighted that the LGBT community was heterogeneous and that factors such as age, race, class, economic status, education all influenced the individual and their perspective and expectations of services (for example Pugh 2010 [13], Ashworth 2012 [17] Hafford-Letchfield 2014 [18])

Nine documents specifically concerned training/education with respect to older LGBT people (although of course some of these documents could apply to non-older people, for example people with early onset dementia, or in a care home due to a physical disability rather than due to age related issues). Three documents were specifically about trans people and five specifically excluded trans people unless they identified as lesbian, gay or bisexual, as the concern of these documents was sexual orientation rather than gender identity. Finally, 11 documents stated that they were including trans people, but not always with any specific content about specific trans needs.

### 3.2.5. Pedagogical Methods

Pedagogical methods were varied. Only one document provided ready to use training materials that could be implemented alongside a facilitator's handbook [27]. Another document provided the wherewithal to produce training by indicating which pages in the pack should be turned into PowerPoint slides and which exercises to use [13]. Among the documents, 11 provided case studies for discussion or examples of best practice (both individual and organisational best practice). Some provided tips or examples, for instance, how to ask open questions. Many documents used direct quotations from LGBT people as to their experience of how non-inclusivity made them feel or their experiences of discrimination within health and social care services (for example LGBT Partnership 2016b [23]).

### 4. Discussion

#### 4.1. Main Findings

There have been no previous systematic reviews of UK education of health and social care professionals in LGBT issues or of evaluations of those training packages. Three action research projects were found which successfully addressed LGBT issues with some NHS cervical screening staff, breast cancer nurses, and private residential care home staff. The three projects in Group 1 were all participatory action research projects and these types of projects are known to have potential biases such as experimenter bias—a process where the researchers performing the research influence the results, in order to portray a certain outcome. However, participatory action research leads to co-production of outcomes with the clients so can have more insightful impact on the communities involved. In total, 16 training packages or sets of materials specifically targeting UK health and social care staff were found. Some of these training materials were from the same organisation or partnership but had different sources, were orientated towards different groups, e.g., dementia, health or health and social care, and contain different materials. The organisations were mostly LGBT-specific and so were very knowledgeable about the sector.

There are a number of position statements from UK health and care organisations, all addressing the need for training staff in health and social care [29–34]. Whilst these position statements draw attention to the inadequate state of current care, none of them offer further detail on how to improve experiences of LGBT patients and service users.

The issue for discussion here is that despite the availability of appropriate training programmes for post qualifying staff, recommendations to undertake training, best practice examples and statements of good intent, LGBT people continue to report that they are experiencing discrimination or direct prejudice from health and/or social care services. We must therefore ask the reasons as to why this might be the case.

As Peel (2007) cited in Westwood and Knocker (2016) [35] identified, "training stems from the belief that 'negative attitudes and behaviours towards lesbians and gay men can be challenged through education". A systematic review of studies evaluating how to change heterosexuals' attitudes towards homosexuals found 17 empirical studies of mixed designs [36]. Most of the studies used educational interventions and/or contact with homosexuals to change heterosexuals' prejudices. Careful analysis of the included studies listed in that systematic review suggests that interventions were effective if they involved direct interaction between the heterosexuals and a homosexual peer or lecturer that they already knew, and many of the purely educational interventions without personal interaction were ineffective. Also, emotive films such as "The Life and Times of Harvey Milk" were effective whereas a video depictive homosexual lifestyles and celebrating Gay Pride was not. Therefore, training materials incorporating more personalised attitudes and behaviour change techniques would be more likely to be effective with health and social care staff than the currently available materials.

Given the documents identified in this review and the expectation of training provision by organisations such as the Care Quality Commission (CQC), it would appear that training has not yet resulted in the desired outcomes. As we have seen, a lot of information is provided in the included documents, including legal responsibilities, organisational expectations, appropriate language to use and general awareness training concerning LGBT lives, and experience. Such training tends towards providing knowledge and, to a certain extent, related competencies rather than trainees' abilities to employ emotional intelligence and to empathise with LGBT people. Oxman et al. (1995), reviewing the effectiveness of 102 educational interventions in health settings, question whether and how professional practice can be improved concluding that there are no 'magic bullets' [37]. They also conclude that there is a need to identify the reasons for sub-optimal performance and the barriers to change. In terms of changing practice in general practice, Wensing et al. (1998) concluded that interventions which simply employed knowledge transfer were less effective than interventions that also used social influence and management support; "knowledge transfer was necessary but insufficient to achieve change in practice routines" [38].

The LGBT training sessions recommended were all for periods of half or full day. Westwood and Knocker (2016) [35], when considering training to support those working with LGBT people who have a diagnosis of dementia, suggest that such training might become simply a tick box exercise such that managers can demonstrate to inspectors that staff have undertaken relevant training. There is relatively little evidence of training being evaluated, other than for the action research studies included in Group 1, and where evaluation is mentioned as having taken place this has tended to be at the end of the day of training rather than after time has elapsed. In this respect, any evaluation is likely to have a recency effect and it would be more useful explore whether trainees attitudes change following social immersion back with their peer group.

A frequent staff response to training such as this is that it is unnecessary as "we treat everyone the same". Such an attitude demonstrates an inability to understand that treating everyone the same does not result in everyone receiving an equally good service. Person-centred treatment is cited throughout the documents as being essential, but in reality this will have little impact if staff have a poor understanding of the impact of interventions, treatments and ambience on LGBT individuals. The relevance of LGBT to general health issues (as opposed to sexual health) is not acknowledged. Similarly, there is acknowledgement within the documents that the LGBT community is not homogeneous and that a huge variety of other factors—such as race, ethnicity, class, gender, economic status, disability, etc.—all impact on the individual's experience. It is unclear whether this emphasis on intersectionality as an important aspect of the interaction between professionals and service users/patients results in changes in practice.

*4.2. Strengths and Limitations*

Strengths include the development of a protocol, extensive searches for any relevant UK studies and inclusion of studies from a variety of sources, including grey literature. The main limitations are the difficulty of developing themes in this area from a variety of different types of training materials. We acknowledge that the thematic analysis is of a basic descriptive nature. Although every effort was made to find all relevant training materials some may have been missed. However, it is unlikely that any missed training materials would have been influential in the themes developed. We acknowledge that the included papers in Group 2 are not fully published and peer reviewed papers, but educational materials are rarely, if ever, published and peer reviewed. As grey literature, developed by committed activists or charities, they may be biased towards the LGBT sector but are made by people very knowledgeable about this sector. Also, they are aimed at staff education rather than promotion of research findings. Some researcher bias may have influenced our theme selection and their development, but our thematic analysis attempts to develop themes in an unbiased way as possible.

*4.3. Implications for Policymakers*

Many health and social care staff exhibit poor behaviour towards LGBT patients and service users. This is contrary to the expectations of the NHS Constitution and positions statements of relevant organisations. For example, the Royal College of Nursing is committed to reducing health exclusion and inequalities, challenging stigma, and unlawful discrimination in health care [34]. Guidelines exist on how expected behaviour of staff, but these do not seem to have been audited regarding LGBT issues. It is unclear how the excellent policy aims will be achieved, since there have been core training standards available since 2006 [8] but these do not seem to be used widely. Better training for health and social care staff is needed.

*4.4. Implications for Research*

There has been no research evaluating how best to encourage UK health and social care professionals to deliver appropriate care to LGBT patients or clients. Large, well conducted studies are needed to establish the effectiveness and appropriateness of current curricular developments such as the new training package for staff supporting young LGBTQ people in care [39]. Training materials incorporating more evidence-based attitude and behaviour change techniques should be developed and then evaluated to ensure their effectiveness with health and social care staff in a wide variety of settings.

## 5. Conclusions

Given that there is a wealth of resources available for training health and social care staff in the UK, some of which has been available for over a decade, it seems surprising that surveys such as the Unhealthy Attitudes Survey [3] and The National LGBT Survey [1] are still finding that some LGBT patients and service users face heteronormativity, inappropriate care, and occasional overt homophobia from health and social care staff. It is also worrying that, given that the materials are produced by very knowledgeable organisations, it is even more worrying that they do not appear to be positively influencing staff attitudes and behaviours. It seems evident that either the training packs that have been developed are not being used, or that they are being used but are not sufficiently effective. Training materials incorporating more evidence-based attitude and behaviour change techniques should be developed and evaluated properly. It is important for LGBT patients and service users to know that they will not face ignorance or hostility from any health and social care staff. Until staff are properly trained and aware of the issues, this will continue to occur.

**Author Contributions:** The authors were involved as follows: Project steering committee—all; development of protocol—C.M. and C.B.; searches—C.M. and C.B.; analysis of results—R.H. and C.M.; writing paper—C.M., R.H., and S.R.; editing paper—all.

**Funding:** The study arose from an initial project undertaken during a part-funded summer placement at Anglia Ruskin University but was otherwise unfunded.

**Conflicts of Interest:** The authors declare no conflicts of interest.

**Disclosure Summary:** The authors had no financial support for this work; no financial relationships with any organisations that might have an interest in the submitted work in the previous 3 years; no other relationships or activities that could appear to have influenced the submitted work.

**Details of Ethics Approval:** Not required.

# References

1. Government Equalities Office (GEO). *National LGBT Survey Research Report*; UK Government Department for Education: Manchester, UK, 2018.
2. Hudson-Sharp, N.; Metcalf, H. *Inequality among Lesbian, Gay Bisexual and Transgender Groups in the UK: A Review of Evidence*; National Institute of Economic and Social Research: London, UK, 2016.
3. Somerville, C. *Unhealthy Attitudes*; Stonewall: London, UK, 2015.
4. Richards, C.; Gibson, S.; Jamieson, R.; Lenihan, P.; Rimes, K.; Semlyen, J. *Guidelines for Psychologists Working with Gender, Sexuality and Relationship Diversity*; British Psychological Society: Leicester, UK, 2019.
5. Government Equalities Office (GEO). *LGBT Action Plan*; UK Government: London, UK, 2018.
6. Elliott, M.N.; Kanouse, D.E.; Burkhart, Q.; Abel, G.A.; Lyratzopoulos, G.; Beckett, M.K.; Schuster, M.A.; Roland, M. Sexual minorities in England have poorer health and worse health care experiences: A national survey. *J. Gen. Intern. Med.* **2014**, *30*, 9–16. [CrossRef] [PubMed]
7. Urwin, S.; Whittaker, W. Inequalities in family practitioner use by sexual orientation: Evidence from the English General Practice Patient Survey. *BMJ Open* **2016**, *6*, e011633. [CrossRef] [PubMed]
8. Cree, W.; O'Corra, S. *Core Training Standards for Sexual Orientation, Making National Health Services Inclusive for LGB People*; UK DoH SOGIAG: London, UK, 2006.
9. Hafford-Letchfield, T.; Simpson, P.; Willis, P.B.; Almack, K. Developing inclusive residential care for older lesbian, gay, bisexual and trans (LGBT) people: An evaluation of the Care Home Challenge action research project. *Health Soc. Care Community* **2018**, *26*, e312–e320. [CrossRef] [PubMed]
10. Willis, P.; Almack, K.; Hafford-Letchfield, T.; Simpson, P.; Billings, B.; Mall, N. Turning the co-production corner: Methodological reflections from an action research project to promote LGBT inclusion in care homes for older people. *Int. J. Environ. Res. Public Health* **2018**, *15*, 695. [CrossRef] [PubMed]
11. Fish, J. Co-producing knowledge about lesbian and bisexual women in breast cancer: Messages for nursing professionals from a knowledge exchange project. *J. Res. Nurs.* **2016**, *21*, 225–239. [CrossRef]
12. Carter, L.; Hedges, L.; Congdon, C. Using diversity interventions to increase cervical screening of lesbian and bisexual women. *J. Psychol. Issues Organ. Cult.* **2013**, *3*, 133–145. [CrossRef]
13. Pugh, S.; McCartney, W.; Ryan, J. *With the Older lesbian, Gay Men, Bisexual and Transgendered People's Network In Moving Forward: Working with and for Older Lesbians, Gay Men, Bisexuals &Transgendered People: Training and Resource Pack*; University of Salford: Salford, UK, 2010.
14. Taylor, J. *Working with Older Lesbian, Gay and Bisexual People: A Guide for Care and Support Services*; Stonewall: London, UK, 2015.
15. Opening Doors (London) & Camden Age UK (2011). *Supporting older Lesbian, Gay, Bisexual & Transgender People: A Checklist for Social Care Providers*; Opening Doors (London) & Camden Age UK: London, UK.
16. Social Care Institute for Excellence. Implications for Lesbian, Gay Bisexual and Transgender (LGBT) People. 2011. Available online: www.scie.org.uk (accessed on 11 November 2019).
17. Ashworth, A. *Sexual Orientation: A Guide for the NHS*; Stonewall: London, UK, 2012.
18. Hafford-Letchfield, T. *Working with lesbian, gay, bisexual and transgender older people*; Community Care Inform: London, UK, 2014.
19. Pride Cymru & Age Cymru. *How to be LGBT+ Friendly: Guide for Care Homes*; Pride Cymru & Age Cymru: Cardiff, UK, 2015.

20. LGB&T Partnership, VODG & NCF. *Dementia Care and LGBT Communities: A Good Practice Paper*; National Care Forum: Coventry, UK, 2016.
21. Barker, M.J.; Overton, R.; Durr, P.; Rolfe, L.; Williams, H.; Walters, C.; Richards, C. *LGB&T People & Mental Health: Guidance for Services and Practitioners*; LGB&T Partnership: London, UK, 2015.
22. Mind. *Lesbian, Gay, Bisexual, Trans and Queer Good Practice Guide*; Mind Out and Mind: London, UK, 2016.
23. LGB&T Partnership. *Out Loud: LGBT Voices in Health & Social Care: A Narrative Account of LGBT Needs*; National LGB&T Partnership: London, UK, 2016.
24. LGB&T Partnership. *Best Practice in Providing Healthcare to Lesbian, Bisexual and Other Women Who Have Sex with Women*; National LGB&T Partnership: London, UK, 2016.
25. LGB&T Partnership. *Lesbian, Gay, Bisexual & Trans Health Priorities*; National LGB&T Partnership: London, UK, 2017.
26. LGB&T Partnership. *A Whole Systems Approach to Tackling Inequalities in Health for Lesbian, Gay, Bisexual & Trans (LGBT) People: A Toolkit*; National LGB&T Partnership: London, UK, 2018.
27. European Commission. *Health4LGBTI Trainer's Manual and 4 packs Reducing Health Inequalities experienced by LGBTI People: What is Your Role as a Professional?* European Commission: Brussels, Belgium, 2018.
28. Knocker, S.; Smith, A. *Safe to be Me: Meeting the Needs of Older Lesbians, Gay, Bisexual and Transgender People Using Health and Social Care Services: A Resource Pack for Professionals*; Age UK: London, UK, 2018.
29. Royal College of Nursing and Unison. Not just a friend. In *Best Practice Guidance on Healthcare for Lesbian, Gay, and Bisexual Service Users and Their Families*; Royal College of Nursing and Unison: London, UK, 2004.
30. British Medical Association. *Sexual Orientation in the Workplace*; BMA: London, UK, 2005.
31. NHS Scotland and Stonewall Scotland. *Fair for All—The Wider Challenge Good LGBT Practice in the NHS*; NHS Inclusion Project: Glasgow, UK, 2005.
32. Health Professions Council. *Equality and Diversity Scheme*; HPC: London, UK, 2007.
33. Commission for Social Care Inspection. Putting people first: Equality and diversity matters 1. In *Providing Appropriate Services for Lesbian, Gay and Bisexual and Transgender People*; CSCI: London, UK, 2008.
34. Royal College of Nursing. *Caring for Lesbian, Gay, Bisexual and Trans Clients or Patients: Guide for Nurses and Health Care Support Workers on Next of Kin Issues*; RCN: London, UK, 2016.
35. Westwood, S.; Knocker, S. One-day training courses on LGBT* awareness–are they the answer? In *Lesbian, Gay, Bisexual and Trans* Individuals Living with Dementia: Concepts, Practice and Rights*; Westwood, S., Price, E., Eds.; Abingdon: Routledge, UK, 2016; pp. 155–167.
36. Tucker, E.; Potocky-Tripodi, M. Changing heterosexuals' attitudes towards homosexuals: A systematic review of the empirical literature. *Res. Soc. Work Pract.* **2006**, *16*, 176–190. [CrossRef]
37. Oxman, A.D.; Thomson, M.A.; Davis, D.A.; Haynes, R.B. No magic bullets: A systematic review of 102 trials of interventions to improve professional practice. *Can. Med Assoc. J.* **1995**, *153*, 1423–1431.
38. Wensing, M.; Van der Weijden, T.; Grol, R. Implementing guidelines and innovations in primary care. Which interventions are effective? *Br. J. Gen. Pract.* **1998**, *40*, 991–997.
39. Collaboration for Leadership in Applied Health Research & Care (CLAHRC) East of England. Supporting LGBTQ Young People In Care: co-devising research-led training materials for multi-professional practice. Available online: https://www.clahrc-eoe.nihr.ac.uk/2017/04/supporting-lgbtq-young-people-care-co-devising-research-led-training-materials-multi-professional-practice/ (accessed on 28 October 2019).

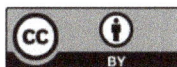

© 2019 by the authors. Licensee MDPI, Basel, Switzerland. This article is an open access article distributed under the terms and conditions of the Creative Commons Attribution (CC BY) license (http://creativecommons.org/licenses/by/4.0/).

International Journal of
*Environmental Research
and Public Health*

MDPI

Article

# Interpersonal Sensitivity and Loneliness among Chinese Gay Men: A Cross-Sectional Survey

Dongdong Jiang [1,†], Yitan Hou [1,†], Xiangfan Chen [1], Rui Wang [1], Chang Fu [2], Baojing Li [1], Lei Jin [3], Thomas Lee [4] and Xiaojun Liu [1,2,*]

[1] School of Health Sciences, Wuhan University, 115# Donghu Road, Wuhan 430071, China; dongdjiang@whu.edu.cn (D.J.); houyitan@whu.edu.cn (Y.H.); chenxiangfan@whu.edu.cn (X.C.); elvin_wang@whu.edu.cn (R.W.); baojingli@whu.edu.cn (B.L.)
[2] Global Health Institute, Wuhan University, 115# Donghu Road, Wuhan 430071, China; 2015103050006@whu.edu.cn
[3] Department of Sociology, The Chinese University of Hong Kong, RM 431, Sino Building, Shatin, Hong Kong, China; ljin@cuhk.edu.hk
[4] Office of Public Health Studies, University of Hawaii at Manoa, Honolulu, HI 96822, USA; tlee3@hawaii.edu
* Correspondence: xiaojunliu@whu.edu.cn; Tel.: +86-027-6875-9118
† These authors contributed equally to this work.

Received: 23 March 2019; Accepted: 4 June 2019; Published: 8 June 2019

**Abstract:** To understand the current status of, and factors related to interpersonal sensitivity (IS) and loneliness among Chinese gay men. The Chinese version SCL-90-R was used to evaluate the status of IS, and the short-form UCLA Loneliness scale (ULS-8) was used for assessing loneliness level. Associations between demographics and IS were examined by chi-square tests and multivariable logistic regress analysis. Linear regression was used to assess the correlations between demographic factors and IS and loneliness. Dating practices and venues were summarized by multiple responses. Gay men who screened positive IS was identified in 36%. Age ($OR_{25-29} = 8.731$, 95% CI 2.296 to 33.139), education level ($OR_{college} = 0.037$, 95% CI 0.046 to 0.911), being the only-child at home ($OR_{yes} = 4.733$, 95% CI 2.293 to 9.733), monthly income ($OR_{>7000} = 0.228$, 95% CI 0.055 to 0.944), numbers of current sexual partners ($OR_1 = 0.285$, 95% CI 0.129 to 0.629; $OR_2 = 0.109$ 95% CI 0.027 to 0.431) were related to IS. IS was also associated with a higher score of ULS-8 ($\beta = 6.903$, $p < 0.001$). Other variables associated with the score of ULS-8 included: living in a non-nuclear family ($\beta = 0.998$, $p = 0.020$), being a college student ($\beta = -1.556$, $p = 0.044$), having a higher monthly income ($\beta$ for 3000–5000 yuan = $-1.177$, $p = 0.045$; $\beta$ for over 7000 yuan = $-2.207$, $p = 0.002$), having sexual partners (all $\beta < 1$, $p < 0.001$), being the only-child ($\beta = 1.393$, $p = 0.005$). Nearly half of the sample (46.78%) reported that they looked for dating partners on the Internet or dating apps. IS and loneliness are positively correlated. Our study suggests that more humanistic care and social support should be given to Chinese gay men.

**Keywords:** Chinese gay men; interpersonal sensitivity; loneliness; influencing factors

## 1. Introduction

Previous studies suggested that chronic loneliness may cause changes in the cardiovascular, immune, and nervous systems [1]. Additionally, the experience of loneliness can induce continual pain and is highly likely to turn into mental illness or exacerbate the psychological dysfunction [2–4]. Loneliness could be manifested through external behaviors, such as aggressive behavior [5], alcohol abuse and suicidal behavior [6]. Rokach et al. found that loneliness was influenced by age and culture background [7]. Segrin et al. proved that the reach of family influence on loneliness was still evident even if when considering more distal family relationships [8]. Interpersonal relationship is the most studied variable affecting loneliness. It is suggested that poor-quality relationships and loneliness were closely related [9], while Cheng et al. also indicated that interpersonal relationships were negatively correlated with loneliness [10]. These studies suggest the possibility of a strong association between interpersonal relationships and loneliness.

There are many types of interpersonal relationships, including interpersonal attachment, interpersonal rejection, and interpersonal sensitivity (IS). As a major measuring indicator of interpersonal relationships, IS refers to the propensity to perceive and elicit criticism and rejection from others [11], which serves as the ability of adaption to social function [12]. It has been well documented that IS is positively associated with depression [13] as well as a central feature of social anxiety disorder [14]. Currently, the association between IS and loneliness is still unclear. Related studies conducted to determine the correlations of IS found that parental over-protection could increase IS [15]. Existing research also indicated that a higher level of IS was associated with the lower quality of life and greater mental distress [16,17]. However, there was no relevant research reporting on the association between IS and loneliness. Additionally, relevant studies were mainly carried out among the young adults [17], school students [9,10], and the elderly [3,16]. Little attention has been paid to sexual minorities groups.

Research about gay men and/or lesbians was mainly conducted in developed countries. Previous studies on same-sex group usually focused on the cause of homosexuality [18], social support [19], sexual behavior [20], and sexual health [21,22]. In recent years, the focus has shifted to better understanding of mental health in the gay men and/or lesbians. However, few contributions exist regarding sex-related research from developing and underdeveloped countries and regions, such as Asia and Africa, because of history, religion and policy. Very little research exists on gay men and/or lesbians in China, with most Chinese researchers focusing on the spread and prevention of sexually transmitted diseases (STDs), such as HIV infection, particularly for those men who have sex with men (MSM) [23,24]. This leaves a huge gap in the literature regarding mental health amongst Chinese gay men.

Traditional Chinese culture highly emphasizes family inheritance and reproduction. Homosexuals, especially gay men may face greater misunderstanding and prejudice [25,26]. Thus, great pressure from society and family may be imposed on Chinese gay men. In addition, Chinese society is a 'RenQing society', which means Chinese people highly value interpersonal relationships. It could be hard for Chinese gay men to cope with pressures and discrimination in personal relationship. A survey revealed only 21% of Chinese accepted gay men and/or lesbians [27]. Moreover, China currently has no specific laws or policies to guarantee gay men's legal rights [28]. Chinese gay men may confront with overwhelming social discrimination, family backlash and a lack of legal protection. We suspect that, under this social dilemma, Chinese gay men may be more likely to suffer from psychological problems [25,29], like IS and loneliness. Therefore, the purposes of this study were to investigate the reality and influencing factors of IS and loneliness among Chinese gay men, and to further examine the relationship between them.

## 2. Materials and Methods

### 2.1. Inclusion and Exclusion Criteria of Participants

Participants were recruited both online and offline. Respondents were recruited according to the following inclusion criteria: (1) males, (2) individuals who voluntarily participated in this survey, (3) self-identified as a gay. The exclusion criteria of potential participants were as follows: (1) male persons who engaged in sexual activity with other men, but did not sexually self-identified as gay, (2) bisexuals, (3) individuals who have been diagnosed with a mental illness.

*2.2. Procedures*

We utilized a cross-sectional design, and it was conducted from November to December, 2017. We informed the respondents that our survey was conducted anonymously and that the questionnaire did not include respondents' personal contact information. To increase the diversity of participants, online questionnaire links were sent by web-based live chat applications designed specifically for gay men, such as Blued, Gaypark and Aloha. We also shared survey links to online chat communities for gay men in MoMo, QQ and WeChat. Investigators from the Chinese Center for Disease Control and Prevention (China CDC) conducted the offline survey in their pilot sites. All questionnaires were filled by participants themselves. We adopted a one-on-one online anonymous chat style and self-administered questionnaire combining with a face-to-face interview in official pilot sites, receiving 298 online questionnaires and 78 offline questionnaires, respectively. We conducted a logic error-check inference on the online questionnaires and screened the consistent answers or the blank content to ensure accuracy. We excluded 9 online questionnaire responses, with an effective rate of 96.98%. The offline questionnaires completed by the national CDC were valid and met the inclusion and exclusion criteria. After data collection, we used EpiData 3.1 software (The EpiData Association, Odense, Denmark) to create the database for the offline questionnaires. To make sure the accuracy of the database, we adopted double entry and logical validation.

*2.3. Instruments*

The questionnaire used in this study consists of the following three parts:

2.3.1. Demographic Information

Questions regarding demographics include participants' age, household registration, education level, family structure, and monthly income. We also asked if the participant is the only-child in the family, and their years of self-identifying sexual orientation, number of current sexual partners and sexual orientation disclosure status.

2.3.2. Measurement of Loneliness

The short-form UCLA Loneliness scale (ULS-8) contains 8 items selected from the revised UCLA Loneliness Scale of Hays and Dimatteo [30,31]. A 4-point Likert scale (1 = never, 2 = seldom, 3 = sometimes, 4 = always) was adopted and two items were reverse-coded prior to analyses. The ULS-8 was confirmed to have good reliability and validity by many scholars [32,33].

2.3.3. Measurement of IS

The SCL-90 intends to measure symptom intensity on nine different subscales, including somatization, obsessive-compulsive, interpersonal sensitivity, depression, anxiety, hostility, phobic anxiety, paranoid ideation, psychoticism. Ninety items of the questionnaire utilize a five-point Likert scale (1 = not at all, 2 = a little bit, 3 = moderately, 4 = quite a bit, 5 = extremely) [34]. The average scores for each item were reported with higher scores of the SCL-90-R indicating greater risk for mental health issues. Many Chinese scholars have proved good reliability and validity of the Chinese version SCL-90-R [35–38]. Our study adopted the dimension of IS (contains nine items), and the participants' total average score of IS ≥ 3 was identified as positive.

*2.4. Statistical Analysis*

All analyses were conducted using SPSS software, version 22.0 (SPSS Inc., Chicago, IL, USA), with a significance level of 0.05. Chi-square tests were used to explore the bivariate relationships between demographic factors (age, household registration, educational level, etc.) and IS. Multivariable logistic regression was conducted to analyze the influencing factors between IS and demographic characteristics. And *t*-tests were employed to detect the differences between each item (including total scores) of ULS-8 loneliness scale and IS detection. The multiple linear regression model adjusted for potential confounders, including educational level, family structure, one-child or not at home, monthly income, years of identifying sexual orientation, numbers of current sexual partners, disclose sexual orientation or not. Respondents also selected all possible dating practices and venues.

*2.5. Ethical Statements*

This study was proceeded on the basis of the Declaration of Helsinki. Permission was obtained from the School of Health Science IRB of Wuhan University (MS2017024). The China CDC also reviewed this study, and offered great help in the offline data collection process.

## 3. Results

*3.1. Descriptions of Sample Characteristics*

Descriptive statistics for all measures are presented according to IS screening status in Table 1. A total of 131 participants (35.69% of the total sample) tested positive for IS. Chi-square tests illustrated that age ($\chi^2$ = 54.653, $p$ < 0.001), educational level ($\chi^2$ = 29.118, $p$ < 0.001), being the only-child at home ($\chi^2$ = 99.941, $p$ < 0.001), monthly income ($\chi^2$ = 62.552, $p$ < 0.001), current sexual partner numbers ($\chi^2$ = 69.885, $p$ < 0.001) and situation of opening sexual orientation ($\chi^2$ = 75.155, $p$ < 0.001) were significantly associated with IS.

**Table 1.** Demographic information of participants by interpersonal sensitivity status ($n$ = 367).

| Demographics | Negative | Positive | $\chi^2$ | *p*-Value |
|---|---|---|---|---|
| | *n* = 236 (64.31%) | *n* = 131 (35.69%) | | |
| Age | | | 54.653 | <0.001 |
| <20 | 56 (76.71) | 17 (23.29) | | |
| 20–24 | 54 (72.00) | 21 (28.00) | | |
| 25–29 | 31 (35.63) | 56 (64.37) | | |
| 30–34 | 29 (53.70) | 25 (46.30) | | |
| ≥35 | 66 (84.62) | 12 (15.38) | | |
| Household registration | | | 0.860 | 0.354 |
| Countryside | 107 (61.85) | 66 (38.15) | | |
| City | 129 (66.49) | 65 (33.51) | | |
| Educational level | | | 29.118 | <0.001 |
| Junior high school and lower | 12 (33.33) | 24 (66.67) | | |
| High school | 55 (53.92) | 47 (46.08) | | |
| College | 138 (73.02) | 51 (26.98) | | |
| Post-graduate and higher | 31 (77.50) | 9 (22.50) | | |
| Family structure | | | 0.035 | 0.851 |
| Nuclear family | 159 (64.63) | 87 (35.37) | | |
| Others | 77 (63.64) | 44 (36.36) | | |
| Being the only-child at home | | | 99.941 | <0.001 |
| No | 178 (86.41) | 28 (13.59) | | |
| Yes | 58 (36.02) | 103 (63.98) | | |
| Monthly income (RMB) | | | 62.552 | <0.001 |
| <3000 | 99 (70.71) | 41 (29.39) | | |
| 3001–5000 | 30 (32.61) | 62 (67.39) | | |
| 5001–7000 | 42 (67.74) | 20 (32.26) | | |
| >7000 | 65 (89.04) | 8 (10.96) | | |
| Years of identifying sexual orientation | | | 2.941 | 0.401 |
| ≤3 | 58 (57.43) | 43 (42.57) | | |
| 4–6 | 49 (66.22) | 25 (33.78) | | |
| 7–9 | 43 (66.15) | 22 (33.85) | | |
| ≥10 | 86 (67.72) | 41 (32.28) | | |

**Table 1.** *Cont.*

| Demographics | Negative | Positive | $\chi^2$ | *p*-Value |
|---|---|---|---|---|
| | **n = 236 (64.31%)** | **n = 131 (35.69%)** | | |
| Numbers of current sexual partners | | | 69.885 | <0.001 |
| 0 | 59 (40.97) | 85 (59.03) | | |
| 1 | 90 (81.08) | 21 (18.92) | | |
| 2 | 52 (94.55) | 3 (5.45) | | |
| ≥3 | 35 (61.40) | 22 (38.60) | | |
| Disclose sexual orientation or not | | | 75.155 | <0.001 |
| Confidential | 95 (45.45) | 114 (54.55) | | |
| Open | 141 (89.24) | 17 (10.76) | | |

Note: RMB 3000, 5000, and 7000 equal about USD 434, 724, and 1013, respectively using an exchange rate of USD to RMB 1 to 6.91.

### 3.2. The Factors Affecting IS

Table 2 lists the adjusted odds ratios (ORs) obtained from multivariable logistic regression model with the 95% confidence intervals (CIs). The results showed that gay men who aged 25–29 were more likely to present with IS, as compared with gay men who were under 20 years old (OR = 8.731, CI: 2.296–33.199). Gay men who had a college degree (OR = 0.204, CI: 0.046–0.911) were less likely to be detected as positive for IS, as compared with those who had junior high school education or lower. We also found that gay men who were the only-child at home had a higher risk in IS (OR = 4.733, CI: 2.293–9.773). When compared with those whose monthly incomes were less than 3000 yuan, gay men with a monthly income over 7000 yuan showed lower possibilities in having IS (OR = 0.228, CI: 0.055–0.944). In addition, gay men having at least one sexual partner were also less likely to be detected as positive for IS.

**Table 2.** Logistic regression analysis of influencing factors of interpersonal sensitivity.

| Variables (Control Group) | β | S.E | *p*-Value | OR | 95% CI for OR |
|---|---|---|---|---|---|
| Age (<20) | | | | | |
| 20–24 | 0.511 | 0.495 | 0.303 | 1.666 | 0.631–4.399 |
| 25–29 | 2.167 | 0.681 | 0.001 | 8.731 | 2.296–33.199 |
| 30–34 | 1.000 | 0.773 | 0.195 | 2.719 | 0.598–12.369 |
| ≥35 | −1.543 | 0.801 | 0.054 | 0.214 | 0.044–1.028 |
| Household registration (Countryside) | | | | | |
| City | −0.509 | 0.373 | 0.173 | 0.601 | 0.289–1.250 |
| Educational level (Junior high school and lower) | | | | | |
| High school | −1.048 | 0.692 | 0.130 | 0.351 | 0.090–1.361 |
| College | −1.588 | 0.762 | 0.037 | 0.204 | 0.046–0.911 |
| Post-graduate and higher | −1.700 | 0.949 | 0.073 | 0.183 | 0.028–1.173 |
| Family structure (Nuclear family) | | | | | |
| Others | 0.196 | 0.375 | 0.601 | 1.216 | 0.583–2.536 |
| Being the only-child at home (No) | | | | | |
| Yes | 1.555 | 0.370 | <0.001 | 4.733 | 2.293–9.773 |
| Monthly income (RMB) (<3000) | | | | | |
| 3001–5000 | 0.718 | 0.473 | 0.129 | 2.050 | 0.811–5.179 |
| 5001–7000 | −0.958 | 0.604 | 0.113 | 0.384 | 0.117–1.254 |
| >7000 | −1.479 | 0.725 | 0.041 | 0.228 | 0.055–0.944 |
| Years of identifying sexual orientation (≤3) | | | | | |
| 4–6 | −0.672 | 0.477 | 0.159 | 0.511 | 0.201–1.301 |
| 7–9 | −0.885 | 0.638 | 0.166 | 0.413 | 0.118–1.442 |
| ≥10 | −0.145 | 0.626 | 0.817 | 0.865 | 0.253–2.953 |
| Numbers of current sexual partners (0) | | | | | |
| 1 | −1.257 | 0.405 | 0.002 | 0.285 | 0.129–0.629 |
| 2 | −2.219 | 0.702 | 0.002 | 0.109 | 0.027–0.431 |
| ≥3 | 0.059 | 0.530 | 0.912 | 1.060 | 0.375–2.996 |
| Disclose sexual orientation or not (Confidential) | | | | | |
| Open | −0.778 | 0.411 | 0.058 | 0.459 | 0.205–1.027 |

Note: RMB 3000, 5000, and 7000 equal about USD 434, 724, and 1013, respectively using an exchange rate of USD to RMB 1 to 6.91; β = Coefficient; S.E = Standard Error; OR = Odds Ratio; CI = Confidence Interval.

### 3.3. Scores of Total Loneliness and Its Eight Items

Table 3 recorded that all ULS-8 items were associated with positive rate of IS. Each item's score and total scores of those who screened positive for IS were higher than those who screened negative. Total ULS-8 scores of subjects who screened negative and positive for IS in loneliness were 15.08 and 25.45, respectively.

**Table 3.** Assessment results of each item of ULS-8 ($\bar{x} \pm s$).

| Items of ULS-8 | Negative | Positive | t/t' | p-Value |
| --- | --- | --- | --- | --- |
| I lack companionship. | 2.10 ± 0.82 | 3.50 ± 0.65 | −16.70 | <0.001 |
| There is no one I can turn to. | 1.83 ± 0.87 | 2.95 ± 0.66 | −13.78 | <0.001 |
| I feel left out. | 1.92 ± 0.81 | 3.37 ± 0.67 | −17.41 | <0.001 |
| I feel isolated from others. | 1.89 ± 0.82 | 3.35 ± 0.64 | −17.64 | <0.001 |
| I am unhappy being so withdrawn. | 1.84 ± 0.82 | 3.29 ± 0.72 | −16.97 | <0.001 |
| People are around me but not with me. | 1.79 ± 0.78 | 3.34 ± 0.60 | −21.22 | <0.001 |
| I am an outgoing person. | 1.75 ± 0.93 | 2.78 ± 0.71 | −11.93 | <0.001 |
| I can find companionship when I want it. | 1.95 ± 0.94 | 2.89 ± 0.58 | −11.78 | <0.001 |
| Total scores | 15.08 ± 4.37 | 25.45 ± 3.77 | −23.83 | <0.001 |

### 3.4. Factors Associated with Loneliness, and the Relationship of Loneliness and IS

Similar with the unadjusted results showed in Table 4, the adjusted results displayed in Table 4 identified that participants who were screened positive for IS showed a higher score in loneliness ($\beta = 6.903$, S.E $= 0.537$, $p < 0.001$).

Among the demographic characteristic factors, being the only-child (yes, $\beta = 1.393$, S.E $= 0.490$, $p = 0.005$) and family structure (others, $\beta = 0.998$, S.E $= 0.425$, $p = 0.020$) were positively associated with the loneliness. Whereas the education level (college, $\beta = -1.556$, S.E $= 0.769$, $p = 0.044$), monthly income (3001–5000, $\beta = -1.177$, S.E $= 0.585$, $p = 0.045$; $> 7000$, $\beta = -2.207$, S.E $= 0.722$, $p = 0.002$), numbers of current sexual partners (1, $\beta = -2.852$, S.E $= 0.518$, $p < 0.001$; 2, $\beta = -2.075$, S.E $= 0.648$, $p = 0.001$; ≥3, $\beta = -2.276$, S.E $= 0.626$, $p < 0.001$), and situation of disclosing the sexual orientation (open, $\beta = -1.637$, S.E $= 0.505$, $p = 0.001$) were negatively associated with the loneliness.

**Table 4.** Estimated adjusted associations (β and 95% CI) of loneliness by interpersonal sensitivity and other factorss.

| Variables | Unstandardized Coefficients | | Standardized Coefficients | *t* | *p*-Value | 95% CI for β | Collinearity Statistics | |
|---|---|---|---|---|---|---|---|---|
| | β | S.E | Beta | | | | Tolerance | VIF |
| Interpersonal sensitivity (negative = control group) | 6.903 | 0.537 | 0.511 | 12.866 | <0.001 | (5.848, 7.959) | 0.528 | 1.894 |
| Education level (≤Junior high school = control group) | | | | | | | | |
| High school | −0.969 | 0.730 | −0.067 | −1.327 | 0.185 | (−2.405, 0.467) | 0.326 | 3.067 |
| College | −1.556 | 0.769 | −0.120 | −2.024 | 0.044 | (−3.068, −0.044) | 0.236 | 4.232 |
| ≥Post-graduate | −1.607 | 0.982 | −0.077 | −1.637 | 0.103 | (−3.537, 0.324) | 0.373 | 2.683 |
| Family structure (nuclear family = control group) | 0.998 | 0.425 | 0.072 | 2.346 | 0.020 | (0.161, 1.834) | 0.873 | 1.146 |
| Being the only-child at home (No = control group) | 1.393 | 0.490 | 0.107 | 2.847 | 0.005 | (0.431, 2.356) | 0.591 | 1.692 |
| Monthly income (RMB) (≤3000 = control group) | | | | | | | | |
| 3001–5000 | −1.177 | 0.585 | −0.079 | −2.014 | 0.045 | (−2.327, −0.028) | 0.543 | 1.840 |
| 5001–7000 | −0.161 | 0.658 | −0.009 | −0.245 | 0.807 | (−1.454, 1.132) | 0.575 | 1.740 |
| >7000 | −2.207 | 0.722 | −0.136 | −3.058 | 0.002 | (−3.627, −0.788) | 0.420 | 2.380 |
| Numbers of current sexual partners (0 = control group) | | | | | | | | |
| 1 | −2.852 | 0.518 | −0.202 | −5.508 | <0.001 | (−3.870, −1.834) | 0.617 | 1.621 |
| 2 | −2.075 | 0.648 | −0.114 | −3.201 | 0.001 | (−3.350, −0.800) | 0.652 | 1.534 |
| ≥3 | −2.276 | 0.626 | −0.127 | −3.638 | <0.001 | (−3.506, −1.045) | 0.680 | 1.472 |
| Disclose the sexual orientation or not (confidential = control group) | −1.637 | 0.505 | −0.125 | −3.242 | 0.001 | (−2.630, −0.644) | 0.558 | 1.791 |

$F = 42.834$, $R^2 = 0.696$, $0 < p < 0.001$

Note: RMB 3000, 5000, and 7000 equal about USD 434, 724, and 1013, respectively using an exchange rate of USD to RMB 1 to 6.91.; β = Coefficient; S.E = Standard Error

*3.5. Measurement of Dating Practices and Is Detection Amongst Chinese Gay Men*

The dating practices of Chinese gay men were presented in Table 5 and Figure 1. Almost half of the responses (46.78%) used the internet or dating apps, of whom 115 participants were screened positive in IS. Gay bar or dance hall was the second commonly selected venue. Only 6.45% of the responses indicated that their frequent meeting places were at bathhouses. The proportion of gay men who detected positive for IS in internet/dating app, gay bars/dance halls, tea house/clubs, bathhouses, parks/toilets/lawns, others was 36.86%, 47.52%, 48.75%, 44.18%, 46.55%, 38.36%, respectively.

**Table 5.** Multiple responses of dating venues or ways to Chinese gay men.

| Dating Venues or Ways | Responses | | Percent of Cases |
|---|---|---|---|
| | Total | % | |
| Internet/Dating Apps | 312 | 46.78 | 85.01 |
| Gay Bars/Dance Halls | 101 | 15.14 | 27.52 |
| Tea Houses/Clubs | 80 | 11.99 | 21.80 |
| Bathhouses | 43 | 6.45 | 11.72 |
| Parks/Toilets/Lawns | 58 | 8.70 | 15.80 |
| Others | 73 | 10.94 | 19.89 |
| Total | 667 | 100 | 181.74 |

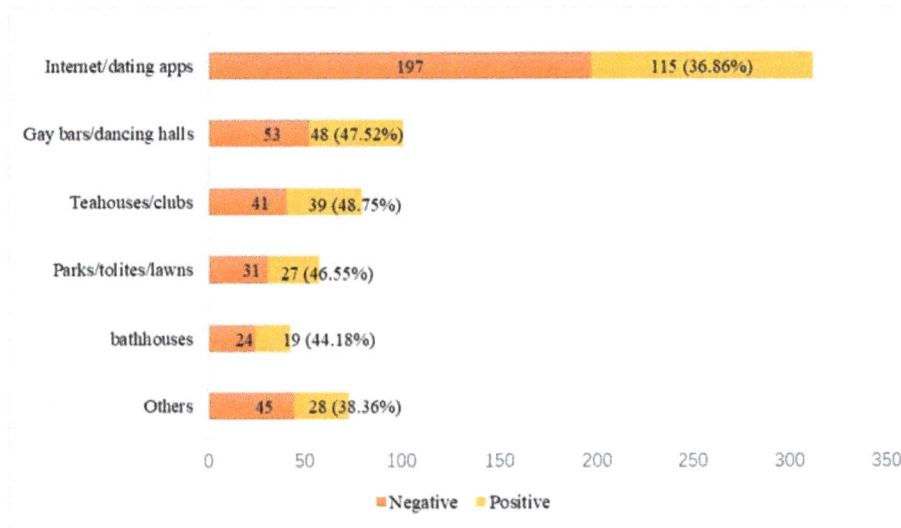

**Figure 1.** Dating venues and IS detection among Chinese gay men.

## 4. Discussion

Gay is still a sensitive topic in China, and many Chinese, especially the elderly, look down upon gay men because of the deep-rooted traditional morals that overemphasize fertility and patriarchy [29], causing mental health issues in Chinese gay men. The current research attempts to build a bridge between natural science and social science by providing a baseline understanding of mental health issues in Chinese gay men.

This study revealed that gay men who aged 25–29 had higher positive rate of IS, which is in line with a previous study that declared mood-related IS in younger ages was more common across the lifespan [39]. People aged 25–29 in China usually have joined the workforce, considering young sexual minorities have a greater risk of experiencing continuous discrimination, violence and rejection [40], and relationship at work is positively associated with mental health [41], thus gay men may be afraid of disclosing their sexual orientation which could lead to IS. Educational background is widely seen as a major indicator of measuring mental health, which was also confirmed by our study. Gay men with college degree are less likely to be detected positive in IS. Tong et al. suggested that people with junior high school education or lower have higher scores in IS than those with undergraduate degrees [42], indicating that those with higher education may have a decreased chance to be susceptible to IS. In our study, we also found that gay men in China with college level felt less lonely than those with junior high school degree or lower. It is possible that individuals with higher education are less likely to suffer from mental health problems [29]. People who receive higher education may have greater knowledge and skills to handle IS and other mental problems.

Our study reported that gay men who were the only child at home were more likely to be detected positive in IS, as compared with gay men with siblings. This may be explained by the conflicts between the pressures of Chinese traditional filial piety and disclosure of sexual orientation. Furthermore, our study indicated that gay men who were the only child at home were detected higher levels of loneliness. Fu et al. believed an obvious difference existed in mental health between twins and only-child [43]. Gay men who are the only child may face even more pressure. They may fear to disclose their sexual orientation. Ryan et al. suggested that it was risky for gay men to disclose their sexual orientation because of prejudice and family rejection [44]. In the worst cases, rejection from family may result in the risk of suicide and substance misuse [45]. Given that the one-child policy in China was implemented nearly 40 years ago, the number of people who are gay men among the only-child families is considerable. It is necessary to increase related public education to make the society, especially family members, understand and accept this vulnerable group [28]. This would reduce the pressure on gay men, allowing them to face their sexual orientation and avoid the risk of disclosing sexual orientation to their family.

In our research samples, the number of gay men who kept their sexual orientation confidential was almost 7 times than that of those who openly shared their sexual orientation. Research conducted by San Francisco State University revealed that family rejection was significantly associated with poorer health outcomes for LGB young adults [46]. It is generally agreed that disclosing sexual orientation to others is beneficial for gay men and their relationships, but most parents tend to react with shock, disappointment and shame [47]. Disclosure of sexual orientation is most likely to result in a family crisis and create rifts between family members [48]. We did not find whether open sexual orientation or keep it confidential was associated with IS, but those who wholly open their sexual orientation felt less loneliness than those who keep it confidential.

The majority (80%) dating practices of Chinese gay men are done through the Internet. We also found that gay men who detected positive in IS chose online dating, accounting for a fewer proportion than offline dating. We speculate that it is because the internet allows anonymity during the early communication process, which could make gay men reduce the possibility of rejection in making virtual friends and get comfort in the virtual world. A current study indicated that online interaction could fill a void in the offline world and play an important role in the daily lives of people who live with HIV/AIDS [49]. This situation can also apply to gay men. Therefore, it is necessary for the society to increase acceptance and build more public venues to reduce the isolation of Chinese gay men [50]. The relevant government departments, especially public health institutions, need to provide financial support and offer counseling to raise Chinese gay men's psychologically healthy level.

Previous studies confirmed that adolescents from single parent and blended families were more likely to be lonely and had worse health status compared with adolescents from intact families [51,52]. Our study demonstrated that risks of experiencing loneliness in non-nuclear family structures (one-parent, blended or united families) were higher than nuclear families among Chinese gay men. It is a common phenomenon that Chinese adults aged over 22 years old have reached the legal age of marriage, and their parents may urge them to get married as soon as possible. It could be even worse for adolescents from non-nuclear family, for they may face pressure from both their parents and brothers and/or sisters.

We found that gay men who earn over 7000 yuan had lower IS positive rate. Esmina et al. noted that socio-economic factors such as the level of income could be the predictors of psychological symptoms [53]. We assume that high income may meet gay men's material possessions and lead to a more equal identity to talk about their sexual orientation. In line with previous findings [54,55], loneliness among Chinese gay men in our study was reduced with higher personal monthly income. Our paper also revealed that IS among Chinese gay men was significantly affected by the number of current sexual partners. To some degree, gay men are always in need of finding sexual partners [56]. Sexual behaviors can increase emotional contact and alleviate insecurity [57], which may relieve their IS. In addition, sexual partners can also decrease Chinese gay men's loneliness. As our research has shown, few gay men were willing to open their sexual orientation. But sex partners can provide access to converse, which may reduce the level of loneliness.

Our study reported that gay men with positive detection in IS felt much more loneliness than those with negative detection. Butler et al. found that IS and interpersonal skills were negatively correlated [58]. Duygu et al. and Mccabe et al. also reported that IS was related to negative coping styles [59,60]. Gay men with high IS may have difficulties in dealing with interpersonal communication and give some negative feedback to people around them, because they do not want their sexual orientation to be found. Previous studies have reported that IS was a susceptible factor for depression and anxiety [13,14], while depression and anxiety were also closely related to loneliness [61]. Therefore, it is essential to encourage Chinese gay men to conduct psychological counseling when they realize the symptoms of these mental illnesses. Social media should help to increase the dissemination of sex-related knowledge and public acceptance to Chinese gay men, which could decrease the risk of STDs and protect the right of gay men [62].

As the first study addressing IS and loneliness among gay men in mainland China, the following limitations of this study should be noted. First, we used non-random sampling, including convenient sampling and snowball sampling, which may lead to some bias. Moreover, finding enough gay men samples is quite difficult, because most gay men in China are used to hiding their sexual orientation in order to avoid social discrimination, stigma and pressure from family [25,26]. In fact, many of them refused to participate, and most gay men might just ignore our online messages. Only those agreed to take part in our survey were included in the analysis. It is possible that those who completely voluntarily involved in this study may be more open-minded and with a better mental state. Therefore, the research outcome of Chinese gay men's IS and loneliness could be underestimated. Sending survey links online can limit access to certain sample populations, for only those who use the related apps and surf the Internet could join this survey. Results showed most participants were young and received a certain education. Finally, the non-response rate was not able to assess. Thus, the results of this study should be cited with caution.

## 5. Conclusions

This study first clearly reveals that IS and loneliness are positively correlated in Chinese gay men. We also found gay men who aged 25–29 and are the only-child at home could be more likely to be detected IS positive. College degree, monthly income over 7000 yuan and sexual partners are the protective factors of decreasing IS positive rates. The factors lead to loneliness for Chinese gay men are living in a non-nuclear family, being the only-child at home. While being a college student, having a higher monthly income, having sexual partners, opening sexual orientation can reduce the risk of loneliness of Chinese gay men. Results of this paper suggest that we need to be more aware of the Chinese gay men's mental health, especially their feelings of IS and loneliness. To minimize the level of IS and loneliness, actions should be taken in the care for the Chinese gay men. The government should encourage everyone, especially family members, to give more support and humanistic care to Chinese gay men. The social environment should be more open and inclusive. Psychological counseling centers should be established to provide mental health evaluation. More dating sites should be built to increase the chance to attend group communication.

**Author Contributions:** Firstly, all authors have approved the content of the submitted manuscript. Conceptualization, X.L.; Formal analysis, D.J. and X.L.; Investigation, D.J., Y.H., X.C., R.W., B.L.; Writing—original draft preparation, D.J. and Y.H.; Writing—review and editing, C.F., L.J., T.L. and X.L.; Validation, D.J., Y.H. and X.L.

**Funding:** This research received no external funding.

**Acknowledgments:** The lead agency of this study is Global Health Institute, Wuhan University. We would like to express our great appreciation to Ning Wang, a distinguished Professor from National Center for AIDS/STD Control and Prevention, China CDC, for he and his research team helped in data collection. We also wish to thank members of the Equality Research Society of Gender and Sexual Orientation, Wuhan University Medical Students' Association, for their support and collaboration in forwarding and spreading our online survey links to the potential target population. Furthermore, we gratefully acknowledge the assistance and cooperation from the research participants who contributed their time and effort for this study. The authors would also like to thank Jiayi Zhou from Wuhan University, for her assistance in regard to the English language-editing of this paper.

**Conflicts of Interest:** The authors declare no conflict of interest.

## References

1. Miller, G. Why Loneliness Is Hazardous to Your Health. *Science* **2011**, *331*, 138–140. [CrossRef] [PubMed]
2. Nilsson, B.; Lindström, U.A.; Nåden, D. Is loneliness a psychological dysfunction? A literary study of the phenomenon of loneliness. *Scand. J. Caring Sci.* **2006**, *20*, 93–101. [CrossRef] [PubMed]
3. Alpass, F.M.; Neville, S. Loneliness, health and depression in older males. *Aging Ment. Health* **2003**, *7*, 212–216. [CrossRef] [PubMed]
4. Cacioppo, J.T.; Patrick, W. *Loneliness: Human Nature and the Need for Social Connection*; Norton & Company: New York, NY, USA, 2008; pp. 71–89.
5. Chen, X.; He, Y.; DeOliveira, A.M.; Coco, A.L.; Zappulla, C.; Kaspar, V.; Schneider, B.; Valdivia, I.A.; Tse, H.C.; Desouza, A. Loneliness and social adaptation in Brazilian, Canadian, Chinese and Italian children: A multi-national comparative study. *J. Child. Psychol. Psychiatry* **2004**, *45*, 1373–1384. [CrossRef] [PubMed]
6. Liu, D.; Yu, X.; Wang, Y.; Zhang, H.; Ren, G. The impact of perception of discrimination and sense of belonging on the loneliness of the children of Chinese migrant workers: A structural equation modeling analysis. *Int. J. Ment. Health Syst.* **2014**, *8*, 52. [CrossRef] [PubMed]
7. Rokach, A. The effect of age and culture on the causes of loneliness. *Soc. Behav. Personal.* **2007**, *35*, 169–186. [CrossRef]
8. Segrin, C.; Burke, T.J.; Dunivan, M. Loneliness and poor health within families. *J. Soc. Pers. Relat.* **2012**, *29*, 597–611. [CrossRef]
9. Vanhalst, J.; Luyckx, K.; Goossens, L. Experiencing Loneliness in Adolescence: A Matter of Individual Characteristics, Negative Peer Experiences, or Both? *Soc. Dev.* **2014**, *23*, 100–118. [CrossRef]
10. Cheng, H.; Furnham, A. Personality, peer relations, and self-confidence as predictors of happiness and loneliness. *J. Adolesc.* **2002**, *25*, 327–339. [CrossRef]
11. Siegel, S.D.; Molton, I.; Penedo, F.J.; Llabre, M.M.; Kinsinger, D.P.; Traeger, L.; Schneiderman, N.; Antoni, M.H. Interpersonal sensitivity, partner support, patient–physician communication, and sexual functioning in men recovering from prostate carcinoma. *J. Pers. Assess.* **2007**, *89*, 303–309. [CrossRef] [PubMed]
12. Carney, D.R.; Harrigan, J.A. It Takes One to Know One: Interpersonal Sensitivity Is Related to Accurate Assessments of Others' Interpersonal Sensitivity. *Emotion* **2003**, *3*, 194–200. [CrossRef] [PubMed]
13. Masillo, A.; Day, F.; Laing, J.; Howes, O.; Fusar-Poli, P.; Byrne, M.; Bhattacharyya, S.; Fiori, N.P.; Girardi, P.; McGuire, P.K.; et al. Interpersonal sensitivity in the at-risk mental state for psychosis. *Psychol. Med.* **2012**, *42*, 1835–1845. [CrossRef] [PubMed]
14. Harb, G.C.; Heimberg, R.G.; Fresco, D.M.; Schneier, F.R.; Liebowitz, M.R. The psychometric properties of the Interpersonal Sensitivity Measure in social anxiety disorder. *Behav. Res. Ther.* **2002**, *40*, 961–979. [CrossRef]
15. Otani, K.; Suzuki, A.; Matsumoto, Y.; Kamata, M. Parental overprotection increases interpersonal sensitivity in healthy subjects. *Compr. Psychiatry* **2009**, *50*, 54–57. [CrossRef] [PubMed]
16. Wedgeworth, M.G.; Larocca, M.; Chaplin, W.F.; Scogin, F. The role of interpersonal sensitivity, social support, and quality of life in rural older adults. *Geriatr. Nurs.* **2017**, *38*, 22–26. [CrossRef] [PubMed]

17. Bhutani, R.; Sudhir, P.M.; Philip, M. Teasing experiences, interpersonal sensitivity, self-schema and psychological distress in youth: An exploratory study. *Psychol. Stud.* **2014**, *59*, 241–251. [CrossRef]
18. James, W.H. Two hypotheses on the causes of male homosexuality and paedophilia. *J. Biosoc. Sci.* **2006**, *38*, 745–761. [CrossRef] [PubMed]
19. Schmidt, C.K.; Miles, J.R.; Welsh, A.C. Perceived discrimination and social support: The influences on career development and college adjustment of LGBT college students. *J. Career Dev.* **2011**, *65*, 1098–1106. [CrossRef]
20. Torres, H.; Delonga, K.; Lee, S.; Gladstone, K.A.; Barrad, A.; Huckaby, S.; Koopman, C.; Gore, F.C. Socio-Contextual Factors: Moving Beyond Individual Determinants of Sexual Risk Behavior among Gay and Bisexual Adolescent Males. *J. LGBT Youth* **2013**, *10*, 173–185. [CrossRef] [PubMed]
21. Hegazi, A.; Pakianathan, M. LGBT sexual health. *Medicine* **2018**, *46*, 300–303. [CrossRef]
22. Shover, C.L.; Beymer, M.R.; Unger, E.M.; Javanbakht, M.; Bolan, R.K. Accuracy of Presumptive Gonorrhea Treatment for Gay, Bisexual, and Other Men Who Have Sex with Men: Results from a Large Sexual Health Clinic in Los Angeles, California. *LGBT Health* **2018**, *5*, 139–144. [CrossRef] [PubMed]
23. Xu, J.; Yu, H.; Tang, W.; Leuba, S.I.; Zhang, J.; Mao, X.; Wang, H.; Geng, W.; Jiang, Y.; Shang, H. The Effect of Using Geosocial Networking Apps on the HIV Incidence Rate among Men Who Have Sex With Men: Eighteen-Month Prospective Cohort Study in Shenyang, China. *J. Med. Internet Res.* **2018**, *20*, e11303. [CrossRef] [PubMed]
24. Mi, G.; Wu, Z.; Zhang, B.; Zhang, H. Survey on HIV/AIDS-related high risk behaviors among male sex workers in two cities in China. *AIDS* **2007**, *21* (Suppl. 8), S67–S72. [CrossRef] [PubMed]
25. Choi, K.H.; Steward, W.T.; Miège, P.; Hudes, E.; Gregorich, S.E. Sexual Stigma, Coping Styles, and Psychological Distress: A Longitudinal Study of Men Who Have Sex with Men in Beijing, China. *Arch. Sex. Behav.* **2016**, *45*, 1483–1491. [CrossRef] [PubMed]
26. Liu, H.; Yang, H.; Li, X.; Wang, N.; Liu, H.; Wang, B.; Zhang, L.; Wang, Q.; Stanton, B. Men Who Have Sex with Men and Human Immunodeficiency Virus/Sexually Transmitted Disease Control in China. *Sex. Transm. Dis.* **2006**, *33*, 68–76. [CrossRef]
27. The Global Divide on Homosexuality. Pew Research Center. 2013. Available online: http://www.pewglobal. org/2013/06/04/the-global-divide-on-homosexuality/ (accessed on 27 May 2014).
28. Melissa, S. A Review of Homosexuality in China: Urban Attitudes toward Homosexuality in Light of Changes in the One-Child Policy. Available online: http://works.bepress.com/melissa_sim/1/ (accessed on 4 April 2014).
29. Liu, X.; Jiang, D.; Chen, X.; Tan, A.; Hou, Y.; He, M.; Lu, Y.; Mao, Z. Mental Health Status and Associated Contributing Factors among Gay Men in China. *Int. J. Environ. Res. Public Health* **2018**, *15*, 1065. [CrossRef]
30. Hays, R.D.; Dimatteo, M.R. A short-form measure of loneliness. *J. Pers. Assess.* **1987**, *51*, 69–81. [CrossRef]
31. Russell, D.; Peplau, L.A.; Cutrona, C.E. The Revised UCLA Loneliness Scale: Concurrent and Discriminant Validity Evidence. *J. Pers. Soc. Psychol.* **1980**, *39*, 472–480. [CrossRef]
32. Zhou, L.; Li, Z.; Hu, M.; Xiao, S. Reliability and validity of ULS-8 loneliness scale in elderly samples in a rural community. *Zhong Nan Da Xue Xue Bao Yi Xue Ban* **2012**, *37*, 1124–1128. (In Chinese)
33. Wu, C.H.; Yao, G. Psychometric analysis of the short-form UCLA Loneliness Scale (ULS-8) in Taiwanese undergraduate students. *Pers. Indiv. Differ.* **2008**, *44*, 1762–1771. [CrossRef]
34. Derogatis, L.R.; Rickels, K.; Rock, A.F. The SCL-90 and the MMPI: A step in the validation of a new self-report scale. *Br. J. Psychiatry* **1976**, *128*, 280–289. [CrossRef] [PubMed]
35. Wang, Z.Y. *Symptom Checklist (SCL-90)*; Shanghai Psychiatry: Shanghai, China, 1984; pp. 68–70. (In Chinese)
36. Tan, H.; Lan, X.M.; Yu, N.L.; Yang, X.C. Reliability and validity assessment of the revised symptom checklist 90 for alopecia areata patients in China. *J. Dermatol.* **2015**, *42*, 975–980. [CrossRef] [PubMed]
37. Zhang, J.; Zhang, X. Chinese college students' scl-90 scores and their relations to the college performance. *Asian J. Psychiatry* **2013**, *6*, 134–140. [CrossRef] [PubMed]
38. Yang, H.; Gao, J.; Wang, T.; Yang, L.; Liu, Y.; Shen, Y.; Gong, J.; Dai, W.; Zhou, J.; Gu, J.; et al. Association between adverse mental health and an unhealthy lifestyle in rural-to-urban migrant workers in Shanghai. *J. Formos Med. Assoc.* **2017**, *116*, 90–98. [CrossRef] [PubMed]
39. Schaakxs, R.; Comijs, H.C.; Lamers, F.; Beekman, A.T.; Penninx, B.W. Age-related variability in the presentation of symptoms of major depressive disorder. *Psychol. Med.* **2017**, *47*, 543–552. [CrossRef] [PubMed]

40. Cohen, J.M.; Blasey, C.; Barr, T.C.; Weiss, B.J.; Newman, M.G. Anxiety and Related Disorders and Concealment in Sexual Minority Young Adults. *Behav. Ther.* **2016**, *47*, 91–101. [CrossRef] [PubMed]

41. Rydstedt, L.W.; Head, J.; Stansfeld, S.A.; Woodley, J.D. Quality of workplace social relationships and perceived health. *Psychol. Rep.* **2012**, *110*, 781–790. [CrossRef]

42. Tong, X.Y.; Qi, Y. Influence of the differences of role, gender, educational level and resident place on mental health in the relatives of stroke patients. *Chin. J. Clin. Rehabil.* **2005**, *9*, 14–15. (In Chinese)

43. Fu, Y.; Meng, H. The difference of personality, mental health and family environment between twin child and only child in China. *Eur. Psychiat.* **2012**, *27*, 1. [CrossRef]

44. Ryan, C.; Huebner, D.; Diaz, R.M.; Sanchez, J. Family Rejection as a Predictor of Negative Health Outcomes in White and Latino Lesbian, Gay, and Bisexual Young Adults. *Pediatrics* **2009**, *123*, 346–352. [CrossRef]

45. Klein, A.; Golub, S.A. Family Rejection as a Predictor of Suicide Attempts and Substance Misuse among Transgender and Gender Nonconforming Adults. *LGBT Health* **2016**, *3*, 193–199. [CrossRef] [PubMed]

46. San Francisco State University. Family Rejection of Lesbian, Gay and Bisexual Children Linked to Poor Health in Childhood. ScienceDaily. Available online: www.sciencedaily.com/releases/2008/12/081229080901.htm (accessed on 31 December 2008).

47. Lasala, M.C. Lesbians, gay men, and their parents: Family therapy for the coming-out crisis. *Fam. Process.* **2000**, *39*, 67–81. [CrossRef] [PubMed]

48. Mitrani, V.B.; DeSantis, J.P.; Mccabe, B.E.; Deleon, D.A.; Gattamorta, K.A.; Leblanc, N.M. The Impact of Parental Reaction to Sexual Orientation on Depressive Symptoms and Sexual Risk Behavior among Hispanic Men Who Have Sex with Men. *Arch. Psychiatr. Nurs.* **2017**, *31*, 352–358. [CrossRef] [PubMed]

49. Han, X.; Li, B.; Qu, J.; Zhu, Q. Weibo friends with benefits for people live with HIV/AIDS? The implications of Weibo use for enacted social support, perceived social support and health outcomes. *Soc. Sci. Med.* **2018**, *211*, 157–163. [CrossRef] [PubMed]

50. Elizabeth, M.C.; Bálint, N.; Bernie, H.; Aaron, K.; Antonia, C.; Michelle, B. "Everybody Puts Their Whole Life on Facebook": Identity Management and the Online Social Networks of LGBTQ Youth. *Int. J. Environ. Res. Public Health* **2018**, *15*, 1078.

51. AntognoliToland, P.L. Parent-child relationship, family structure, and loneliness among adolescents. *Adolesc. Fam. Health* **2001**, *2*, 20–26.

52. Stickley, A.; Koyanagi, A.; Koposov, R.; Blatný, M.; Hrdlička, M.; Schwab-Stone, M.; Ruchkin, V. Loneliness and its association with psychological and somatic health problems among Czech, Russian and U.S. adolescents. *BMC Psychiatry* **2016**, *16*, 1–11. [CrossRef]

53. Avdibegović, E.; Hasanović, M.; Hodzić, M.; Selimbašić, Z. Psychological symptoms among workers employed in companies undergoing privatization in postwar Bosnia and Herzegovina. *Coll. Antropol.* **2011**, *35*, 993–999.

54. Wang, G.; Zhang, X.; Wang, K.; Li, Y.; Shen, Q.; Ge, X.; Hang, W. Loneliness among the rural older people in Anhui, China: Prevalence and associated factors. *Int. J. Geriatr. Psychiatry* **2011**, *26*, 1162–1168. [CrossRef]

55. Hacihasanoglu, R.; Yildirim, A.; Karakurt, P. Loneliness in elderly individuals, level of dependence in activities of daily living (ADL) and influential factors. *Arch. Gerontol. Geriatr.* **2012**, *54*, 61–66. [CrossRef]

56. Bauermeister, J.A.; Leslie-Santana, M.; Johns, M.M.; Pingel, E.; Eisenberg, A. Mr. Right and Mr. Right Now: Romantic and Casual Partner-Seeking Online Among Young Men Who Have Sex with Men. *AIDS Behav.* **2011**, *15*, 261–272. [CrossRef] [PubMed]

57. Meston, C.M.; Buss, D.M. Why humans have sex. *Arch. Sex. Behav.* **2007**, *36*, 477–507. [CrossRef] [PubMed]

58. Butler, J.C.; Doherty, M.S.; Potter, R.M. Social antecedents and consequences of interpersonal rejection sensitivity. *Pers. Indiv. Differ.* **2007**, *43*, 1376–1385. [CrossRef]

59. Hiçdurmaz, D.; Öz, F. Interpersonal sensitivity, coping ways and automatic thoughts of nursing students before and after a cognitive-behavioral group counseling program. *Nurse Educ. Today* **2016**, *36*, 152–158. [CrossRef] [PubMed]

60. Mccabe, R.E.; Blankstein, K.R.; Mills, J.S. Interpersonal Sensitivity and Social Problem-Solving: Relations with Academic and Social Self-Esteem, Depressive Symptoms, and Academic Performance. *Cogn. Ther. Res.* **1999**, *23*, 587–604. [CrossRef]

61. Lim, M.H.; Rodebaugh, T.L.; Zyphur, M.J.; Gleeson, J.F. Loneliness over time: The crucial role of social anxiety. *J. Abnorm. Psychol.* **2016**, *125*, 620–630. [CrossRef]

62. Chen, X.; Elliott, A.L.; Wang, S. Cross-country Association of Press Freedom and LGBT freedom with prevalence of persons living with HIV: Implication for global strategy against HIV/AIDS. *Glob. Health Res. Policy* **2018**, *3*, 6. [CrossRef]

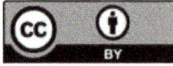

© 2019 by the authors. Licensee MDPI, Basel, Switzerland. This article is an open access article distributed under the terms and conditions of the Creative Commons Attribution (CC BY) license (http://creativecommons.org/licenses/by/4.0/).

International Journal of
*Environmental Research and Public Health*

MDPI

*Article*

# Romantic Attraction and Substance Use in 15-Year-Old Adolescents from Eight European Countries

András Költő [1,2,*], Alina Cosma [3], Honor Young [4], Nathalie Moreau [5], Daryna Pavlova [6], Riki Tesler [7], Einar B. Thorsteinsson [8], Alessio Vieno [9], Elizabeth M. Saewyc [10] and Saoirse Nic Gabhainn [1]

[1]  Health Promotion Research Centre, School of Health Sciences, National University of Ireland Galway, University Road, H91 TK33 Galway, Ireland
[2]  Institute of Psychology, ELTE Eötvös Loránd University, Izabella utca 46, 1064 Budapest, Hungary
[3]  Department of Interdisciplinary Social Science, Faculty of Social and Behavioural Sciences, Utrecht University, P.O. Box 80.140, 3508 TC Utrecht, The Netherlands
[4]  Centre for the Development and Evaluation of Complex Interventions for Public Health Improvement, Cardiff School of Social Sciences, Cardiff University, 1–3 Museum Place, CF10 3BD Cardiff, UK
[5]  Independent Researcher, 1180 Brussels, Belgium
[6]  Department for Monitoring and Evaluation of Social Projects, Ukrainian Institute for Social Research after Oleksandr Yaremenko, 26 Panasa Myrnogo Str., Of. 211, 01011 Kyiv, Ukraine
[7]  The Department of Health Systems Management, Ariel University, Ramat HaGolan St 65, 40700 Ariel, Israel
[8]  School of Psychology, Faculty of Medicine and Health, University of New England, Armidale, NSW 2351, Australia
[9]  Department of Developmental and Social Psychology, University of Padova, 8 via Venezia, 35131 Padova, Italy
[10] Stigma and Resilience Among Vulnerable Youth Centre (SARAVYC), School of Nursing, University of British Columbia, T222-2211 Wesbrook Mall, Vancouver, BC V6T 2B5, Canada
*   Correspondence: andras.kolto@nuigalway.ie

Received: 30 July 2019; Accepted: 19 August 2019; Published: 23 August 2019

**Abstract:** Sexual minority youth are at higher risk of substance use than heterosexual youth. However, most evidence in this area is from North America, and it is unclear whether the findings can be generalized to other cultures and countries. In this investigation, we used data from the 2014 Health Behaviour in School-aged Children (HBSC) study to compare substance use in same- and both-gender attracted 15-year-old adolescents from eight European countries ($n = 14{,}545$) to that of their peers who reported opposite-gender attraction or have not been romantically attracted to anyone. Both-gender attracted, and to a lesser extent, same-gender attracted adolescents were significantly more likely to smoke cigarettes, consume alcohol, get drunk and use cannabis, or be involved in multiple substance use in the last 30 days compared to their opposite-gender attracted peers. Those adolescents who have not been in love had significantly lower odds for substance use than all other youth. The pattern of results remained the same after adjusting for country, gender and family affluence. These findings are compatible with the minority stress and romantic stress theories. They suggest that sexual minority stigma (and love on its own) may contribute to higher substance use among adolescents in European countries.

**Keywords:** adolescents; romantic attraction; same-gender attraction; both-gender attraction; sexual minority youth; substance use; alcohol consumption; drunkenness; tobacco; cannabis; HBSC

## 1. Introduction

Many young people who identify as Lesbian, Gay, Bisexual (LGB), other sexual or gender minority (for example Queer, Transgender or Intersex), or report being attracted to same- or both-gender partners, have poorer health than their peers who identify as heterosexual, cisgender or as exclusively attracted to members of the opposite gender [1,2]. The studies show a large variation in the use of (biological) sex or (socially constructed) gender. They also employ various sexual identity terms or classify youth based on other dimensions of sexual orientation, such as gender of sexual or love partner(s). In this study, we use the term 'gender' to describe whether the respondents identified themselves as boys or girls. The 'sexual minority youth' (SMY) term is used, as this is the most inclusive, unless we refer to studies that used more specific terminology (such as LGB).

Extensive research indicates that SMY are more likely to engage in substance use [3,4]. However, the validity of the evidence is limited by the fact that most investigations have been conducted in North America. There are just a few sporadic observations from other countries, and cross-cultural comparisons are largely missing. This study aimed to describe and compare substance use frequency across patterns of romantic attraction, in nationally representative samples of 15-year-old adolescents from eight European countries and regions with various geographical location, history, and levels of tolerance towards sexual minorities.

### 1.1. Tobacco Use

While LGB youths appear to start smoking at a later age than the general population, compared to their heterosexual peers they are significantly more likely to use various (and multiple) tobacco products, as well as to report smoking in the past month, or being current smokers [5–8]. Smoking patterns were influenced by sexual identity, gender, race or ethnicity, and their interactions [8–10]. In some studies, significant differences were found between sexual minority girls and boys, or bisexual youths and those identifying as lesbian or gay. Such findings indicate the importance of mapping the relative risk of SMY boys and girls separately.

Cross-sectional and longitudinal studies have concluded that psychological distress in SMY was associated with smoking [11,12]. Sexual minority adolescents were significantly more likely to report smoking in the past year compared to heterosexual youth in a large-sample U.S. national prospective cohort study, after adjusting for gender, age, race/ethnicity, and family income. However, SMY youth living in states where the social environment was less stigmatizing toward LGB people had a significantly lower relative risk for smoking than those who lived in a state imposing stronger structural stigma. The stigmatizing environment did not have a differential effect on heterosexual youth [13]. This indicates that besides micro-environmental influences, macro-level societal indicators may also be associated with substance use in SMY. Therefore, it is important to investigate cross-cultural variations in the associations between sexual minority status and substance use or other risk behaviors, ideally including sexual minority young people from various countries and cultures.

### 1.2. Alcohol Consumption and Drunkenness

Sexual minority adolescents are more likely than heterosexual youth to drink alcohol and get drunk [3,14]. LGB young people report earlier alcohol initiation and sharper drinking trajectories into adulthood than heterosexual youth [15]. The experience of sexual minority belonging in adolescence may shape alcohol-related behaviors in later age [16]. Some argue that consuming any amount of alcohol and excessive drinking (i.e., heavy episodic drinking) may diverge, for instance for cultural reasons [17], therefore they should be examined separately.

While there was a general decline in adolescent alcohol use in the United States and Europe over the last decade [18], the alcohol-related disparities between heterosexual and SMY have remained stable or even widened [19]. More recent findings demonstrate that pluri-sexual males (having both-gender sexual partners or identifying as bisexual) have higher risk for earlier onset and persistent use of alcohol than those with monosexual behavior (having exclusively opposite- or same-gender partners) or identifying as heterosexual or gay [20].

### 1.3. Cannabis Use

SMY are at an increased risk of cannabis use [21–23]. A systematic review of Canadian studies revealed that cannabis use is consistently higher in SMY than in heterosexual respondents, with sexual minority young men and bisexual youth having greater risk than young women or those identifying as lesbian or gay [24]. Furthermore, trends observed in cannabis use in SMY are similar to those in alcohol and tobacco use. Between 1999 and 2013, a population-based US study found that while cannabis use had decreased overall, the disparities between some SMY subgroups (in lesbian and bisexual females) and their heterosexual counterparts remained stable [25].

Potential explanatory pathways for the association between SMY status and cannabis use are comparable to those of alcohol and tobacco use. Internalized homophobia and community connectedness were both positively associated with cannabis use in LGB young people [26]. These effects may be attributed to minority stress, and greater community connectedness may be associated with greater conformity to social norms within the LGB community that are more permissive toward substance use.

### 1.4. Minority and Romantic Stress: Explanation for Different Types and Combinations of Substance Use?

In addition to the single substance studies cited above, there is a large corpus of evidence on multiple or poly-substance use and the association with mental health outcomes in SMY. These studies examine alcohol, tobacco and cannabis or other drugs [20,25,27], alcohol and cigarettes [28], drugs and alcohol [29,30], tobacco, methamphetamine use and suicidal ideation [31], or meta-analyses where different types of substance use were pooled [3,4].

In a systematic review of 18 studies [3], it was found that LGB youth were around three times more likely, compared to their heterosexual peers, to be involved in any type of substance use. The effects were larger in bisexual compared to lesbian/gay young people, and in females compared to males. When one large-effect size study was removed from the pool, no significant differences were observed between studies conducted in the United States or elsewhere, which suggests that the disparity may be universal across different countries and cultures. Another systematic review of 12 studies revealed that the strongest risk factors for substance use (smoking cigarettes, consuming alcohol, cannabis, cocaine and ecstasy) in SMY were LGB-related or general victimization, lack of supportive environments, psychological stress, internalizing/externalizing behaviors, negative responses to coming out, and housing status [4].

The disparities between SMY and heterosexual youth's substance use can be explained by the minority stress theory which argues that experiences of discrimination, victimization, and stigma are prevalent due to a pervasive homophobic culture [32,33]. The existing literature points out that sexual orientation-based bullying and harassment at school contributes to SMY disparities in all forms of substance use. Hatzenbuehler's [34] extension of minority stress suggests that due to stigmatization, sexual (and gender) minority individuals experience chronic stress, which in the long term may lead to deficits in emotion regulation and negative affect. To cope with these, sexual minority individuals may turn to alcohol (and other substance) use [4,12,35].

Consistent with the ecological framework provided by minority stress theory, it is important to examine factors that may predict substance use, particularly societal attitudes and policies regarding sexual minority communities and individuals. Although attitudes toward sexual minorities also are changing in several parts of the world, there are still many countries with strong anti-LGB policies or cultural norms. The negative effects of stigma and discrimination on sexual minority individuals' health, including minority stress, depression, and fear of seeking help are well-documented. However, most of the evidence is from North America [36]. The question remains whether these findings can be generalized to other countries and cultures (i.e., in the European region), given the large variation in societal attitudes, tolerance and acceptance towards gender and sexual minority individuals and issues within Europe [37,38].

The countries involved in our study represent large variation both geographically (from Iceland to North Macedonia), historically (from traditionally Capitalist countries such as Belgium, England, France and Switzerland to post-Communist countries as Bulgaria and Hungary), and in terms of tolerance towards sexual minorities. The latter can be demonstrated by the International Lesbian Gay, Bisexual, Trans and Intersex Association's (https://www.ilga-europe.org/rainboweurope) Rainbow Score, a composite measure reflecting the legal situation and acceptance of gender and sexual minorities in different countries, ranging from 0 (gross violations of human rights) to 100 (full respect of human rights, full equality between sexual and gender minority and heterosexual and cisgender individuals). In the eight countries or regions involved in the present study, the Rainbow Score in 2014, when the data were collected, ranged from 13% in North Macedonia to 82% in the United Kingdom [39].

In a nine-country investigation of substance use in 16–35-year-old LGB and heterosexual individuals, Demant and colleagues [40] argue that cross-cultural comparisons in this area are important because cultural norms and attitudes towards both substances and sexual minority identities show considerable variations across countries with liberal versus more conservative policies and regulations. Until such studies are replicated, we cannot conclude that higher frequency of substance use in SMY is a universal phenomenon. Therefore, in this study we aimed to explore the associations between SMY and different substance use behaviors across different European countries and regions.

Another potential explanation, partly overlapping with the minority stress model, is that love, irrespective of the gender of the partner(s) with whom a young person is in love with, may be associated with stress on its own. Indeed, a cross-cultural study conducted in 17 countries found that adolescents experienced stress related the romantic relationships, especially in Mid- and South-European countries. Overall, around 20% of the adolescents used externalizing coping strategies, such as alcohol and drug use, to cope with these stressors [41]. This prompts the notion that maybe not just same-or both-gender attracted adolescents may be at elevated risk of substance use, but *anyone* who are in love may be at higher risk than those who are not being in love.

*1.5. Dimensions of Sexual Orientation*

The number of young people with same-gender attractions far exceeds those who engage in same-gender sexual behavior or who identify as lesbian, gay or bisexual. This is consistent with findings from large-scale nationally representative studies with adults, where the proportion of individuals with same- or both-gender attraction was much larger than those who identified as LGB [42]. A population-based study in the United Kingdom demonstrated substantial diversity between identity, behavior and attraction in sexual minority adults [43]. Studies have also varied on how they categorized SMY (identity, behavior or attraction), and whether they separated mono- and plurisexual youth. In one study, respondents as young as 9–10 years old were asked whether they consider themselves to be lesbian, gay or bisexual [44]. While acknowledging the importance of all dimensions of sexual orientation, we argue that asking whether adolescents are attracted to girls, boys or both-gender partners may be easier for young people to answer, be more accurate, and can be used to subsequently categorize SMY based on same- or both-gender romantic attraction. This approach may be developmentally more appropriate than employing the identity labels of sexual orientation [45]. Relying on sexual identity as a classifier for SMY may 'mask' or eliminate those young people who are still exploring their sexuality, have same- or both-gender attraction, but do not identify as LGB.

Health disparities in SMY can be found when respondents are classified by same- or both-gender romantic attraction. In a nationally representative study of U.S. adolescents [46], boys romantically attracted to both-gender partners smoked more cigarettes, were more likely to have consumed alcohol while being alone, to have been drunk, and to use illegal drugs (including cannabis) compared to those who had been attracted to the opposite gender. Girls attracted to their same- or both-gender peers were more likely to smoke cigarettes, have been drunk, and have used cannabis or other drugs compared to opposite-gender attracted females. However, their conclusion was that SMY or certain subgroups within this category had a greater risk of substance use than heterosexually identifying or exclusively opposite-gender attracted youth. Therefore, in the current study we anticipate finding significant gender differences in the associations being investigated.

Another U.S. adolescent study demonstrated that sexual identity (i.e., defining oneself as LGB) and sexual behavior (i.e., having exclusively same- or both-gender partners) explained unique and significant sources of variability in tobacco and methamphetamine use and suicidal ideation [31]. In another investigation, same- and both-sex romantic attraction and romantic relationship status were associated with various risk behaviors such as the number of cigarettes smoked in the past month, being drunk in the past year, and cannabis or other drug use [46]. When adolescents were categorized into SMY based not on their identity but either on a history of same-gender attraction or sexual behavior, a sharper increase was observed in their cigarette and cannabis use than in those adolescents with heterosexual identity (or opposite-gender attraction or behavior) [47]. These findings demonstrate that apart from identity, other dimensions of sexual orientation (i.e., behavior or romantic attraction) may also be associated with higher incidence of risk behaviors.

Based on these considerations and empirical evidence, in the present study, romantic attraction will be used to classify sexual minority adolescents and separate adolescents reporting being in love with any gender partners from those who have not been in love.

### 1.6. Aims of the Present Study

We aimed to describe and compare substance use frequency across patterns of romantic attraction, in nationally representative samples of 15-year-old adolescents from eight European countries and regions.

Romantic attraction was operationalized by an item on whether the respondent had already been in love, and if yes, whether the partner who they felt love for was a girl(s), boy(s), or both- a boy and a girl [45]. This approach is in line with the notion that romantic attraction and love are conditional to each other [48]. The responses, combined with the gender of the respondent, enabled us to categorize opposite-, same-, or both-gender attracted respondents, those who have not been attracted to anyone, or who have not responded to the love item. Contrary to most studies that concentrate on those with any type of attraction or sexual identity, we also measured the prevalence of substance use in those who reported not having been in love or who did not respond to this item. Based on previous findings from the literature, we hypothesized that same- and both-gender attracted young people will have significantly higher odds of cigarette smoking, drinking alcohol, being drunk, and cannabis use than their opposite-gender attracted peers or those who reported not having been in love. Our other hypothesis is that those young people who report being in love (with any gender partners) will have higher odds of substance use than those who have not been in love. We anticipated that despite cultural differences in the prevalence of these risk behaviors, higher incidence of substance use will be found in same- and both-gender attracted young people (and those who report being in love) across different countries and regions. Given the differences between sexual minority boys and girls found in many studies, analyses were stratified for gender.

An additional aim was to assess involvement of SMY in multiple risk behaviors (any two or all three of cigarette smoking, alcohol consumption, or cannabis use in the last 30 days). We hypothesized that youth reporting attraction to same- or both-gender partners will be more likely to be involved in using more than one type of substances than those who are exclusively attracted to opposite-gender partners or reported not having been in love.

## 2. Materials and Methods

Data was collected within the 2014 survey round of the Health Behaviour in School-aged Children (HBSC) study, a World Health Organization collaborative cross-national epidemiological study. The HBSC study investigates health-related behaviors and related psychosocial contextual factors in nationally representative samples of 11-, 13- and 15-year-old school children, in four-year study cycles across more than forty countries, covering the geographical areas of Europe, North America, and former Soviet Republics. There were 42 countries that collected data as part of the HBSC international survey in 2014. Out of these, data from eight countries and regions are featured in this paper. A detailed description of HBSC methodology is provided by Inchley et al. [49] and Currie et al. [50]. In HBSC, a survey questionnaire is employed containing (1) items administered in each participating countries in the same format ('mandatory' items), (2) items following the same format, but the national team decides if they will be administered in the questionnaire ('optional' items) and (3) items that are relevant for the health of young people in the given country ('national' items). In the present study, substance use was monitored using mandatory items, while romantic attraction was measured by an optional item. As such, the measure of romantic attraction was included in the national surveys if the research team in the given country or region considered investigating the health of sexual minority youth substantially important. The methodology used by HBSC is described at http://www.hbsc.org/methods/index.html, and details on data access are provided at https://www.uib.no/en/hbscdata.

*2.1. Sample*

Schoolchildren in the 15-year-old age group from eight countries and regions (French Belgium, Bulgaria, Switzerland, England, France, Hungary, Iceland, and North Macedonia) where the national HBSC Research Team included the measure on romantic attraction (see below, Section 2.2) in their national survey. The raw sample contained data from 14,545 respondents (mean age: 15.55 years, $SD = 0.33$, range: 14.58–16.50, percentage girls: 49.8). Listwise deletion was employed (for all predictor, outcome and sociodemographic control variables) to determine the number of respondents featured in the final statistical models. There were 13,504 respondents (92.8%) in the cigarette smoking model; 13,440 respondents (92.4%) in the alcohol consumption model; 13,471 respondents (92.6%) in the drunkenness model; 12,109 respondents (83.3%) in the cannabis use model; and 13,580 respondents (93.4%) in the multiple substance use model. The characteristics of the sample are displayed in Table 1. Since the most respondents were featured in the multiple substance use model, the distribution of the Love item and sociodemographic variables are given for this headcount ($n = 13,580$).

*2.2. Ethical Considerations*

In each country, the HBSC research team sought ethical approval from local or national higher education or health authorities: Boards of School Networks of the Brussel-Wallonia Federation (French Belgium), Ministry of Education and Science (Bulgaria), University of Lausanne, Cantonal Commission for Ethics for the Research on Human Beings (Switzerland), University of Hertfordshire, Ethics Committee for Studies Involving Human Participants (England), Ministry of Education and the French National Commission of Computer Science and Freedom (France), Scientific and Research Ethics Committee of the Medical Research Council (Hungary), Icelandic Data Committee (Iceland), and the Ministry for Education and Ministry for Health (North Macedonia). In the eight countries and regions involved in this study, pupils (as well as their parents and the schools) gave informed consent to participate in the study. Before administering the questionnaire, respondents were instructed that responding to any question or the whole questionnaire was entirely voluntary, and they could withdraw at any time. The questionnaires were anonymous and treated as confidential. Our research procedures are following the WHO Standards and operational guidance for ethics review of health-related research with human participants (https://www.who.int/ethics/research/en/).

Table 1. Characteristics of the sample, overall and by romantic attraction (n = 13,580).

| | OVERALL | | Opposite-Gender Love | | Same-Gender Love | | Both-Gender Love | | Not in Love | | Not Responding | | Assoc. [2] |
|---|---|---|---|---|---|---|---|---|---|---|---|---|---|
| | n | % | n | % (RA) [1] | n | % (RA) | n | % (RA) | n | % (RA) | n | % (RA) | |
| **Love** | | | | | | | | | | | | | |
| Opposite-sex love | 11,024 | 81.2 | | | | | | | | | | | |
| Same-sex love | 219 | 1.6 | | | | | | | | | | | |
| Both-sex love | 248 | 1.8 | | | | | | | | | | | |
| Not in love | 1756 | 12.9 | | | | | | | | | | | |
| Not responding | 333 | 2.5 | | | | | | | | | | | |
| **Country** | | | | | | | | | | | | | p < 0.001, V = 0.173 |
| Belgium (French) | 1779 | 13.1 | 1464 | 13.3 | 27 | 12.3 | 25 | 10.1 | 222 | 12.6 | 41 | 12.3 | |
| Bulgaria | 1542 | 11.4 | 1306 | 11.8 | 61 | 27.9 | 38 | 15.3 | 115 | 6.5 | 22 | 6.6 | |
| Switzerland | 1692 | 12.5 | 1503 | 13.6 | 9 | 4.1 | 21 | 8.5 | 149 | 8.5 | 10 | 3.0 | |
| England | 1442 | 10.6 | 748 | 6.8 | 23 | 10.5 | 37 | 14.9 | 578 | 32.9 | 56 | 16.8 | |
| France | 1658 | 12.2 | 1365 | 12.4 | 34 | 15.5 | 33 | 13.3 | 207 | 11.8 | 19 | 5.7 | |
| Hungary | 1085 | 8.0 | 853 | 7.7 | 4 | 1.8 | 16 | 6.5 | 129 | 7.3 | 83 | 24.9 | |
| Iceland | 2980 | 21.9 | 2707 | 24.6 | 49 | 22.4 | 57 | 23.0 | 151 | 8.6 | 16 | 4.8 | |
| North Macedonia | 1402 | 10.3 | 1078 | 9.8 | 12 | 5.5 | 21 | 8.5 | 205 | 11.7 | 86 | 25.8 | |
| **Gender** | | | | | | | | | | | | | p < 0.001, V = 0.080 |
| Boy | 6732 | 49.6 | 5622 | 51.0 | 96 | 43.8 | 70 | 28.2 | 762 | 43.4 | 182 | 54.7 | |
| Girl | 6848 | 50.4 | 5402 | 49.0 | 123 | 56.2 | 178 | 71.8 | 994 | 56.6 | 151 | 45.3 | |
| **Relative FAS** | | | | | | | | | | | | | p < 0.001, V = 0.037 |
| Lowest 20 percent | 2828 | 20.8 | 2217 | 20.1 | 67 | 30.6 | 63 | 25.4 | 393 | 22.4 | 88 | 26.4 | |
| Medium 60 percent | 8127 | 59.8 | 6618 | 60.0 | 113 | 51.6 | 145 | 58.5 | 1070 | 60.9 | 181 | 54.4 | |
| Highest 20 percent | 2625 | 19.3 | 2189 | 19.9 | 39 | 17.8 | 40 | 16.1 | 293 | 16.7 | 64 | 19.2 | |

[1] % (RA): Proportion within the given romantic attraction category. [2] Assoc.: Association between the given variable and romantic attraction.

*2.3. Measures*

*Romantic attraction* was measured by a standardized item "Have you ever been in love with … ", response options being "A girl or girls", "A boy or boys", "Both girls and boys", "I have never been in love". Girls who reported being in love with boys, and boys who reported being in love with girls were categorized into the opposite-gender love group, while girls who reported being in love with girls and boys reporting love for boys were categorized into the same-gender love group. Respondents reporting being in love with both girls and boys were categorized into the both-gender love group. A fourth group consisted of those respondents reporting having never been in love, while the fifth category included those who did not answer the item. The development and basic descriptive statistics for the question are reported elsewhere [45].

*Substance use:* Four standardized items were used to measure the frequency of substance use in the last 30 days [50,51]. "On how may days (if any) have you smoked cigarettes (tobacco) in the last 30 days?", "On how many days (if any) have you drunk alcohol in the last 30 days?", "Have you ever taken cannabis (hashish, grass, pot) in the last 30 days?" with response options being "Never", "1–2 days", "3–5 days", "6–9 days", "10–19 days", "20–29 days", "30 days (or more)". "Have you ever had so much alcohol that you were really drunk in the last 30 days?", with response options being "Never", "Yes, once", "Yes, 2–3 times", "Yes, 4–10 times", "Yes, more than 10 times". In line with methodological recommendations and reporting practice of the European School Survey Project on Alcohol and Other Drugs (ESPAD) for fifteen-year-olds [51], the four substance use variables were dichotomized into reporting never having used the given substance (never being drunk) *versus* ever. We created a dichotomous variable to express multiple substance use. If the respondent reported any two of cigarette smoking, alcohol consumption and cannabis use in the last 30 days, they were categorized into ever being involved in multiple substance use.

*Gender and age:* Respondents were asked to indicate whether they are a boy or a girl, as well as to report their date of birth (month/year).

*Socioeconomic status* was measured by the Family Affluence Scale (FAS), a six-item composite measure developed by the HBSC network [52–54]. FAS measures material family wealth as an indicator of socio-economic position. It asks about concrete possessions (i.e., number of family cars; computers), characteristics of the home (i.e., having a bedroom for one own; number of bathrooms; owning a dishwasher), and the number of family holidays in the last year. The scores are summed up. The absolute Family Affluence Scale scores (0 = lowest affluence, 13 = highest affluence) were then transformed into a ridit-based trichotomous variable separating children from families within the lowest 20%, the medium 60%, and the highest 20% affluence categories [49].

*2.4. Statistical Analysis*

Data analysis was carried out in IBM SPSS Statistics for Windows, version 25.0 (IBM Corp., Armonk, NY, USA). First, descriptive analyses were conducted for the overall sample and broken down into categories of romantic attraction. Chi-square tests were computed along with Cramér's $V$ effect sizes to check for potential associations between romantic attraction and the sociodemographic and substance use variables. Uni- and multivariate binary logistic regression models were built to map the odds of substance use in adolescents belonging to other romantic attraction categories, compared to those who reported (exclusively) opposite-gender love.

Univariate models were constructed to obtain crude odds ratios (COR) of substance use in different romantic attraction groups. The reference was the group reporting opposite-gender love. Then country, gender and relative FAS grouping were added to the models to obtain adjusted odds ratios (AOR). French Belgium, boys, and adolescents belonging to the lowest family affluence group were set as reference categories. Multivariate analyses were carried out for the entire sample and stratified for gender. Wald statistics indicated that each predictor variable made a significant contribution to the models ($p \leq 0.04$). Model fit was examined. In many cases, the Chi-square tests indicated poor fit ($p > 0.05$), which may be a result of the large (overall) sample size and the imbalance between the compared subgroup sizes. This does not necessarily mean that the model should be discredited [55,56]. No collinearity was observed in the predictor variables. To test the potential confounding effect by interactions between the predictors, we constructed models that included two-way interactions, but these did not improve model fit.

It was at the discretion of the national HBSC teams to decide whether they would weight their data to correct imbalances in the composition of the sample. Data were not weighted if the characteristics of the actual sample corresponded to those of the national sampling frame (e.g., gender or family affluence distribution). The only exception to this was France. It means that from the eight national data sets included in this analysis, weighting was only applied to the French data. Therefore, we have used a weight variable with actual values for the French data and set to 1 for data from other countries.

The HBSC study uses classrooms as sampling units. To check whether cluster-based sampling method impacted the results, we have carried out the analyses using the Complex Samples function in SPSS. Design effects in the multivariate models, indicating the extent to which clustering effect needs to be corrected, were not substantially different from 1 ($0.98 \leq DEFF \leq 1.24$), indicating that clustering had a negligible impact. Therefore, the analyses have not been adjusted for cluster sampling.

## 3. Results

The number of respondents in each substance use group in the binary logistic models was determined by how many answered the given substance use item. As Table 2 shows, most respondents reported on the frequency of smoking item in the last 30 days ($n = 13,504$), while a lower number answered the items on alcohol consumption ($n = 13,440$), drunkenness ($n = 13,471$), and cannabis use ($n = 12,109$). For the multiple substance use model, all responses featured in any two of the single substance use models were collapsed ($n = 13,580$).

### 3.1. Love and Sociodemographic Characteristics

There was a significant association between love and country: $\chi^2(28) = 1625.87$, $p < 0.001$, but with a low effect size: $V = 0.173$ (Table 1). Love was associated with gender of the respondents: $\chi^2(4) = 87.30$, $p < 0.001$, but with a low effect size: $V = 0.080$. More girls reported same-gender love than boys, and the difference was even larger in the case of both-gender love. Girls were also more likely than boys to report not having been in love, but they were less likely than boys not to respond to the item. Love was also associated with family affluence: $\chi^2(8) = 36.46$, $p < 0.001$, but the effect size was negligible: $V = 0.037$.

### 3.2. Romantic Attraction and Substance Use

The prevalence of substance use across different attraction patterns is displayed in Table 2. Respondents reporting both-gender love reported the highest prevalence for each substance use: Cigarette smoking (33.6%), drinking alcohol (51.2%), being drunk (25.1%), and cannabis use in the last 30 days (20.6%). They also reported the highest rate of engagement in multiple substance use in the last 30 days (30.2%). Across all these romantic attraction groups, the lowest rates of engagement with substance use (apart from alcohol use) was reported by those who have never been in love.

Table 2. Frequency of risk behaviors, overall and by romantic attraction.

| | OVERALL | | Opposite-Gender Love | | Same-Gender Love | | Both-Gender Love | | Not in Love | | Not Responding | | Assoc. [2] |
|---|---|---|---|---|---|---|---|---|---|---|---|---|---|
| | n | % | n | % (RA) [1] | n | % (RA) | n | % (RA) | n | % (RA) | n | % (RA) | |
| **Cigarette smoking in the last 30 days** | 13,504 | | | | | | | | | | | | |
| No | 11,097 | 82.2 | 8933 | 81.5 | 150 | 69.4 | 164 | 66.4 | 1580 | 90.3 | 270 | 81.1 | $p < 0.001$, |
| Yes | 2407 | 17.8 | 2025 | 18.5 | 66 | 30.6 | 83 | 33.6 | 170 | 9.7 | 63 | 18.9 | $V = 0.105$ |
| **Alcohol consumption in the last 30 days** | 13,440 | | | | | | | | | | | | |
| No | 8348 | 62.1 | 6656 | 61.0 | 122 | 55.7 | 120 | 48.8 | 1214 | 70.0 | 236 | 70.7 | $p < 0.001$, |
| Yes | 5092 | 37.9 | 4251 | 39.0 | 97 | 44.3 | 126 | 51.2 | 520 | 30.0 | 98 | 29.3 | $V = 0.079$ |
| **Drunkenness in the last 30 days** | 13,471 | | | | | | | | | | | | |
| No | 11,680 | 86.7 | 9463 | 86.5 | 168 | 77.1 | 182 | 74.9 | 1587 | 90.8 | 280 | 87.0 | $p < 0.001$, |
| Yes | 1791 | 13.3 | 1477 | 13.5 | 50 | 22.9 | 61 | 25.1 | 161 | 9.2 | 42 | 13.0 | $V = 0.073$ |
| **Cannabis use in the last 30 days** | 12,109 | | | | | | | | | | | | |
| No | 11,159 | 92.2 | 9149 | 92.2 | 165 | 84.2 | 185 | 79.4 | 1522 | 94.5 | 138 | 91.4 | $p < 0.001$, |
| Yes | 950 | 7.8 | 770 | 7.8 | 31 | 15.8 | 48 | 20.6 | 88 | 5.5 | 13 | 8.6 | $V = 0.083$ |
| **Multiple substance use in the last 30 days [3]** | 13,580 | | | | | | | | | | | | |
| No | 11,499 | 84.7 | 9262 | 84.0 | 165 | 75.3 | 173 | 69.8 | 1610 | 91.7 | 289 | 86.8 | $p < 0.001$, |
| Yes | 2081 | 15.3 | 1762 | 16.0 | 54 | 24.5 | 75 | 30.2 | 146 | 8.3 | 44 | 13.2 | $V = 0.097$ |

[1] % (RA): Proportion within the given romantic attraction category. [2] Assoc.: Association between the given variable and romantic attraction. [3] Any two of cigarette smoking, alcohol consumption or cannabis use in the last 30 days.

### 3.3. Cigarette Smoking across Romantic Attraction

The univariate models indicated that same-gender and both-gender attracted respondents were significantly more likely to smoke in the last 30 days, while those not having been in love were less likely to report this behavior compared to opposite-gender attracted respondents (Table 3). Adjusting the model for country/region, family affluence, and gender did not substantially change the odds (the full model is displayed in supplementary Table S1). Compared to opposite-gender attracted adolescents, those who had been in love with both-gender partners had odds of 2.3, while same-gender attracted had odds of 1.9 for smoking. Those not having been in love had significantly lower odds (AOR = 0.4). Those who did not respond to the love item had statistically similar odds of smoking to those who were opposite-gender attracted. Gender-stratified analyses demonstrated that both-gender attracted boys and girls had somewhat higher odds of smoking (AOR = 2.8 and 2.1, respectively) than the same-gender attracted boys and girls (AOR = 2.4 and 1.6, respectively), but these differences were not statistically different. Those who reported never having been in love were significantly less likely to smoke (boys' AOR = 0.5; girls' AOR = 0.4) compared to opposite-gender attracted youth.

### 3.4. Alcohol Consumption across Romantic Attraction

Same-gender attracted youth did not have higher odds of alcohol consumption in the last 30 days than those reporting love with opposite-gender partners, but both-gender attracted youth had significantly higher odds, whereas those not attracted and non-responders had significantly lower odds (Table 3). The unadjusted model and model adjusted for country/region, family affluence, and gender yielded a similar pattern (the full model can be found in supplementary Table S2). Compared to their opposite-gender attracted peers, those who reported love for both-gender partners had odds of 1.8 for alcohol consumption, while those reporting never having been in love or not responding to the love item had odds of 0.5. However, analyses stratified for gender showed that only same-gender attracted boys (AOR = 1.7) and both-gender attracted girls (AOR = 2.2) were significantly more likely to have had alcohol in the last 30 days. Both boys and girls who reported never being in love or who did not respond to the item on love had significantly lower odds of alcohol consumption.

### 3.5. Drunkenness across Romantic Attraction

In the univariate model, same- and both-gender attracted youth were significantly more likely to report drunkenness in the last 30 days than opposite-gender attracted respondents, while those who had been in love less likely (Table 3). The same pattern was found in the multivariate model adjusted for country/region, family affluence, and gender (the full model can be found in supplementary Table S3). Compared to opposite-gender attracted youth, those reporting same-gender attraction had of 1.8 times, and both-gender love odds of 2.2 (both significantly higher) for drunkenness, while never attracted (AOR = 0.5) and non-responding youth (AOR = 0.7) had significantly lower odds. Same-gender attracted boys were significantly more likely to report drunkenness (AOR = 2.4) but same-gender attracted girls were not (AOR = 1.4). No gender differences were observed in the other groups.

**Table 3.** Crude and adjusted odds for the four types of substance use, overall and by gender.

| | Univariate Model | | | Multivariate Model (Overall) | | | Multivariate Model Stratified for Gender | | | | | |
| --- | --- | --- | --- | --- | --- | --- | --- | --- | --- | --- | --- | --- |
| | | | | | | | Boys (n = 6693) | | | Girls (n = 6811) | | |
| | COR [1] | p | (95% CI) | AOR [2] | p | (95% CI) | AOR | p | (95% CI) | AOR | p | (95% CI) |
| **Cigarettes in the last 30 days** | (n = 13,504) | | | (n = 13,504) | | | | | | | | |
| Opposite-gender love | 1 | | | 1 | | | 1 | | | 1 | | |
| Same-gender love | 2.00 | <0.001 | (1.48–2.69) | 1.85 | <0.001 | (1.34–2.55) | 2.36 | <0.001 | (1.46–3.82) | 1.57 | <0.001 | (1.02–2.41) |
| Both-gender love | 2.28 | <0.001 | (1.74–2.99) | 2.31 | <0.001 | (1.71–3.13) | 2.80 | <0.001 | (1.65–4.75) | 2.10 | <0.001 | (1.44–3.04) |
| Not in love | 0.47 | <0.001 | (0.40–0.56) | 0.44 | <0.001 | (0.37–0.52) | 0.53 | <0.001 | (0.41–0.70) | 0.38 | <0.001 | (0.30–0.48) |
| Not responding | 1.08 | 0.599 | (0.81–1.43) | 0.89 | 0.450 | (0.67–1.20) | 1.12 | 0.584 | (0.75–1.65) | 0.68 | 0.093 | (0.44–1.07) |
| **Alcohol in the last 30 days** | (n = 13,440) | | | (n = 13,440) | | | | | | | | |
| Opposite-gender love | 1 | | | 1 | | | 1 | | | 1 | | |
| Same-gender love | 1.27 | 0.093 | (0.96–1.66) | 1.20 | 0.230 | (0.89–1.63) | 1.66 | 0.036 | (1.03–2.66) | 0.97 | 0.880 | (0.64–1.46) |
| Both-gender love | 1.67 | <0.001 | (1.29–2.15) | 1.80 | <0.001 | (1.33–2.43) | 1.08 | 0.784 | (0.64–1.81) | 2.15 | <0.001 | (1.50–3.08) |
| Not in love | 0.67 | <0.001 | (0.60–0.75) | 0.52 | <0.001 | (0.46–0.59) | 0.56 | <0.001 | (0.47–0.67) | 0.49 | <0.001 | (0.42–0.58) |
| Not responding | 0.66 | 0.001 | (0.52–0.84) | 0.48 | <0.001 | (0.38–0.62) | 0.57 | 0.001 | (0.41–0.79) | 0.37 | <0.001 | (0.26–0.56) |
| **Drunkenness in the last 30 days** | (n = 13,471) | | | (n = 13,471) | | | | | | | | |
| Opposite-gender love | 1 | | | 1 | | | 1 | | | 1 | | |
| Same-gender love | 1.92 | <0.001 | (1.39–2.67) | 1.81 | 0.001 | (1.28–2.55) | 2.42 | <0.001 | (1.48–3.96) | 1.38 | 0.204 | (0.84–2.28) |
| Both-gender love | 2.20 | <0.001 | (1.63–2.96) | 2.19 | <0.001 | (1.59–3.02) | 1.93 | 0.016 | (1.13–3.31) | 2.25 | <0.001 | (1.51–3.34) |
| Not in love | 0.65 | <0.001 | (0.55–0.77) | 0.51 | <0.001 | (0.43–0.61) | 0.55 | <0.001 | (0.42–0.72) | 0.47 | <0.001 | (0.37–0.60) |
| Not responding | 0.98 | .879 | (0.70–1.36) | 0.68 | 0.021 | (0.48–0.94) | 0.71 | 0.120 | (0.46–1.09) | 0.63 | .090 | (0.37–1.07) |
| **Cannabis in the last 30 days** | (n = 12,109) | | | (n = 12,109) | | | | | | | | |
| Opposite-gender love | 1 | | | 1 | | | 1 | | | 1 | | |
| Same-gender love | 2.21 | <0.001 | (1.48–3.31) | 2.16 | 0.001 | (1.39–3.36) | 2.90 | 0.001 | (1.57–5.38) | 1.62 | 0.142 | (0.85–3.09) |
| Both-gender love | 3.19 | <0.001 | (2.30–4.44) | 3.57 | <0.001 | (2.48–5.13) | 4.12 | <0.001 | (2.33–7.30) | 3.20 | <0.001 | (1.99–5.15) |
| Not in love | 0.68 | 0.001 | (0.54–0.85) | 0.62 | <0.001 | (0.48–0.79) | 0.71 | 0.048 | (0.51–1.00) | 0.53 | 0.001 | (0.36–0.77) |
| Not responding | 1.18 | 0.581 | (0.66–2.10) | 1.05 | 0.979 | (0.57–1.93) | 1.10 | 0.821 | (0.50–2.40) | 1.01 | 0.990 | (0.38–2.65) |

[1] COR: Crude odds ratios. [2] AOR: Odds ratios adjusted for region, gender, and relative family affluence. Boldface indicates statistically significant differences in (p < 0.05) odds for the given substance use in the given group, as compared to the reference group.

### 3.6. Cannabis Use across Romantic Attraction

In the univariate model, same- and both-gender attracted adolescents were significantly more likely, while those who had not been in love were significantly less likely to report cannabis use in the last 30 days compared to their opposite-gender attracted peers (Table 3). After adjusting for country/region, family affluence, and gender, a similar pattern was observed (the full model can be found in supplementary Table S4). Compared to those reporting opposite-gender love, those who had been in love with same-gender partners had odds of 2.2 and those in love with both-gender partners had odds of 3.6 (both significantly higher) of reporting cannabis use, while those who had never been in love had significantly lower odds (AOR = 0.6); the odds of non-responders were not significantly different from their opposite-gender attracted peers. Same-gender attracted boys' odds were significantly higher (AOR = 2.9) but same-gender attracted girls had similar odds (AOR = 1.6) for cannabis use as their opposite-gender attracted peers. Both-gender attracted boys and girls had higher odds than those reporting opposite-gender attraction (boys' AOR = 4.1, girls' AOR = 3.2), whereas never having been in love was associated with significantly lower odds in both boys (AOR = 0.7) and girls (AOR = 0.5).

### 3.7. Multiple Substance Use across Romantic Attraction

The comparison of participants reporting multiple substance use among those with different patterns of attraction yielded analogous results to those found with use of single substances (Table 4). In both the univariate model and the model adjusted for country/region, family affluence and gender (the full model can be found in supplementary Table S5), same- and both-gender attracted adolescents had higher odds of using any two or all three substances than opposite-gender attracted young people, while not being in love was associated with significantly lower odds. Non-respondents had a similar likelihood to their opposite-gender attracted peers of reporting multiple substance use. However, in the gender-stratified analyses, only same-gender attracted boys had significantly higher odds of multiple substance use (AOR = 2.1; $p = 0.02$), while among girls, the difference was not statistically significant (AOR = 1.4; $p = 0.16$). When compared to opposite-gender attracted youth, both-gender attraction was associated with significantly higher odds of multiple substance use for both boys (AOR = 2.8) and girls (AOR = 2.2), while those not having been in love had significantly lower odds (boys' AOR = 0.5, girls' AOR = 0.4). Girls not responding to the love item also had significantly lower odds of multiple substance use (AOR = 0.6, $p = 0.04$), but not boys (AOR = 0.9, $p = 0.65$).

**Table 4.** Crude and adjusted odds for multiple substance use, overall and by sex (n = 13,580).

| | Univariate Model | | | Multivariate Model (Overall) | | | Multivariate Model Stratified for Sex | | | | | |
| --- | --- | --- | --- | --- | --- | --- | --- | --- | --- | --- | --- | --- |
| | | | | | | | Boys (n = 6693) | | | Girls (n = 6811) | | |
| | COR[1] | p | (95% CI) | AOR[2] | p | (95% CI) | AOR | p | (95% CI) | AOR | p | (95% CI) |
| Multiple substance use in the last 30 days[3] | | | | | | | | | | | | |
| Opposite-gender love | 1 | | | 1 | | | 1 | | | 1 | | |
| Same-gender love | **1.79** | <0.001 | (1.30–2.46) | **1.68** | 0.003 | (1.20–2.35) | **2.12** | 0.002 | (1.33–3.64) | 1.39 | 0.161 | (0.88–2.20) |
| Both-gender love | **2.34** | <0.001 | (1.77–3.09) | **2.43** | <0.001 | (1.79–3.31) | **2.78** | <0.001 | (1.64–4.70) | **2.24** | <0.001 | (1.54–3.27) |
| Not in love | **0.47** | <0.001 | (0.39–0.56) | **0.44** | <0.001 | (0.36–0.53) | **0.53** | <0.001 | (0.40–0.70) | **0.38** | <0.001 | (0.29–0.49) |
| Not responding | 0.84 | 0.291 | (0.60–1.16) | 0.74 | 0.081 | (0.53–1.03) | 0.90 | 0.651 | (0.58–1.41) | **0.59** | 0.044 | (0.35–0.99) |

[1] COR: Crude odds ratios. [2] AOR: Odds ratios adjusted for region, gender, and relative family affluence. Boldface indicates statistically significant differences in (p < 0.05) odds for the given substance use in the given group, as compared to the reference group. [3] Based on cigarettes, alcohol or cannabis in the last 30 days.

## 4. Discussion

This study aimed to explore the association between different romantic attraction patterns and substance use across national representative samples of adolescents from eight European countries and regions with various geographical location, history and level of tolerance towards sexual minorities. Our findings indicate higher risks for both same- and both-gender attracted youth to engage in substance use. This pattern was observed for single (cigarette smoking, alcohol consumption, drunkenness, and cannabis use) and multiple substance use (any two or more of cigarette smoking, alcohol consumption, or cannabis use), thus supporting findings from existing international literature. The fact that the pattern of the odds ratios remained very similar after controlling for gender, country/region and relative family affluence suggests that the elevated vulnerability of SMY to be engaged in substance use is a universal phenomenon, at least across the eight investigated European countries. These findings imply that as well as differentiating between heterosexual and homosexual or bisexual orientation, separating monosexual (heterosexual or gay/lesbian) and plurisexual (bisexual) identities may also reveal health disparities. Expanding the investigation to those who have not been in love revealed that, to a certain extent, reporting being in love (irrespective the gender of the love partner) was associated with higher odds of substance use than not having been in love. These results can be integrated with the minority stress and romantic stress theoretical models.

### 4.1. Gender and Attraction

Differences in alcohol, drunkenness, cannabis and multiple substance use were found across the groups of same- and both-gender attracted boys and girls. Regarding alcohol and drunkenness, same-gender attracted boys were at somewhat (but not to a significant extent) higher risk than both-gender attracted boys. Among girls, both-gender attraction was associated with higher risk for all five substance use indicators compared to same-gender attraction. This finding is in line with other studies showing that bisexual or both-gender attracted youths are among the highest risk of all SMY groups in relation to substance use [8,20,24], and even they are not homogenous in terms of risk [57].

### 4.2. Socioeconomic Status, Country and Attraction

Both family affluence and country/region were significant predictors in all multivariate models, however both unadjusted and adjusted substance use models follow very similar patterns. This indicates that the association between romantic attraction and substance use is not substantially influenced by family background or country/region of residence, at least in the eight European countries featured in our study. While lower socioeconomic status is associated with greater likelihood of reporting substance use [58], some argue that minority stress exacerbates the involvement of all SMYs in substance use, against which racial (or socio-economic) factors are not protective [11]. In other words, sexual minority status may be more strongly associated with substance use than socio-economic status. The observation that the risks of substance use among SMY is similar across regions and countries reinforces existing findings in this area, from single European countries [59–63] or from cross-cultural investigations [21].

### 4.3. Love: A 'Sweet Poison'?

In line with our hypotheses, we have observed that those young people who reported never having been in love had significantly lower (0.4–0.7 times) odds of any single or multiple substance use than their opposite-gender attracted peers. This was found in the general models as well as in those disaggregated for gender. In other words, it seems that never having been in love is protective against substance use. This finding is in line with available evidence that romantic relationships (irrespective of the gender of the partner) may be associated with stress in adolescence [64], thus support the concept of romantic stress. Involvement in romantic relationships may be stressful for young people for a variety of reasons. These include separation and individuation from family, cultural expectations, conflicts with the romantic partner, and a double standard of love and sexual initiation for boys and girls [41,65]. As mentioned in Section 1.4, some participants might have been engaged in substance use (e.g., alcohol and drug consumption) to cope with romantic stress [41]. The romantic partner's substance use habits may also be predictive of the adolescents' own substance use [66]. Time spent with peers is predictive of substance use [67], and a similar association might be there with romantic partners. Further studies are needed to disentangle the separate effects of minority and romantic stress in SMY.

*4.4. Non-Responders*

Not responding to the item on love was not associated with higher odds of cigarette smoking, drunkenness, and cannabis use, but was associated with lower odds for alcohol use (in both boys and girls) and for multiple substance use (in girls) than for those who reported opposite-gender attraction. Adolescents may have various motives for not answering survey questions related to sexual orientation. They may be reluctant or unwilling to assume a socially stigmatized identity label, or it may reflect personal, cultural, religious, or political resistance to being categorized or defined by their sexuality [42]. We do not know participants' motives for not responding to the item, but we speculate that this is not associated with elevated stress (based on the above-mentioned findings on the association of stress and frequent substance use). When developing the item on love, a few young people told our research team that they felt it is too private [68]. Further qualitative studies are needed to better understand young people's motivations for not answering questions of this nature.

*4.5. Limitations*

Our findings are limited by the fact that the study was cross-sectional, therefore no causal or temporal inferences can be made. Given the low subsample sizes in countries, we could not carry out country-stratified analyses. However, from the fact that country as a control variable (as gender and family affluence) did not substantially change the pattern of the results, we infer that SMY may be at elevated risk regardless of their gender, family background and country of residence, at least in these eight European countries/regions.

We have concentrated on feelings of love for opposite-, same- or both-gender partners, which may not totally correspond to self-identified sexual orientation, erotic desire or sexual behavior [42,43].

Finally, we used a binary variable (boy or girl) to categorize adolescents' gender, which does not reflect trans, non-binary or other gender minority groups. The links between gender, biological sex and sexual orientation constitute a very complex issue [69]. The HBSC International Network is currently working on how the survey can be more inclusive of both gender and sex diversity.

*4.6. Reducing Risk and Promoting Resilience in Sexual Minority Youth*

How can we reduce the risk associated with romantic attraction (compared to those who have not been in a romantic relationship) and the risk associated with both- and same-gender attraction compared to those who are attracted to opposite-gender partners? Love is experienced by many young people; professionals working with adolescents in health or social care, or educational settings, should be aware of the potential stressful effects of romantic relationships and minority stress, and be prepared to discuss these intimate matters with young people. Promoting healthy romantic relationships, both for SMY and heterosexual youth, may reduce (romantic) stress and have a positive impact on peer norms. Direct measures to promote health and resilience in SMY, such as 'gay-straight alliances' or 'gender-sexuality alliances' [70], media-based interventions to address sexual orientation related prejudice [71] or introducing safe school policies [72] have a documented beneficial effect on the health of not just SMY, but on heterosexual adolescents as well. Risk prevention and enhancing resilience and well-being in SMY should be part of national youth health strategies [73]. Some suggest that researchers and practitioners should consider how to shift from a victimizing and pathologizing narrative, which describes sexual minority individuals as 'vulnerable' [74]. A more positive view on sexual (and gender) minority people include, for instance, resilience, compassion, and tolerance towards members of other minorities [75]. Despite the hardships sexual minority young people experience, they have the potential to express their identity and love and lead healthy and happy lives.

*4.7. Future Directions*

Dimensions of sexual orientation, involvement in romantic attractions, minority stress, risk behaviors and psychosocial factors constitute a complex causal 'web'. Future studies are needed to map how bullying involvement and social support shape substance use and other risky and health promoting behaviors, and various health outcomes in SMY. Using a positive approach, such research projects may also map health-protective factors and resources in sexual minority youth.

## 5. Conclusions

Sexual minority youth from eight European countries (identified based on reporting love for same- or both-gender partners) were found to be at higher risk of substance use behaviors than their opposite-gender attracted peers. On the other hand, adolescents who reported not having been in love were at lower risk of these substance use behaviors. These results support the assertion that romantic experiences on their own might be stressful for adolescents across different cultures, and that sexual minority status is associated with higher risk of substance use even after controlling for country/region, socio-economic status and gender. Targeted policy actions are needed to reduce risk and promote well-being and resilience in SMY, and further cross-national research needs to be conducted to better understand how dimensions of sexual orientation impact the health of young people.

**Supplementary Materials:** The following are available online at http://www.mdpi.com/1660-4601/16/17/3063/s1. Data collected in the 2013/2104 round of HBSC can be accessed following registration at https://www.uib.no/en/hbscdata. The supplementary tables can be downloaded from: https://osf.io/d38px/?view_only=690caa0ccc3545eea8e7c32cf93f41fc.

**Author Contributions:** Conceptualization, A.K.; data curation, A.K.; formal analysis, A.K.; funding acquisition, E.B.T., E.M.S. and S.N.G.; investigation, A.K., A.C., H.Y., N.M., D.P., R.T., E.B.T., A.V., E.M.S. and S.N.G.; methodology, A.K., A.C., N.M., D.P., R.T., E.B.T. and A.V.; project administration, A.K.; supervision, E.M.S. and S.N.G.; validation, A.K., A.C., H.Y., N.M., D.P., R.T., A.V. and S.N.G.; writing—original draft, A.K., D.P., R.T. and A.V.; writing—review & editing, A.K., A.C., H.Y., N.M., E.B.T., E.M.S. and S.N.G.

**Funding:** HBSC Belgium (FWB) is funded by the Wallonia-Brussels Federation (FWB), the Office of Birth and Childhood (ONE), the Walloon Region and the Brussels-Capital Region. HBSC Bulgaria is funded by UNICEF-Bulgaria. HBSC England is funded by the Department of Health and Social Care. HBSC France is funded by Santé Publique France and OFDT (French Monitoring Centre for Drug Use and Addiction). HBSC Hungary is funded by ELTE Eötvös Loránd University. HBSC Iceland is funded by grants from the Icelandic Directorate of Health, KEA and the University of Akureyri. North Macedonia is funded by the United Nations Population Fund/United Nations Development Programme. HBSC Switzerland is funded by the Swiss Federal Office of Public Health and most of the Swiss cantons. The study was funded in part by grant #FDN 154335 from the Canadian Institutes of Health Research (Saewyc, PI).

**Acknowledgments:** HBSC is an international study carried out in collaboration with WHO Europe. The International Coordinator of the 2013/2014 survey was Joanna Inchley (University of Glasgow, Scotland) and the Data Bank Manager was Oddrun Samdal (University of Bergen, Norway). The following Principal Investigators of national HBSC Teams gave us permission to use national data from the given country: Katia Castetbon (French Belgium), Lidiya Vasileva (Bulgaria), Fiona Brooks and Ellen Klemera (England), Emmanuelle Godeau (France), Lina Kostarova-Unkovska (North Macedonia), Ágnes Németh (Hungary), Arsaell Arnarsson (Iceland), and Marina Delgrande Jordan and Hervé Kuendig (Switzerland). We are grateful for HBSC Communications Officer Joseph Hancock and our colleagues in the HBSC Sexual Health Focus Group for their help. For details on HBSC, see http://www.hbsc.org.

**Conflicts of Interest:** The authors declare no conflict of interest.

## References

1.  Semlyen, J.; King, M.; Varney, J.; Hagger-Johnson, G. Sexual orientation and symptoms of common mental disorder or low wellbeing: Combined meta-analysis of 12 UK population health surveys. *BMC Psychiatry* **2016**, *16*, 67. [CrossRef] [PubMed]

2.  Hafeez, H.; Zeshan, M.; A Tahir, M.; Jahan, N.; Naveed, S. Health Care Disparities Among Lesbian, Gay, Bisexual, and Transgender Youth: A Literature Review. *Cureus* **2017**, *9*, e1184. [CrossRef] [PubMed]
3.  Marshal, M.P.; Friedman, M.S.; Stall, R.; King, K.M.; Miles, J.; Gold, M.A.; Bukstein, O.G.; Morse, J.Q. Sexual orientation and adolescent substance use: A meta-analysis and methodological review. *Addiction* **2008**, *103*, 546–556. [CrossRef] [PubMed]
4.  Goldbach, J.; Tanner-Smith, E.; Bagwell, M.; Dunlap, S. Minority stress and substance use in sexual minority adolescents: A meta-analysis. *Prev. Sci.* **2014**, *15*, 350–363. [CrossRef] [PubMed]
5.  Austin, S.B.; Ziyadeh, N.; Fisher, L.B.; Kahn, J.A.; Colditz, G.A.; Frazier, A.L. Sexual Orientation and Tobacco Use in a Cohort Study of US Adolescent Girls and Boys. *Arch. Pediatr. Adolesc. Med.* **2004**, *158*, 317–322. [CrossRef]
6.  Dai, H. Tobacco Product Use among Lesbian, Gay, and Bisexual Adolescents. *Pediatrics* **2017**, *139*, e20163276. [CrossRef]
7.  Lee, J.; Griffin, G.K.; Melvin, C.L. Tobacco use among sexual minorities in the USA, 1987 to May 2007: A systematic review. *Tob. Control* **2009**, *18*, 275–282. [CrossRef]
8.  Corliss, H.L.; Rosario, M.; Birkett, M.A.; Newcomb, M.E.; Buchting, F.O.; Matthews, A.K. Sexual Orientation Disparities in Adolescent Cigarette Smoking: Intersections With Race/Ethnicity, Gender, and Age. *Am. J. Public Health* **2014**, *104*, 1137–1147. [CrossRef]
9.  Watson, R.J.; Lewis, N.M.; Fish, J.N.; Goodenow, C. Sexual minority youth continue to smoke cigarettes earlier and more often than heterosexuals: Findings from population-based data. *Drug Alcohol Depend.* **2018**, *184*, 64–70. [CrossRef]
10. Fish, J.N.; Turner, B.; Phillips, G.; Russell, S.T. Cigarette Smoking Disparities between Sexual Minority and Heterosexual Youth. *Pediatr* **2019**, *143*, e20181671. [CrossRef]
11. Newcomb, M.E.; Heinz, A.J.; Birkett, M.; Mustanski, B. A Longitudinal Examination of Risk and Protective Factors for Cigarette Smoking among Lesbian, Gay, Bisexual and Transgender Youth. *J. Adolesc. Health* **2014**, *54*, 558–564. [CrossRef] [PubMed]
12. Rosario, M.; Schrimshaw, E.W.; Hunter, J. Cigarette smoking as a coping strategy: Negative implications for subsequent psychological distress among lesbian, gay, and bisexual youths. *J. Pediatr. Psychol.* **2011**, *36*, 731–742. [CrossRef] [PubMed]
13. Hatzenbuehler, M.; Jun, H.J.; Corliss, H.; Austin, S. Structural stigma and cigarette smoking in a prospective cohort study of sexual minority and heterosexual youth. *Ann. Behav. Med.* **2014**, *47*, 48–56. [CrossRef] [PubMed]
14. Talley, A.E.; Hughes, T.L.; Aranda, F.; Birkett, M.; Marshal, M.P. Exploring Alcohol-Use Behaviors among Heterosexual and Sexual Minority Adolescents: Intersections with Sex, Age, and Race/Ethnicity. *Am. J. Public Health* **2014**, *104*, 295–303. [CrossRef] [PubMed]
15. Garofalo, R.; Wolf, R.C.; Kessel, S.; Palfrey, J.; Durant, R.H. The Association between Health Risk Behaviors and Sexual Orientation Among a School-based Sample of Adolescents. *Pediatrics* **1998**, *101*, 895–902. [CrossRef] [PubMed]
16. Fish, J.N.; Pasley, K. Sexual (Minority) Trajectories, Mental Health, and Alcohol Use: A Longitudinal Study of Youth as They Transition to Adulthood. *J. Youth Adolesc.* **2015**, *44*, 1508–1527. [CrossRef] [PubMed]
17. Donath, C.; Gräßel, E.; Baier, D.; Pfeiffer, C.; Karagülle, D.; Bleich, S.; Hillemacher, T. Alcohol consumption and binge drinking in adolescents: Comparison of different migration backgrounds and rural vs. urban residence—A representative study. *BMC Public Health* **2011**, *11*, 84. [CrossRef] [PubMed]
18. Vieno, A.; Altoè, G.; Kuntsche, E.; Elgar, F.J. Do public expenditures on health and families relate to alcohol abstaining in adolescents? Multilevel study of adolescents in 24 countries. *Drug Alcohol Rev.* **2018**, *37*, S120–S128. [CrossRef]
19. Fish, J.N.; Baams, L. Trends in Alcohol-Related Disparities between Heterosexual and Sexual Minority Youth from 2007 to 2015: Findings from the Youth Risk Behavior Survey. *LGBT Health* **2018**, *5*, 359–367. [CrossRef]
20. Talley, A.E.; Turner, B.; Foster, A.M.; Phillips, G. Sexual Minority Youth at Risk of Early and Persistent Alcohol, Tobacco, and Marijuana Use. *Arch. Sex. Behav.* **2019**, *48*, 1073–1086. [CrossRef]
21. Demant, D.; Hides, L.; White, K.M.; Kavanagh, D.J. LGBT communities and substance use in Queensland, Australia: Perceptions of young people and community stakeholders. *PLoS ONE* **2018**, *13*, e0204730. [CrossRef] [PubMed]

22. Gorbach, P.M.; Javanbakht, M.; Shover, C.L.; Bolan, R.K.; Ragsdale, A.; Shoptaw, S. Associations Between Cannabis Use, Sexual Behavior, and Sexually Transmitted Infections/Human Immunodeficiency Virus in a Cohort of Young Men Who Have Sex With Men. *Sex. Transm. Dis.* **2019**, *46*, 105–111. [CrossRef] [PubMed]

23. Goldbach, J.T.; Schrager, S.M.; Dunlap, S.L.; Holloway, I.W. The application of minority stress theory to marijuana use among sexual minority adolescents. *Subst. Use Misuse* **2015**, *50*, 366–375. [CrossRef] [PubMed]

24. Blais, M.; Bergeron, F.A.; Duford, J.; Boislard, M.A.; Hebert, M. Health outcomes of sexual-minority youth in Canada: An overview. *Adolesc. Saude* **2015**, *12*, 53–73. [PubMed]

25. Watson, R.J.; Goodenow, C.; Porta, C.; Adjei, J.; Saewyc, E. Substance use among sexual minorities: Has it actually gotten better? *Subst. Use Misuse* **2018**, *53*, 1221–1228. [CrossRef] [PubMed]

26. Goldbach, J.; Fisher, B.W.; Dunlap, S. Traumatic Experiences and Drug Use by LGB Adolescents: A Critical Review of Minority Stress. *J. Soc. Work. Pract. Addict.* **2015**, *15*, 90–113. [CrossRef]

27. Newcomb, M.E.; Ryan, D.T.; Greene, G.J.; Garofalo, R.; Mustanski, B. Prevalence and Patterns of Smoking, Alcohol Use, and Illicit Drug Use in Young Men Who Have Sex with Men. *Drug Alcohol Depend.* **2014**, *141*, 65–71. [CrossRef] [PubMed]

28. Marshal, M.P.; King, K.M.; Stepp, S.D.; Hipwell, A.; Smith, H.; Chung, T.; Friedman, M.S.; Markovic, N. Trajectories of alcohol and cigarette use among sexual minority and heterosexual girls. *J. Adolesc. Health* **2012**, *50*, 97–99. [CrossRef]

29. Lea, T.; Reynolds, R.; de Wit, J. Alcohol and club drug use among same-sex attracted young people: Associations with frequenting the lesbian and gay scene and other bars and nightclubs. *Subst. Use Misuse* **2013**, *48*, 129–136. [CrossRef]

30. Balsam, K.F.; Molina, Y.; Lehavot, K. Alcohol and Drug Use in Lesbian, Gay, Bisexual, and Transgender (LGBT) Youth and Young Adults. In *Principles of Addiction*; Elsevier: Amsterdam, The Netherlands, 2013; pp. 563–573.

31. Matthews, D.D.; Blosnich, J.R.; Farmer, G.W.; Adams, B.J. Operational definitions of sexual orientation and estimates of adolescent health risk behaviors. *LGBT Health* **2014**, *1*, 42–49. [CrossRef]

32. Meyer, I.H. Prejudice, Social Stress, and Mental Health in Lesbian, Gay, and Bisexual Populations: Conceptual Issues and Research Evidence. *Psychol. Bull.* **2003**, *129*, 674–697. [CrossRef] [PubMed]

33. Meyer, I.H. Prejudice and Discrimination as Social Stressors. In *The Health of Sexual Minorities*; Springer Science and Business Media: New York, NY, USA, 2007; pp. 242–267.

34. Hatzenbuehler, M.L. How Does Sexual Minority Stigma "Get Under the Skin"? A Psychological Mediation Framework. *Psychol. Bull.* **2009**, *135*, 707–730. [CrossRef] [PubMed]

35. Lea, T.; De Wit, J.; Reynolds, R. Minority Stress in Lesbian, Gay, and Bisexual Young Adults in Australia: Associations with Psychological Distress, Suicidality, and Substance Use. *Arch. Sex. Behav.* **2014**, *43*, 1571–1578. [CrossRef] [PubMed]

36. Hughes, T.L.; Wilsnack, S.C.; Kantor, L.W. The influence of gender and sexual orientation on alcohol use and alcohol-related problems: Toward a global perspective. *Alcohol Res.* **2016**, *38*, 121–132. [PubMed]

37. Saewyc, E.M. Research on adolescent sexual orientation: Development, health disparities, stigma and resilience. *J. Res. Adolesc.* **2011**, *21*, 256–272. [CrossRef]

38. Bränström, R.; van der Star, A. More knowledge and research concerning the health of lesbian, gay, bisexual and transgender individuals is needed. *Eur. J. Public Health* **2016**, *26*, 208–209. [CrossRef]

39. ILGA-Europe. *Annual Review of the Human Rights Situation of Lesbian, Gay, Bisexual, Trans and Intersex People in Europe*; ILGA-Europe: Brussels, Belgium, 2014.

40. Demant, D.; Hides, L.; Kavanagh, D.J.; White, K.M.; Winstock, A.R.; Ferris, J. Differences in substance use between sexual orientations in a multi-country sample: Findings from the Global Drug Survey 2015. *J. Public Health (Oxf.)* **2017**, *39*, 532–541. [CrossRef]

41. Seiffge-Krenke, I.; Bosma, H.; Chau, C.; Çok, F.; Gillespie, C.; Loncaric, D.; Molinar, R.; Cunha, M.; Veisson, M.; Rohail, I. All they need is love? Placing romantic stress in the context of other stressors: A 17-nation study. *Int. J. Behav. Dev.* **2010**, *34*, 106–112. [CrossRef]

42. Savin-Williams, R.C.; Cohen, K.M. Development of Same-Sex Attracted Youth. In *The Health of Sexual Minorities: Public Health Perspectives on Lesbian, Gay, Bisexual and Transgender Populations*; Meyer, I.H., Northridge, M.E., Eds.; Springer US: Boston, MA, USA, 2007; pp. 27–47.

43. Geary, R.S.; Tanton, C.; Erens, B.; Clifton, S.; Prah, P.; Wellings, K.; Mitchell, K.R.; Datta, J.; Gravningen, K.; Fuller, E.; et al. Sexual identity, attraction and behaviour in Britain: The implications of using different dimensions of sexual orientation to estimate the size of sexual minority populations and inform public health interventions. *PLoS ONE* **2018**, *13*, e0189607. [CrossRef]

44. Calzo, J.P.; Blashill, A.J. Child Sexual Orientation and Gender Identity in the Adolescent Brain Cognitive Development Cohort Study. *JAMA Pediatr.* **2018**, *172*, 1090–1092. [CrossRef]

45. Költő, A.; Young, H.; Burke, L.; Moreau, N.; Cosma, A.; Magnusson, J.; Windlin, B.; Reis, M.; Saewyc, E.M.; Godeau, E.; et al. Love and Dating Patterns for Same- and Both-Gender Attracted Adolescents Across Europe. *J. Res. Adolesc.* **2018**, *28*, 772–778. [CrossRef] [PubMed]

46. Russell, S.T.; Driscoll, A.K.; Truong, N. Adolescent Same-Sex Romantic Attractions and Relationships: Implications for Substance Use and Abuse. *Am. J. Public Health* **2002**, *92*, 198–202. [CrossRef] [PubMed]

47. Marshal, M.P.; Friedman, M.S.; Stall, R.; Thompson, A.L. Individual trajectories of substance use in lesbian, gay and bisexual youth and heterosexual youth. *Addiction* **2009**, *104*, 974–981. [CrossRef] [PubMed]

48. Diamond, L.M. What does sexual orientation orient? A biobehavioral model distinguishing romantic love and sexual desire. *Psychol. Rev.* **2003**, *110*, 173–192. [CrossRef] [PubMed]

49. Inchley, J.; Currie, D.; Young, T.; Samdal, O.; Torsheim, T.; Augustson, L.; Mathisen, F.; Aleman-Diaz, A.; Molcho, M.; Weber, M.; et al. Growing up Unequal: Gender and Socioeconomic Differences in Young people's Health and Well-Being. In *Health Behaviour in School-Aged Children (HBSC) Study. International Report from the 2013/2014 Survey*; WHO Regional Office for Europe: Copenhagen, Denmark, 2016.

50. Health Behaviour in School-Aged Children (HBSC). *Study Protocol: Background, Methodology and Mandatory Items for the 2013/14 Survey*; Currie, C., Inchley, J., Molcho, M., Lenzi, M., Veselska, Z., Wild, F., Eds.; Child and Adolescent Health Research Unit (CAHRU), University of St. Andrews: St. Andrews, UK, 2014.

51. Guttormsson, U.; Leifman, H.; Kraus, L.; Molinaro, S.; Monshouwer, K.; Trapencieres, M.; Vincente, J.; Englund, A.; Svensson, J. *ESPAD 2015: Methodology*; European Monitoring Centre for Drugs and Drug Addiction (EMCDDA) and The European School Survey Project on Alcohol and Other Drugs (ESPAD): Lisbon, Portugal, 2016.

52. Currie, C.; Molcho, M.; Boyce, W.; Holstein, B.; Torsheim, T.; Richter, M. Researching health inequalities in adolescents: The development of the Health Behaviour in School-Aged Children (HBSC) Family Affluence Scale. *Soc. Sci. Med.* **2008**, *66*, 1429–1436. [CrossRef] [PubMed]

53. Schnohr, C.; Makransky, G.; Kreiner, S.; Torsheim, T.; Hofmann, F.; De Clercq, B.; Elgar, F.; Currie, C. Item response drift in the Family Affluence Scale: A study on three consecutive surveys of the Health Behaviour in School-aged Children (HBSC) survey. *Measurement* **2013**, *46*, 3119–3126. [CrossRef]

54. Torsheim, T.; Cavallo, F.; Levin, K.A.; Schnohr, C.; Mazur, J.; Niclasen, B.; Currie, C.; The FAS Development Study Group. Psychometric validation of the revised family affluence scale: A latent variable approach. *Child Indic. Res.* **2016**, *9*, 771–784. [CrossRef]

55. Allison, P.D. Measures of Fit for Logistic Regression. In Proceedings of the SAS Global Forum, Washington, DC, USA, 23–26 March 2014.

56. Barrett, P. Structural equation modelling: Adjudging model fit. *Pers. Individ. Differ.* **2007**, *42*, 815–824. [CrossRef]

57. Feinstein, B.A.; Turner, B.C.; Beach, L.B.; Korpak, A.K.; Phillips, G. Racial/Ethnic Differences in Mental Health, Substance Use, and Bullying Victimization Among Self-Identified Bisexual High School-Aged Youth. *LGBT Health* **2019**, *6*, 174–183. [CrossRef]

58. Adler, N.E.; Boyce, T.; Chesney, M.A.; Cohen, S.; Folkman, S.; Kahn, R.L.; Syme, S.L. Socioeconomic status and health: The challenge of the gradient. *Am. Psychol.* **1994**, *49*, 15–24. [CrossRef]

59. Arnarsson, A.; Sveinbjornsdottir, S.; Thorsteinsson, E.B.; Bjarnason, T. Suicidal risk and sexual orientation in adolescence: A population-based study in Iceland. *Scand. J. Public Health* **2015**, *43*, 497–505. [CrossRef] [PubMed]

60. Thorsteinsson, E.B.; Loi, N.M.; Sveinbjornsdottir, S.; Arnarsson, A. Sexual orientation among Icelandic year 10 adolescents: Changes in health and life satisfaction from 2006 to 2014. *Scand. J. Psychol.* **2017**, *58*, 530–540. [CrossRef] [PubMed]

61. Clarke, A.; Beenstock, J.; Lukacs, J.N.; Turner, L.; Limmer, M. Major risk factors for sexual minority young people's mental and physical health: Findings from a county-wide school-based health needs assessment. *J. Public Health (Oxf.)* **2018**, fdy167. [CrossRef] [PubMed]

62. Amos, R.; Manalastas, E. Mental Health, Social Adversity and Health Outcomes in Sexual Minority Adolescents Aged 14 Years: Findings from the Millennium Cohort Study (MCS6). In Proceedings of the BPS Psychology of Sexualities Annual Conference, London, UK, 4–5 July 2019.

63. Kuyper, L.; De Roos, S.; Iedema, J.; Stevens, G. Growing Up With the Right to Marry: Sexual Attraction, Substance Use, and Well-Being of Dutch Adolescents. *J. Adolesc. Health* **2016**, *59*, 276–282. [CrossRef] [PubMed]

64. Collins, W.A.; Welsh, D.P.; Furman, W. Adolescent romantic relationships. *Annu. Rev. Psychol.* **2008**, *60*, 631–652. [CrossRef] [PubMed]

65. Moreau, N.; Költő, A.; Young, H.; Maillochon, F.; Godeau, E. Negative feelings about the timing of first sexual intercourse: Findings from the Health Behaviour in School-aged Children study. *Int. J. Public Health* **2019**, *64*, 219–227. [CrossRef] [PubMed]

66. Aikins, J.W.; Simon, V.A.; Prinstein, M.J. Romantic Partner Selection and Socialization of Young Adolescents' Substance Use and Behavior Problems. *J. Adolesc.* **2010**, *33*, 813–826. [CrossRef] [PubMed]

67. Barnes, G.M.; Hoffman, J.H.; Welte, J.W.; Farrell, M.P.; Dintcheff, B.A. Adolescents' time use: Effects on substance use, delinquency and sexual activity. *J. Youth Adolesc.* **2007**, *36*, 697–710. [CrossRef]

68. Young, H.; Költő, A.; Reis, M.; Saewyc, E.M.; Moreau, N.; Burke, L.; Cosma, A.; Windlin, B.; Gabhainn, S.N.; Godeau, E. Sexual health questions included in the Health Behaviour in School-aged Children (HBSC) study: An international methodological pilot investigation. *BMC Med. Res. Methodol.* **2016**, *16*, 169. [CrossRef]

69. Fausto-Sterling, A. Gender/Sex, Sexual Orientation, and Identity Are in the Body: How Did They Get There? *J. Sex Res.* **2019**, *56*, 529–555. [CrossRef]

70. Li, G.; Wu, A.D.; Marshall, S.K.; Watson, R.J.; Adjei, J.K.; Park, M.; Saewyc, E.M. Investigating site-level longitudinal effects of population health interventions: Gay-Straight Alliances and school safety. *SSM Popul. Health* **2019**, *7*, 100350. [CrossRef] [PubMed]

71. Burk, J.; Park, M.; Saewyc, E.M. A Media-Based School Intervention to Reduce Sexual Orientation Prejudice and Its Relationship to Discrimination, Bullying, and the Mental Health of Lesbian, Gay, and Bisexual Adolescents in Western Canada: A Population-Based Evaluation. *Int. J. Environ. Res. Public Health* **2018**, *15*, 2447. [CrossRef] [PubMed]

72. Russell, S.T.; Kosciw, J.; Horn, S.; Saewyc, E.M. Safe schools policy for LGBTQ students. *SRCD Soc. Policy Rep.* **2010**, *24*, 1–25. [CrossRef]

73. DCYA. *LGBTI+ National Youth Strategy 2018–2020*; Department of Children and Youth Affairs: Dublin, Ireland, 2018.

74. Fineman, M.A. Vulnerability, Resilience, and LGBT Youth Symposium: LGBT youth: Reconciling pride, family, and community. *Temple Political Civ. Rights Law Rev.* **2013**, *23*, 307–330.

75. Riggle, E.D.B.; Rostosky, S.S. *A Positive View of LGBTQ: Embracing Identity and Cultivating Well-Being*; Rowman & Littlefield Publishers, Inc.: Lanham, MD, USA, 2012.

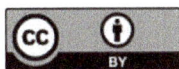

© 2019 by the authors. Licensee MDPI, Basel, Switzerland. This article is an open access article distributed under the terms and conditions of the Creative Commons Attribution (CC BY) license (http://creativecommons.org/licenses/by/4.0/).

International Journal of
*Environmental Research and Public Health*

MDPI

*Article*

# The Needs of LGBTI People Regarding Health Care Structures, Prevention Measures and Diagnostic and Treatment Procedures: A Qualitative Study in a German Metropolis

Ute Lampalzer *, Pia Behrendt, Arne Dekker, Peer Briken and Timo O. Nieder[iD]

Institute for Sex Research, Sexual Medicine and Forensic Psychiatry, University Medical Center
Hamburg-Eppendorf, 20246 Hamburg, Germany; p.behrendt@uke.de (Pi.B.); dekker@uke.de (A.D.);
briken@uke.de (P.B.); t.nieder@uke.de (T.O.N.)
* Correspondence: u.lampalzer@uke.de

Received: 25 July 2019; Accepted: 16 September 2019; Published: 22 September 2019

**Abstract:** (1) Background: Studies indicate that lesbian, gay, bisexual, transgender and intersex (LGBTI) people constantly face challenges and disadvantages in the health care system that prevent them from getting the best possible patient-centered care. However, the present study is the first to focus on LGBTI-related health in a major German metropolis. It aimed to investigate health care structures, prevention measures and diagnostic as well as treatment procedures that LGBTI individuals need in order to receive appropriate patient-centered health care and health promotion. (2) Methods: Following a participatory approach, five expert interviews with LGBTI people with multiplier function, i.e., people who have a key role in a certain social milieu which makes them able to acquire and spread information in and about this milieu, and three focus groups with LGBTI people and/or health professionals were conducted. Qualitative data were analyzed according to the principles of content analysis. (3) Results: The specific needs of LGBTI individuals must be recognized as a matter of course in terms of depathologization, sensitization, inclusion, and awareness. Such an attitude requires both basic knowledge about LGBTI-related health issues, and specific expertise about sufficient health care services for each of the minorities in the context of sex, sexual orientation and gender identity. (4) Conclusions: For an appropriate approach to LGBTI-centered health care and health promotion, health professionals will need to adopt a better understanding of specific soft and hard skills.

**Keywords:** diversity; gender; health care system; homosexuality; LGBTI

---

## 1. Introduction

"The mission of the International Psychology Network for Lesbian, Gay, Bisexual, Transgender and Intersex Issues (IPsyNet) is to facilitate and support the contributions that the discipline of psychology makes to a global understanding of human sexuality and gender diversity so as to ensure the health and well-being of people around the world who identify, or are perceived as, lesbian, gay, bisexual, transgender, intersex, queer, or sexually and gender diverse people (LGBTIQ+)" [1]. The IPsyNet consists of psychological organizations from different countries from around the world and their Statement on LGBTIQ+ Concerns states: "LGBTIQ+ identities and expressions are normal and healthy variations of human functioning and relationships" [1]. In line with this, guidelines, policy statements, and human rights initiatives emphasized in recent years that ignorance, discrimination, stigmatization and lack of knowledge are major problems in the health care of lesbian, gay, bisexual, transgender and intersex (LGBTI) people. The term transgender is used as an umbrella term for people whose gender identity does not (completely) correspond with their sex characteristics (e.g., people who identify as trans, transsexual, nonbinary, or genderqueer). Intersex is used as an umbrella term to denote a number of different variations (chromosomal, gonadal, hormonal, and phenotypical) in a person's innate bodily characteristics that do not all correspond with one or the same sex. LGB people can be cisgender (meaning that they feel that their gender is congruent with their sex characteristics), transgender, and intersex people. Guidelines, policy statements, and human rights initiatives aimed at tackling health disparities [2,3] to better ensure the health and well-being of LGBTI people [1,4], and called for LGBTI people's right to health [5–9]. The APA "Guidelines for Psychological Practice with Lesbian, Gay, and Bisexual Clients" highlight the need to understand the effects of stigma and the recognition of the unique experiences and challenges of lesbian, gay and bisexual clients [2]. The "Agenda 2030 for LGBTI Health and Well-Being" calls for commitment "to end stigma and discrimination based on sexual orientation, gender identity and expression, and sex characteristics ( ... ) in the provision of health care services, including prevention, promotion, and treatment" [4]. "HIV & Aids", "Mental Health & Well-Being", "Drug & Alcohol Use", "Sexual & Reproductive Health", "Universal Health Coverage", "Access to Affordable Medicines", and "Training of the Health Workforce" are named as important issues in LGBTI health and well-being [4]. Furthermore, a wide range of empirical research shows that these issues are specifically relevant for LGBTI individuals [9–30]. In summary, there is a call for equal opportunities for LGBTI individuals and heterosexual cisgender people in health care treatment on the one hand, as well as a need for specific patient-centered services for LGBTI individuals on the other hand.

Although many issues affect all LGBTI groups, it is nonetheless important to differentiate between gender identity and sexual orientation: "( ... ) gender identity and sexual orientation are distinct but interrelated constructs. ( ... ) *Sexual orientation* is defined as a person's sexual and/or emotional attraction to another person ( ... ), compared with *gender identity*, which is defined by a person's felt, inherent sense of gender" [3].

Medical guidelines for gender incongruence, gender dysphoria, and transgender health emphasize the need to take psychological, physical, social, and cultural aspects into consideration in the context of diagnostic and treatment procedures. Transition-related health care, such as mental health care (e.g., assistance to explore one's gender identity), endocrine care (e.g., sex hormones), surgeries (e.g., breast and/or genital reconstructive surgery), and so forth, should be tailored to the individual's needs [31–33]. Medical guidelines for the management of individuals with intersex conditions demand good medical care (e.g., careful clinical and biochemical evaluation, genetic counselling, longitudinal assessment). They also point out the importance of informed consent and psychosocial support, including peer support, mental health care, and communication skills training for health professionals [34–37]. Care for intersex and transgender clients requires interdisciplinary cooperation between different medical disciplines and mental health services [38,39]. Thus, medical and mental health care needs are strongly interlinked.

Several international and national qualitative studies have already investigated the health care needs of LGBTI people [9,17–22]. However, the present study is the first to investigate the health care needs of LGBTI people in Hamburg, a major German metropolitan city. Thus, it is still unknown whether the results of existing studies also prove true for health care in Hamburg. The present study is part of a larger research project about the challenges and problems with health promotion and health care for LGBTI people in Hamburg, Germany [40–42]. In 2017, the senate of Hamburg adopted an action plan for gender and sexual diversity, which contained eleven areas of activity for people between childhood and ninety years of age. The plan was a token of tolerance and openness in Hamburg. Financial resources were provided for 90 measures. With regards to content, the plan's aims were information, education, sensitization, making different concepts of living more common, and the protection of rights [43]. The present study is part of this action plan.

According to the relevant specialist literature, access to care, discrimination, knowledge and dissemination of knowledge about LGBTI health, as well as awareness and sensitivity regarding LGBTI communities, are prominent issues concerning the health care needs of LGBTI people [44,45]. These issues are reflected in the topics of the expert interviews and focus groups. The present study focuses on health care structures, prevention measures, and diagnostic and treatment procedures. Therefore, the research question is: what health care structures, prevention measures, and diagnostic as well as treatment procedures do LGBTI individuals need in order to receive needs-based health care and health promotion? The common needs of LGBTI individuals as well as the specific needs of each target group (L, G, B, T, and I) will be addressed.

## 2. Materials and Methods

This study was conducted at the Institute for Sex Research, Sexual Medicine and Forensic Psychiatry at the University Medical Center Hamburg-Eppendorf as part of a gender equality policy framework program of the Free and Hanseatic City of Hamburg (FHH). It took place from April 2017 to January 2018 and was approved by the ethics committee of the Chamber of Psychotherapists Hamburg (04/2017-PTK-HH).

The present study took a qualitative approach. We were interested in specific and detailed experiences of professionals and/or clients in the health care system and aimed at discovering and understanding how the participants view their living conditions under these circumstances. Thus, a person-centered and participatory approach seemed to be appropriate to learn more about factors influencing LGBTI health in Hamburg [46,47]. The main purpose was to collect what problems and challenges LGBTI people face in Hamburg's health care.

Data comprised five expert interviews with LGBTI people conducted in June and July 2017 and three focus groups with three to six participants in September 2017. Prior to participation, participants were provided with information about this study, including the approximate length of time for participation, data protection, and the goals of this study. Afterwards, they were asked to give informed consent. All audio recordings were transcribed and pseudonymized. Personal data that would have enabled inferences about specific interviewees were not recorded. Participants were able to withdraw from this study during and after their participation without explanation. They would have been identified by an individual code generated at the beginning of the interviews. No one withdrew from participation.

According to Denzin's [48] basic types of triangulation, the present study ensured data triangulation via multiple data sources, i.e., experts who were interviewed because of their function as multiplier key people and people in their role as private individuals who took part in focus groups. Investigator triangulation was accomplished via integrating three researchers in the process of data collection, data analysis and interpretation. Methodological triangulation was assured when using two different qualitative methods of data collection, i.e., expert interviews and focus groups.

### 2.1. Expert Interviews

Based on current research literature, an interview guideline (Appendix A) was developed including the most prominent issues [42]:

1.     What kind of observable disadvantages in specific treatment/advice situations exist?

In the context of information about specific groups of the LGBTI community:

2.     To what extent does a lack of knowledge about each group persist?
3.     How available is the information on specific groups?

For the expert interviews, professional key people of the focused target groups were recruited in the Hamburg area, who in addition to their own health care experiences knew of the experiences of other people in the respective group with medical and mental health professionals (as a multiplier, i.e., as a person who is able to acquire and spread information in and about their milieu). Email requests were sent to relevant counselling centers, specialized practices, interest groups, authorities and self-help organizations. Finally, participants were recruited from BiNe e. V. (expert for bisexual people (EB)), Charlotte e. V. (expert for lesbian women (EL)), Hein and Fiete (expert for gay men (EG)), Intersexuelle Menschen e. V. (expert for intersexual people (EI)) and Magnus-Hirschfeld-Zentrum (mhc) (expert for transgender people (ET)). The interviews took place at the Institute for Sex Research or, if desired, at the workplace or home of the experts and lasted between 43 and 72 minutes. All of the interviews were conducted by the same researcher of the team (U.L.) to ensure a comparable standard. A second researcher of the team (Pi.B.) took part as a participant observer to reveal potential differences in the approach of the interviewees and decrease potential biases in the further research process.

Data were analyzed using the software tool ATLAS.ti, following the iterative process of qualitative content analysis [49]: the interviews were read several times by three researchers (U.L., Pi.B., T.O.N.). Based on the research questions, these three researchers built a system of categories by initial coding and rechecking the interview material. In the end, the results were put together thematically in order to frame the main and subcategories. Frequent comparisons and adjustments of the results by the three independent assessors ensured the interrater reliability of the results.

*2.2. Focus Groups*

Based on qualitative data of the expert interviews conducted previously, a discussion guide was developed which covered the following three main topics:

1. How should each of the LGBTI-groups be addressed so that they can use the health system when needed?
2. With what attitude should skilled professionals approach their clients from the LGBTI groups?
3. To what extent does the community influence the use of health care?

The focus groups were conducted in the same way as the expert interviews (see above); representatives of the LGBTI groups and experts from professional practice were contacted. Since the focus was on personal experiences, the function as a multiplier key person was not a prerequisite for participation. Therefore, one participant was recruited by visiting a regular meeting for bisexual people and another responded via an advertisement on an internet platform. The focus groups involved three to six people aged between 30 and 63 years (focus group 1 included, by their own definition, a queer lesbian cis woman (F1L), a gay cis man (F1G), and a hetero bisexual inter man (F1B); focus group 2 included a questioning cis woman, a lesbian woman (F2L), a gay transman (F2T), and a hetero–pansexual cis inter man (F2I); focus group 3 included a heterosexual cis woman, a lesbian woman (F3L), a gay man (F3G), a bisexual woman (F3B), a gay transman (F3T) and an intersex man (F3I)). (Since the overarching project [42] also addressed heterosexual cisgender people, a questioning cis woman and a heterosexual cis woman also took part in the focus groups. However, the present evaluation refers solely to statements made by LGBTI people.)

The focus groups took place at the Institute for Sex Research and were moderated by the principal investigator (T.O.N.) and the research fellow (U.L.). The student assistant (Pi.B.) documented the process as a participating observer in order to ensure that possible biases due to the personalities of the moderators were revealed and decreased in the further process of investigation. The discussions lasted between 93 and 105 minutes.

The evaluation procedure of this data was the same as for the expert interviews. The already existing category system of the expert interviews was used for the evaluation, which consequently was again checked for its suitability, validated and extended by one subcategory (9.4). The results presented in this paper refer to the categories "requests—structures", "availability (lacking)", "prevention measures", "diagnostic procedures", and "treatment procedures", as these are the categories that are directly linked to the research questions of this study. The category system is set out in Table 1. The direct quotes were translated by T.O.N. (Since the original quotes were in German, T.O.N. and an English proofreader looked for the best possible translation).

**Table 1.** Overview of main categories and subcategories.

| Experts and Focus Groups | EL | EG | EB | ET | EI | Focus Group 1: | Focus Group 2: | Focus Group 3: | |
|---|---|---|---|---|---|---|---|---|---|
| **Main and Subcategories** | | | | | | **Approach** | **Attitude** | **Community** | **In Total** |
| 1. Requests—people | 1 | 0 | 0 | 4 | 1 | 6 | 12 | 2 | 26 |
| 2. Requests—structures | 1 | 5 | 6 | 0 | 2 | 10 | 6 | 3 | 33 |
| 3. Training (incl. further education) | 2 | 4 | 0 | 0 | 2 | 11 | 10 | 4 | 33 |
| 4. Public image | 2 | 4 | 1 | 1 | 1 | 10 | 1 | 11 | 31 |
| 5. Treatment procedures | 3 | 1 | 2 | 4 | 3 | 12 | 12 | 3 | 40 |
| 6. Diagnostic procedures | 0 | 3 | 1 | 7 | 2 | 7 | 0 | 0 | 20 |
| 7. Discrimination | 6 | 4 | 0 | 1 | 6 | 11 | 7 | 6 | 41 |
| 8. Living worlds/situations/realities | | | | | | | | | |
| 8.1 Acceptance | 0 | 4 | 2 | 0 | 0 | 3 | 3 | 5 | 17 |
| 8.2 Coming-out | 0 | 3 | 1 | 0 | 0 | 2 | 2 | 1 | 9 |
| 8.3 Diversity of life forms | 0 | 3 | 3 | 1 | 0 | 1 | 0 | 2 | 10 |
| 8.4 Life stages | 0 | 2 | 1 | 0 | 0 | 2 | 0 | 1 | 6 |
| 8.5 Sex | 1 | 6 | 1 | 0 | 1 | 0 | 0 | 0 | 9 |
| 8.6 Scene/Community | 0 | 2 | 3 | 0 | 0 | 2 | 0 | 11 | 18 |
| 9. Networks | | | | | | | | | |
| 9.1 Address lists | 1 | 1 | 1 | 0 | 1 | 0 | 0 | 2 | 6 |
| 9.2 Interlocking | 0 | 4 | 0 | 0 | 0 | 0 | 0 | 1 | 5 |
| 9.3 Referral | 0 | 1 | 0 | 2 | 0 | 0 | 0 | 1 | 4 |
| 9.4 Mouth-to-mouth | 0 | 0 | 0 | 0 | 0 | 3 | 0 | 4 | 7 |
| 10. Openness/Willingness to communicate | 4 | 4 | 0 | 1 | 1 | 7 | 12 | 23 | 52 |
| 11. Economics | 0 | 3 | 0 | 0 | 1 | 1 | 4 | 0 | 9 |
| 12. Prevention measures | 1 | 2 | 0 | 3 | 1 | 0 | 0 | 1 | 8 |
| 13. Sensitization (Attitude) | 3 | 0 | 3 | 5 | 1 | 16 | 24 | 19 | 71 |
| 14. Sexually transmitted infections | 4 | 6 | 0 | 0 | 0 | 4 | 0 | 4 | 18 |
| 15. (In-)Visibility | 2 | 0 | 0 | 1 | 1 | 6 | 4 | 6 | 20 |
| 16. Availability (lacking) | 3 | 1 | 4 | 5 | 4 | 3 | 7 | 6 | 33 |
| 17. Bias/prejudices | 1 | 1 | 2 | 1 | 0 | 1 | 0 | 2 | 8 |
| In total | 35 | 64 | 31 | 36 | 28 | 118 | 104 | 118 | 534 |

## 3. Results

Four issues were identified by the interviewees and will be presented in more detail: 1. health care structures, 2. human resources, 3. prevention measures, and 4. diagnostic and treatment procedures.

### 3.1. Health Care Structures

Interviewees of all LGBT groups complained about too little psychosocial and/or psychotherapeutic care offered for LGBTI issues.

**EG:** "There is a severe shortage of psychologists and psychiatrists in Hamburg [especially compared to Hamburg's well-established network of specialized medical practices for HIV/STI, UL]."

Interviewees from all LGBTI groups demanded more contact points in the health care system specialized for the group's specific needs.

**F2B:** "A bisexual person is not interested in gay counselling [ … ] or a lesbian coffee shop or similar".

The introduction of an LGBTI certificate for health care professionals who are trained in LGBTI issues was proposed as an approach for making LGBTI people's access to adequate health care easier.

**F1G:** "[ … ] the largest operator of seniors' and nursing homes in Munich just started a model project [ … ] and presents the rainbow flag on its website [ … ]. Unfortunately, this does not mean much, as it is still unknown how gays, lesbians, inter- and trans-people are approached. It is different in Holland. They have a certification procedure [ … ], which is also examined by a third party."

**F1I:** "This has to be accepted by both sides, the community and [health care professionals]."

Lesbian interviewees voiced the need for more information materials concerning lesbian health care concerns so that lesbians are sensitized accordingly and make use of health care services appropriate to their needs. F1L also expressed the need for more research in the field of lesbian health. In addition, she recommended implementing a permanent contact person who knew about LGBTI health and could be asked for advice in medical centers.

**F1L:** "If there are any reasons why they [other professionals] do not address such [LGBTI-related] issues, then I [as an LGBTI person] could do it."

EB explained that there was a lack of visible health care services for bisexual people. He highlighted the need for low-level counseling especially.

**EB:** "A low-level counselling service, that's it. ( … ) Where fears can be reduced by receiving answers to questions that are asked frequently: 'What is happening to me? I am currently changing, do I have to be afraid? ( … ) So that all those who think 'ah, I feel bad', have a service that helps them and makes them feel recognized."

ET also said that there was a lack of low-level health care services. He complained about long waiting times for physician and psychotherapist appointments and also mentioned a lack of couple therapy and gynecological services for transgender people. Furthermore, transgender interviewees stressed the importance of quality control, particularly because transgender people depended on referrals from mental health professionals in order to get treatment for gender dysphoria. F3T pointed to problems with the reimbursement from health insurances.

**F2T:** "You can't chose freely as with a general physician. You are happy when you find the right professional and then you try hard ( … ) to make it work, even though it's actually invasive or unprofessional or just doesn't fit. ( … ) Especially in the field of transgender, where the people concerned depend on getting a referral to go on hormones."

**F3T:** "This simply cannot be accounted for by the health system, because some treatments are linked to gender. Why should a transman go to a gynecologist? That doesn't make any sense at all."

EI, as well as EB, stressed the need for visible health care services, in this case for intersex health care. In this respect, she also highlighted that more peer support was needed, as recommended by the guidelines for intersex care. Moreover, she said that health care services should be evaluated and that quality management was required. Furthermore, she stated that there was no health care service for correct care of a neovagina. F1I complained about the struggle to get the complete patient records of all intersex treatment measures of the past. Similar to F3T, F3I mentioned serious problems with the payment and settlement system.

**F3I:** "Then I went to an endocrinologist and wanted to substitute testosterone, but I was supposed to pay for testosterone myself, because I was assigned female and therefore can't get testosterone. ( … ) At one point, they understood and now they reimburse the costs regularly."

## 3.2. Prevention Measures

For all the different perspectives, cancer prevention was a topic of importance. EL said that in lesbian women the "standard reasons" of heterosexual women for visiting a gynecologist (pregnancy, contraception) did not exist. However, since, for example, the same cancer screening was indicated as for heterosexual women, it was important to provide lesbian women with additional information. EL also mentioned that among lesbian women, the frequency of smoking, alcohol consumption and problem drug use was higher than among heterosexual women—a fact that also shows a need for prevention measures.

EG did not mention cancer prevention but highlighted the need for STI prevention and addiction prevention, also because there was a trend for chemsex (i.e., having sex under the influence of synthetic drugs) in the gay scene. Moreover, he said that the suicide rate was higher among gay men than among heterosexual men and talked about a self-help group called "gay and depressive", thus pointing to the need for suicide and depression prevention.

ET pointed out that in basic health care, he did not know about any prevention programs but only knew about self-organized prevention programs from the transgender activist scene. Transgender interviewees highlighted the need for gynecological and urological prevention measures that were often overlooked with regard to transgender people. In addition, ET expressed the need for prevention of harm, e.g., for transmen who used breast binders.

> **ET:** "What happens after a mastectomy with the breast cancer screening? Will it still be performed or not? ( … ) Urological topics—what about them? Is it clear to people that they still have to take screenings? Are they still actively invited?"

> **ET:** "The whole issue of 'breast binding or not ', i.e., prevention of harm. ( … ) Just to find a good way to deal with the own body."

EI made a plea for adequate counselling regarding degeneration risks for parents of intersex children.

> **EI:** "If I have a child who has a risk, a 32% risk of degeneration of hormone-producing organs ( … ), then I am shocked. But when I am told that my child has a 32% risk of becoming ill with this organ in the second half of his life from the age of 40, then this is a problem that we will have to look at later. But that's what it's all about. Just to give professional counselling."

## 3.3. Diagnostic Procedures

Concerning the diagnostic procedures and issues of openness, heedfulness, physical and psychological health risks of LGBTI people, comorbidities and differential diagnostics were addressed.

F1L advocated authenticity and openness in cases of a lack of expertise, e.g., in the context of LGBTI health. She also pointed to the reality medical doctor having to deal with limited timeslots for each patient.

> **F1L:** "I say 'Okay, this is important, I have to do research, I have to inform myself. Please come back.'"

> **F1L:** "I don't think there's time for that in a regular situation like this. I don't know which physician also asks about the mental state. So, if anybody comes to me and suffers pain, I treat it."

EG stressed that nicotine and alcohol consumption as well as the number of suicides were higher among gay men than among heterosexual men. He pointed out that considering not only medical-physical but also medical-psychological aspects and possibly the need for psychological care was important when seeing gay men.

**EG:** "A relationship that you had for ten years before you were out, and then ends, has a different story than a heterosexual relationship. ( … ) It might express itself in stomach pains and something like that. Then you go to the doctor who treats you with stomach pills. But the symptom is actually a different one—and it's about being sensitive to it."

F1G stated that knowing about a patient's homosexuality might be relevant in the process of diagnostics.

**F1G:** "If there really are specific health problems, I say, 'Okay, I'm homosexual. Please note that. This might be important to know.'"

EB mentioned that especially in the first stages of coming out, there was a higher risk of psychosomatic problems.

**EB:** "So, the most common is definitely depression—and sleep disorders. ( … ) And the coming out is a big topic for many: 'I somehow decide on something. And what do I choose?' And this confusion is great and leads to all sorts of psychosomatic symptoms."

ET highlighted the problem that for transgender people, common standards for males and females might not be applicable and had to be taken into consideration. Moreover, he stressed that precise differential diagnostics and carefully dealing with comorbidities was highly important. In this respect, he also mentioned that there was the danger that somatic health professionals totally ignored psychological aspects.

**ET:** "In the manic phase, is this just the acting-out of trans femininity or does it simply belong in the psychotic sphere? ( … ) Or something like that: That belongs to trans, that belongs to eating disorders, that belongs to fear and panic, that belongs to depression. ( … ) And then to look at the group of diagnoses. ( … ) And the separation of 'Is this acutely related to my transition' ( … )—or is it related to other issues where Trans also plays a role, and I have to interrupt some hormones somehow. ( … ) And with the medical doctors ( … ), I have the feeling that this is still completely different, because they say: 'Well, everything that has to do with the psyche—we just need the referral letter."

Apart from that, ET stressed that a transman's desire to have children should not prevent experts from giving an indication for transgender treatment.

EI stressed a similar issue when expressing that carefully questioning causality was necessary, namely if psychological problems were caused by medical issues, or rather the other way around.

**EI:** "This mental side has its origin very often in a preceding medical treatment [EI for example refers to medically unnecessary surgeries on intersex children in early childhood—such as genital surgeries and gonadectomies with the effect of a need for a lifelong treatment of synthetic sex hormones –, often without a precise patient education even in adulthood]."

F1I mentioned the issue of coming out as intersex towards health professionals and made clear that for some patients it was easy whereas others were shy or ashamed. In addition, he stressed that in the context of intersex being classified as a rare disease, abusive curiosity had to be banned absolutely.

**F1I:** "What also does not work is the demonstration of affected people in the hospital: 'Ah, you are a Klinefelter. Can we see your testicles? Yes, for a moment.' ( … ) I know of cases where that was very distressing."

*3.4. Treatment Procedures*

Regarding treatment procedures, the interviewees on the one hand named contexts in which the sexual orientation should definitely be considered and on the other hand contexts in which it should more or less be ignored. Moreover, the fear of discrimination, the wish for open-mindedness and knowledgeable treatment came up as issues of concern.

EL expressed the need for providing lesbians good support in getting fertility treatment when they asked for it. She stressed that there was a lack of respective services especially in Hamburg:

> **EL:** "Well, in terms of fertility treatment, Hamburg lags behind Munich and Erlangen—and Berlin anyway."

> **EL:** "And there are countries where I assume that they are not lesbian-friendly, but where reproductive medicine is still handled openly and liberally, so there are no barriers."

In the context of pregnancy, F1L underlined that gynecologists should not be more concerned about the family situation of lesbian women than of heterosexual women. She stated that for good health care during pregnancy, sexual orientation was not important.

> **F1L:** "Well, I have two children—and then again: 'Who is the father, how did you do that?' Which doesn't matter at all—nor does it matter in health care during pregnancy."

EG stressed that psychotherapists who treated gay men should be able to openly talk about sexuality, e.g., anal intercourse, because in case of tabooing the gay man's sexuality, effective psychotherapeutic treatment was impossible. Statements of F1G pointed to the fact that there were cases of medical treatments where sexual orientation was irrelevant, e.g., treatment of hemorrhoids at the proctologist, dental treatment, and influenza treatment, cases where it was relevant, e.g., for getting prophylaxis against hepatitis C, and cases where it might be relevant but should not be because otherwise it might be discrimination.

> **F1G:** "The treatment and examination [i.e., prostate biopsy], ( . . . ) everything was no problem. I didn't notice anything afterwards, ( . . . ) whether he was more reserved or treated me differently."

> **F1G:** "Well, in the hospital it was obvious to the staff that a man only has men visiting. But that didn't have any negative effects."

EB highlighted that a psychotherapist who treated a bisexual person could not hold the (wrong) view that bisexuality did not exist, a common assumption of the past that still sometimes existed. Apart from that, he stressed that bisexuality was no illness and did not require any treatment, but many bisexual people sought counseling anyways.

ET made a plea to use the whole scope of action in transgender treatment creatively and also trust the clients' abilities to make their own decisions in a self-determined way. He also mentioned that taking the time to 'wait and see' could be important for the process of a transgender person's self-development. In addition, in transgender treatment, he stressed the integration of all physical changes into the need to be cared for sufficiently, e.g., by also offering body therapy. F2T stressed that, if necessary, it was important to consider the effects of transgender treatment, but if not necessary, he did not want to explain anything about it. He mentioned that when he was at the beginning of his transition process, he was relieved that his gynecologist did not let him sit in the waiting room for long.

> **F2T:** "My personality is none of his [the doctor's] business or what my hobbies are or anything like that. But I want to be treated."

> **F2T:** "Still at the very beginning of my transition, I was at the gynecologist's and suddenly it was my turn, otherwise I always had to wait for ages. Well, I guess this is also a situation that usually gets rather uncomfortable when you sit there for an hour in the waiting room."

Intersex interviewees demanded that harmful treatment practices of the past, such as no ensured informed consent before treatment, had be disestablished. EI said that continuous support and practical psychosocial counselling was important in intersex care. Last but not least, she made a claim to always inform about all the treatment options, also the option of non-treatment.

**EI:** "Non-treatment as a treatment option for example ( . . . ), and accompanying it. You have to stand it. This is much more difficult than doing something quickly. ( . . . ) We don't know what we are doing, but we are doing it. Instead of saying: 'No, we don't know what will happen. Your child is so individual, we don't know that at all—and let's wait together, and we'll make sure together that he's fine.'"

F2I stressed the problem of using the right reference values when treating intersex people.

**F2I:** "There are female reference values on my laboratory sheet because I have a female civil status. However, for me the male reference values are more valid because I am under testosterone. ( . . . ) And then it says: 'But this value is too high and it is too low'. And then I had an endocrinologist, to whom I have to explain again with each treatment that this reference value should not be taken as a basis. This is tedious for me."

## 4. Discussion

The purpose of this study was to investigate the needs of LGBTI people regarding health care structures, prevention measures, and diagnostic as well as treatment procedures. Moreover, this study aimed at analyzing needs that affect both all LGBTI people and particular groups (L, G, B, T, and I). All in all, the participants did not differ very much from each other in their positions. Differences were mainly as a result of the examples given by the interviewees.

Consistent with topics included in relevant reference books on LGBT health, the following subjects were brought up: the health-related institutional culture and climate, mental health, health risk behaviors, substance use, suicide risk, internalized homophobia and disclosure, HIV and sexually transmitted infections, cancer, urologic and gynecologic care, interdisciplinary care, and parenting [44, 45]. The following topics, although regarded as relevant in specialized literature [44,45], were not explicitly mentioned: obesity, chronic illnesses, such as hypertension, asthma, and diabetes, intimate partner violence, living with disabilities, racial and ethnic minority populations, and aging. It is probably due to the interview partner's professional and/or personal background that these topics were not the focus. Compared to previous qualitative research on the needs of LGBTI people, the results of the present study are quite comparable. The fear of discrimination, lack of knowledge of health care professionals, higher risk of mental health problems, fear of disclosure, being confronted with unquestioned heteronormative assumptions, importance of visibility, and pathologization were also highlighted as important issues in previous studies conducted in the European Union [17,18], Australia [20], and the United States [19]. By contrast, with research from Zimbabwe, problems of stigmatization, discrimination, ill-informed personnel and lacking access to health care were much less prominent and serious, although also reported in Hamburg [21,22]. Previous evidence is extended by the present study and enriched by further qualitative content, e.g., personal experiences and concrete examples, from Hamburg, Germany.

Hereinafter, the needs voiced in the present study are discussed, classified into the needs of all target groups, the needs of LGB individuals, and the needs of transgender and intersex people.

### 4.1. Needs of all Target Groups

Regarding health care structures, needs expressed by interviewees that affect all LGBTI groups are related to an increase in psychosocial support and mental health care regarding LGBTI issues, contact points specialized on the specific needs of each LGBTI group as well as permanent contact people for LGBTI concerns in medical centers. Additionally, an LGBTI certificate for health care professionals trained in LGBTI issues was recommended.

These results show that LGBTI people receive insufficient attention in health care and wish to be protected from discriminatory practices. Previous research shows that especially subtle forms of discrimination are still common, e.g., via concealment or heteronormative assumptions [9,17,18,50]. The research project HEALTH4LGBTI by the European Union, which was also based on expert interviews and focus groups, revealed that access to appropriate medical services is often impeded for LGBTI people, and that there is a need for visible and identifiable LGBTI-friendly health care services [17].

Concerning prevention measures, the present study shows that there is a need for adequate cancer, STI/HIV, addiction, suicide and depression prevention for all LGBTI groups. This is in line with previous studies indicating that the smoking prevalence among LGBT people is significantly higher than in the general population, with bisexual and transgender people being at the highest risk for tobacco use [51]. Alcohol and drug abuse are also increased in LGBT populations [14,26,52–54]. According to the minority stress model, the higher smoking prevalence results from minority stress caused by internalized homonegativity and victimization that increase psychological distress [28]. LGBTI-tailored tobacco prevention programs, such as cessation classes, are also cancer prevention programs [51].

Apart from substance abuse, minority stress is also associated with a higher risk of mental health problems among LGBT populations, such as depression and suicide ideation [55–61]. Suicide prevention programs should support LGBTI people in developing a sense of belonging and improving self-esteem, e.g., via affirmative approaches and trainings for health care professionals to raise awareness on LGBTI issues [57]. There is evidence that LGBTI people are at increased risk for certain cancers and that screening programs do not sufficiently reach this population [14,17,62–65]. However, there is still a lack of much needed LGBTI cancer research and programs [62]. With regard to STI transmission, current research shows that gay men are at higher risk of HIV than other groups of people, that rates of HIV and other STIs are higher among transgender people than non-transgender people, and that there is a lack of research on the transmission of HIV among lesbian women [65–68]. This underlines the need for more and extended prevention programs indicated by the present study, such as "The Last Drag", the first known smoking cessation program designed for LGBT smokers [51] and other smoking cessation programs for LGBTI people that have proved to be successful [52], or "Start Talking. Stop HIV", a campaign for gay and bisexual men that aims to increase HIV-related communication and knowledge [69].

In the context of diagnostic investigation, treatment and counselling, the present study reveals a wish of LGBTI people for authenticity and openness, e.g., concerning a lack of knowledge, issues of coming-out, and mental stress, and a wish for the depathologization and elimination of ignorance of LGBTI concerns. This goes in line with the results of previous studies indicating a need for affirmative approaches and the training of health professionals [9,17,50,70,71]. Some interventions with LGBT or LGBTI content have already been researched and proven to be successful [72–74].

### 4.2. Needs of LGB People

With regard to health care structures, the present study indicates that there is a need for more information materials on lesbian health issues, more research in the field of lesbian health, more visibility of health care services that explicitly include bisexual people as a target group, and low-level counselling services for bisexual people, especially those who struggle with insecurities after becoming aware of their attraction to both male and female individuals. This contributes to previous research indicating that lesbians have more health risks but use preventive medical care less often and receive less quality care than other women [75,76]. It reflects research indicating that bisexual people represent an often ignored subgroup among gender and sexual minorities [77], that they experience even more health inequalities and minority stress due to biphobia in both heterosexual and gay and lesbian communities [17], and that bisexual women are less likely to disclose their identity than lesbian women [78]. Thus, bisexual people, on the one hand, rarely make themselves visible in health care and, on the other hand, no visible bisexual friendly health care services are offered. This indicates a great need for health care professionals with persistent awareness, an open attitude, and specific knowledge, which are factors that are associated with quality care for lesbian clients [79]. We also know from previous research that disclosure is associated with better outcomes and an improved quality of care [78].

As for prevention measures, the results of this study show that there is a risk of lesbian women to be disregarded concerning cancer screening because they do not go to gynecologists as often as heterosexual women. This is consistent with previous research that points to the increased risk of lesbian and bisexual women of developing cervical cancer compared to other women. The issue of gay and bisexual men being at much higher risk of anal cancer than the general male population was not mentioned in the present study but has to be considered in the development of screening programs, too [17]. The results of the present study also indicate that drug prevention for gay men should address the risks of sexualized drug use (chemsex). According to a study by Pufall et al. [80] chemsex is associated with "self-reported depression/anxiety, smoking, nonsexual drug use, risky sexual behaviours, STIs, and hepatitis C".

In view of treatment procedures, the results of this study point to the need for the elimination of discrimination, so that, for example, lesbian women get the same access to fertility treatment and the same trust in their abilities of being good mothers as heterosexual women, and that gay men are not treated differently from heterosexual men, e.g., at the proctologist. Moreover, this study indicates that health professionals who treat gay men must not be ashamed of talking about anal intercourse and that health professionals who treat bisexual people fully need to accept bisexuality as a distinct sexual orientation.

### 4.3. Needs of Transgender and Intersex People

Concerning health care structures, the present study points to a lack of low-level health care services, couple therapy and gynecological services for transgender people. Moreover, the results show that there is a need for more physicians and psychotherapists who treat transgender people because current waiting times are too long. Both transgender and intersex people express a need for the quality management of health care services and payment and settlement systems of health insurance that do not directly link certain services to a specific gender, e.g., testosterone substitution only to women. Especially for intersex people, there is a need for increasing peer support networks and giving patients access to their complete patient records. This study also reveals a demand for services that offer care for neovaginas. This contributes to research indicating that transgender individuals experience procedures that are necessary for medical transition as arduous, challenging and very complex [8,23,81–83]. It also contributes to findings that reveal barriers for LGBTI people when accessing health care, e.g., due to a lack of specialist mental health services and counselling services, unrecognized needs, a lack of relevant documents and protocols, and the use of pathologizing language and incorrect pronouns [17,18]. Moreover, it is in line with research that indicates a massive lack of counselling services for intersex people and parents of children with intersex conditions and a great wish especially for more peer support [84].

Regarding prevention measures, the results indicate a need for gynecological and urological prevention measures that address transgender and intersex people adequately. Furthermore, this study shows that for transgender people, the prevention of harm is important, e.g., in connection with the use of breast binders. The present study also shows that for intersex people, down-to-earth counselling regarding degeneration risk is relevant, neither exaggerating nor downplaying the risks. This underlines and expands previous research that points to the specific but insufficiently researched cancer risks for transgender people, e.g., due to hormone treatment [85,86], and intersex people, e.g., due to early fetal germ cells [87,88].

In the context of diagnostic investigation and treatment procedures, this study shows that it has to be taken into consideration that the reference values for males and females might not be valid for intersex and transgender people. Moreover, the results indicate a need for careful differential diagnostics, careful management of comorbidities, and careful assessment of interdependencies between somatic health aspects and psychological aspects. Regarding transgender people, this study points to the need for an unbiased treatment indication, the empowerment of clients, adequate support during treatment, and treatment procedures that are individually tailored to the needs of each client, including health care services that ensure the integration of physical changes into the whole self. These findings extend previous studies that indicate that transgender clients are very interested in support according to individual needs and high decision-making power concerning the treatment process [23], and that point to the higher prevalence of mental health problems, especially affective and anxiety disorders, among transgender people than the general population [53,68,89,90]. With regard to intersex people, this study points to a need for preventing abusive curiosity in the context of a rare disease, stopping the harmful treatment practices of the past, informing about all the treatment options, non-treatment included, and providing continuous support and practical psychosocial counselling. This underlines previous research that reveals the need for more knowledge and sensitivity on the part of medical professionals and the need for local medical and psychosocial support structures that are readily accessible [84,91].

### 4.4. Limitations

The findings of the present study might be limited because the pre-understanding of the researchers might have biased the questions that were posed in the interviews and focus groups. In order to counteract such biases, not only scientific studies but also grey and community literature was included in the literature research. In this way, blind spots were supposed to be detected. Since all qualitative studies can only have a limited number of participants, the generalizability of this study's results can be questioned. It is not possible to determine unambiguously whether all typical aspects were mentioned that have an impact on how LGBTI people feel and think regarding health services. However, professional literature and previous research indicate that the challenges and problems that were the subject of discussion are characteristic. Moreover, choosing experts who had a function as key people was supposed to ensure a certain generalizability, as they were familiar with a wide range of counselling experiences and could talk about issues that went far beyond their personal perspective. But certainly, the whole range of concerns of LGBTI people is not represented in this study. For example, women with transition experiences (transgender women) and people who do not have any connections to the LGBTI scene did not take part. Furthermore, certain topics were almost left out, e.g., care for older LGBTI people, questions of intersectionality (e.g., the situation of LGBTI people from a migration background or with disabilities) or the black market of phosphodiesterase type 5 (PDE-5) inhibitors. Specific health concerns of, for instance, pansexual, asexual or questioning people were not considered either. In addition, this study was limited to the Hamburg metropolis, due to the contracting authority. Thus, the experiences of LGBTI people who live in rural areas are not represented. Further research is needed in this respect.

Finally, qualitative content analysis according to Mayring [49] is a rather schematic analysis method so that the underlying pre-understanding of the researchers is not without relevance. This limitation was supposed to be minimized by building the categories inductively.

## 5. Conclusions

The present study demonstrates that, essentially, it is important to recognize LGBTI individuals and their needs. This is about recognizing depathologization and dealing consciously, sensitively and inclusively with LGBTI people in the health system. This can be done by, for example, visibly marking LGBTI expertise (e.g., with a rainbow sticker on the door label), or by actively including LGBTI individuals in cancer prevention programs (e.g., through mandatory invitations to cancer screening for all). Communication training (e.g., for gender-sensitive and integrative use of language), in-service training (e.g., for nursing staff) and sufficient opportunities for LGBTI-competent counselling and psychosocial care are equally important. General health care professionals should have some basic knowledge about LGBTI health issues, such as STI transmission, risks for certain mental problems, and somatic aspects of transgender and intersex clients. Beyond that, more psychotherapeutic services based on affirmative approaches are needed for LGBTI clients. Moreover, there is a lack of health care services with specific expertise for transgender and intersex clients.

**Author Contributions:** Conceptualization, T.O.N., A.D. and P.B.; methodology, T.O.N., A.D. and P.B.; software, U.L. and Pi.B.; validation, T.O.N., U.L. and Pi.B.; formal analysis, T.O.N., U.L. and Pi.B.; investigation, T.O.N., U.L. and Pi.B.; resources, T.O.N., A.D. and P.B.; data curation, T.O.N., U.L. and Pi.B.; writing—original draft preparation, U.L. and Pi.B., T.O.N.; writing—review and editing, T.O.N., A.D. and P.B.; supervision, T.O.N., A.D. and P.B.; project administration, T.O.N.; funding acquisition, T.O.N., A.D. and P.B.

**Funding:** This research was funded by the Departmental Authority for Science, Research and Gender Equality of the Free and Hanseatic City of Hamburg (Behörde für Wissenschaft, Forschung und Gleichstellung der Freien und Hansestadt Hamburg).

**Acknowledgments:** The authors thank all the participants of the expert interviews and focus groups for their openness and dedication. The authors also thank the Departmental Authority for Science, Research and Gender Equality of the Free and Hanseatic City of Hamburg (Behörde für Wissenschaft, Forschung und Gleichstellung der Freien und Hansestadt Hamburg) for funding the project. Moreover, we thank Laura Pietras, MSc for English proofreading.

**Conflicts of Interest:** The authors declare no conflict of interest.

### Appendix A. Interview Guideline: "What Does Diversity Have in Common? On Equality between Women, men and LGBTI People Using Health Care in Hamburg"

Research question: What are the challenges and problems of health promotion and health care for women, men and LGBTI people in Hamburg?

Lead Text

Information on the goals of the study: Questioning the extent to which equality in health promotion and health care is ensured in Hamburg and at which points shortcomings exist which need to be addressed. In particular, investigation whether gender and/or sexual orientation have an impact on health care.

Information on the course of the study: Orientation on the guideline which is to ensure that the interviews are comparable. Introduction of colleague Pia Behrendt who pays attention to the comparability of the interviews and who documents relevant differences. Enquiries are possible so that no topic is omitted. Altogether, it is about exemplary experiences which can reflect personal and typical experiences.

Audio recording information: Consent for transcription and pseudonymization.

Data protection information: No recording of personal data that would enable inferences about specific interviewees.

Now, I would like to start by asking you a few short questions about your role as an expert, on which I am interviewing you today …

| Topic: Expert Function of the Interviewee |
| --- |
| **Research question**: What makes the interviewee an expert? |
| Concrete interview questions |
| We have chosen you against the background of your activities in the context of (institution the interviewee works for) as an expert for health promotion and health care for women/men/lesbian women/gay men/transgender people/intersexual people. Are there any other functions that qualify you as an expert for this topic?<br>Since when do you execute this function(s)?<br>Are there one or more main age groups that you mainly deal with in this function (these functions)?<br>If so, which? |

In the following, I will first ask questions about the experience of concrete treatment or counselling situations, then I will continue with questions about the specific knowledge of the treatment or counselling personnel and finally ask two questions about existing information needs.

Interview part I: observable disadvantages in concrete treatment/advice situations?

**Topic: Relationship Management**

**Research question**: How do the different groups of people experience relationship management on the part of the treatment or counselling personnel?

| Check/Memos | Concrete interview questions | Maintenance questions |
|---|---|---|
| - sensitive language<br>- recognition of individuality<br>- sufficient self-awareness/ reflection on the part of the practitioners/consultants<br>- good ability to talk openly about sexual orientation/sexuality<br>- disclosure of one's own way of life?<br>- promotion of resilience, resources, self-confidence<br>- caring behavior vs. promotion of self-determination | What do you know about how women/men/LGBTI people experience the relationship with the practitioners/consultants?<br>What do you know about how women/men/LGBTI people experience the behavior of practitioners or consultants towards them?<br><br>- concrete (positive and negative) experiences?<br>- concrete suggestions for improvement? | What do you know about how women/men/LGBTI people feel in treatment or counselling situations?<br>What other experiences can you report?<br>What other experiences can you describe? |

**Topic: Practices and Structures**

**Research question**: To what extent do health care practices and structures provide the best possible treatment/counselling for all groups of people?

| Check/Memos | Concrete interview questions | Maintenance questions |
|---|---|---|
| - knowledge of competent contact people (referral)<br>- legal knowledge<br>- formal discrimination * | Do you assume that women/men/LGBTI people always receive the best possible treatment or counselling? What do you attribute this to?<br><br>- concrete (positive and negative) experiences?<br>- concrete suggestions for improvement? | What do you know about when women/men/LGBTI people have been (very) satisfied with treatment or counselling?<br>Or (very) dissatisfied, and why was that? |

* includes disadvantages or exclusion in treatment processes or lack of access to rights and resources (vs. informal discrimination that affects verbal or non-verbal conduct that offends, excludes and impairs the integrity and well-being of the individuals).

| Topic: **Attitude towards the Group of People** | | |
|---|---|---|
| **Research question**: What is the attitude towards the different groups of people? | | |
| Check/Memos | Concrete interview questions | Maintenance questions |
| - affirmative attitude<br>- inclusive thinking<br>- prejudices<br>- LGBTI-friendly environment<br>- general openness for diversity<br>- interpersonal discrimination * | What do you know about the attitudes of treatment and counselling staff towards women/men/LGBTI people?<br><br>- concrete (positive and negative) experiences?<br>- concrete suggestions for improvement? | What (particularly) positive or (particularly) negative experiences are you aware of that have been made by women/men/LGBTI people, and what exactly has happened? |

\* refers, for example, to the mood that is transported verbally, the number of eye contacts, the time taken by the practitioners/consultants.

Interview part II: lack of knowledge about each group of people.

| Topic: **Expertise on the Specific Health Topics of the Respective Groups of People** | | |
|---|---|---|
| **Research question**: To what extent do health care professionals have sufficient expertise on the specific health issues of the groups? | | |
| Check/Memos | Concrete interview questions | Maintenance questions |
| - somatic health issues<br>- mental health issues<br>- knowledge about sexual orientation/sexuality<br>- relevant transmission pathways of HIV/STI<br>- cancer screening<br>- importance of smoking, alcohol, drugs | Do you have the impression that the treatment or counselling staff is sufficiently aware of the specific health concerns of women/men/LGBTI people? What do you attribute this to?<br><br>- concrete (positive and negative) experiences?<br>- concrete suggestions for improvement? | When did you discover or learn that specific knowledge was helpful or necessary - or would have been?<br>Imagine someone has a health question that concerns the person as a woman/man/LGBTI person. Who would you recommend as a contact person? |

| Topic: **Assumptions on Etiology** | | |
|---|---|---|
| **Research question**: What assumptions, which are specifically related to gender and/or sexual orientation, does the treatment or counselling staff have regarding the etiology of diseases/disorders? | | |
| Check/Memos | Concrete interview questions | Maintenance questions |
| - depathologization<br>- etiology of the development of sexual orientation/sex<br>- attitude towards conversion or reparative therapies | When do you have the impression that the health care professional is explaining a so-called disease or disorder with the help of sex or sexual orientation?<br><br>- concrete (positive and negative) experiences?<br>- concrete suggestions for improvement? | What other examples can you think of where gender or sexual orientation is used to explain a disease or disorder? |

| Topic: Life Reality of the Individual Groups of People | | |
|---|---|---|
| **Research question**: To what extent is there an awareness in health care of the reality of life of the various groups of people? | | |
| Check/Memos | Concrete interview questions | Maintenance questions |
| - experiencing otherness<br>- coming out process<br>- community/scene<br>- parenthood | To what extent do you have the impression that the practitioner or counsellor knows enough about the life situation as a woman/man/LGBTI person?<br><br>- concrete (positive and negative) experiences?<br>- concrete suggestions for improvement? | Do you think that the life reality of women/men/LGBTI people is sufficiently taken into account? Why? |

Interview part III: lack of availability of specific information for the relevant group of people.

| Topic: Provision of Target-Group-Specific Information | | |
|---|---|---|
| **Research question**: To what extent is specific information made available for the respective groups of people in the health care system? | | |
| Check/Memos | Concrete interview questions | Maintenance questions |
| - information on target-group-specific treatment/consulting offers<br>- flyers/brochures and the like<br>- access to treatment/counselling<br>- visibility of the groups of people | In your opinion, how well is information provided about health care services that specifically concern you, women/men/LGBTI?<br><br>- concrete (positive and negative) experiences?<br>- concrete suggestions for improvement? | Where do you get information about special health offers for you as a woman/man/LGBTI person? Imagine you have a health-related question that specifically concerns someone as a woman/man/LGBTI person. Where would you look for information?<br>What information do you have about special health care offers for you as a woman/man/LGBTI person? |

| TOPIC: Raising Awareness of Groups of People for Their Own Health Issues | | |
|---|---|---|
| **Research question**: To what extent are there efforts in health care recognizable which aim to sensitize the various groups of people to their health issues? | | |
| Check/Memos | Concrete interview questions → LAST QUESTION | Maintenance questions |
| - availability of information in online sources<br>- availability of information in brochures<br>- information provided by the practitioner/counsellor | How well do you think women/men/LGBTI people feel informed about health-relevant topics (e.g., prevention of diseases) that specifically concern you as a woman/man/LGBTI person?<br><br>- concrete (positive and negative) experiences?<br>- concrete suggestions for improvement? | Where do women/men/LGBTI people get information on health-relevant topics (e.g., prevention of diseases), which especially concern you as a woman/man/LGBTI person? What kind of health-relevant information (e.g., on the prevention of illnesses) do you know that is especially targeted at women/men/LGBTI people? |

Conclusions

Are there still important aspects of the topic that have not been considered enough in the previous interview?

Would you like to add anything else?

## References

1. American Psychological Association. International Psychology Network for Lesbian, Gay, Bisexual, Transgender and Intersex Issues (IPsyNet) Statement on LGBTIQ+ Concerns. Available online: https://www.apa.org/ipsynet/advocacy/policy/statement-english.pdf (accessed on 25 June 2019).
2. American Psychological Association. Practice guidelines for LGB clients. Guidelines for psychological practice with lesbian, gay, and bisexual clients. *Am. Psychol.* **2012**, *67*, 10–42. [CrossRef] [PubMed]
3. American Psychological Association. Guidelines for psychological practice with transgender and gender nonconforming people. *Am. Psychol.* **2015**, *70*, 832–864. [CrossRef] [PubMed]
4. The Global Advocacy Platform to Fast Track the HIV and Human Rights Responses with Gay and Bisexual Men. Agenda 2030 for LGBTI Health and Well-Being. Available online: https://www.aidsdatahub.org/sites/default/files/publication/Agenda_2030_for_LGBTI_Health_and_Well-Being_2017.pdf (accessed on 25 June 2019).
5. Amnesty International. *First, Do No Harm—Ensuring the Rights of Children with Variations of Sex Characteristics in Denmark and Germany*; Amnesty International: London, UK, 2017.
6. Council of Europe. *Discrimination on Grounds of Sexual Orientation and Gender Identity in Europe*, 2nd ed.; Council of Europe: Strasbourg, France; Available online: https://www.coe.int/t/Commissioner/Source/LGBT/LGBTStudy2011_en.pdf (accessed on 25 June 2019).
7. The Council of Europe Commissioner for Human Rights. Human Rights and Intersex People: Issue Paper published by the Council of Europe Commissioner for Human Rights. Available online: https://wcd.coe.int/com.instranet.InstraServlet?command=com.instranet.CmdBlobGet&InstranetImage=2870032&SecMode=1&DocId=2346276&Usage=2 (accessed on 25 June 2019).
8. FRA—European Agency for Fundamental Rights. Being Trans in the European Union. Comparative Analysis of EU LGBT Survey Data. Available online: https://fra.europa.eu/sites/default/files/fra-2014-being-trans-eu-comparative-0_en.pdf (accessed on 25 June 2019).
9. FRA—European Agency for Fundamental Rights. Professionally Speaking: Challenges to Achieving Equality for LGBT People. Available online: https://fra.europa.eu/sites/default/files/fra_uploads/fra-2016-lgbt-public-officials_en.pdf (accessed on 25 June 2019).
10. Albuquerque, G.A.; de Lima Garcia, C.; da Silva Quirino, G.; Alves, M.J.H.; Belém, J.M.; dos Santos Figueiredo, F.W.; da Silva Paiva, L.; do Nascimento, V.B.; da Silva Maciel, É.; Valenti, V.E.; et al. Access to health services by lesbian, gay, bisexual, and transgender persons: Systematic literature review. *BMC Int. Health Hum. Rights* **2016**. [CrossRef] [PubMed]
11. Almeida, J.; Johnson, R.M.; Corliss, H.L.; Molnar, B.E.; Azrael, D. Emotional distress among LGBT youth: The influence of perceived discrimination based on sexual orientation. *J. Youth Adolesc* **2009**, *38*, 1001–1014. [CrossRef] [PubMed]
12. ASRM Ethics Committee. Access to fertility treatment by gays, lesbians, and unmarried persons: A committee opinion. *Fertil. Steril.* **2013**, *100*, 1524–1527. [CrossRef] [PubMed]
13. Council of Europe. Discrimination on Grounds of Sexual Orientation and Gender Identity in Europe. Background Document. Available online: https://rm.coe.int/discrimination-on-grounds-of-sexual-orientation-and-gender-identity-in/16809079e2 (accessed on 25 June 2019).
14. Dean, L.; Meyer, I.H.; Robinson, K.; Sell, R.L.; Sember, R.; Silenzio, V.M.B.; Bowen, D.J.; Bradford, J.; Rothblum, E.; White, J.; et al. Lesbian, gay, bisexual, and transgender health: Findings and concerns. *J. Gay Lesbian Med. Assoc.* **2000**, *4*, 101–151. [CrossRef]
15. Drewes, J.; Kruspe, M. *Schwule Männer und HIV/AIDS 2013: Schutzverhalten und Risikomanagement in den Zeiten der Behandelbarkeit von HIV [Gay men and HIV/AIDS 2013: Protective Behaviour and Risk Management in Times of Treatability of HIV]*; DAH: Berlin, Germany, 2016.
16. Erbenius, T.; Payne, J.G. Unlearning cisnormativity in the clinic: Enacting transgender reproductive rights in everyday patient encounters. *J. Int. Womens Stud.* **2018**, *20*, 17–39.

17.  European Commission. Health4LGBTI, Reducing Health Inequalities Experienced by LGBTI People. Task 1: State-Of-The-Art Study Focusing on the Health Inequalities Faced by LGBTI People; D1.1 State-Of-The-Art Synthesis Report (SSR). Available online: https://ec.europa.eu/health/sites/health/files/social_determinants/docs/stateofart_report_en.pdf (accessed on 25 June 2019).
18.  European Commission. Health4LGBTI. Reducing Health Inequalities Experienced by LGBTI People. Task 2: Qualitative Research—Focus Groups Studies with LGBTI People and Health Professionals. D2.1 Final Overview Report on the Outcomes of the Focus Groups. Available online: https://ec.europa.eu/health/sites/health/files/social_determinants/docs/focusgroup_sr_en.pdf (accessed on 25 June 2019).
19.  Alpert, A.B.; CichoskiKelly, E.M.; Fox, A.D. What lesbians, gay, bisexual, transgender, queer, and intersex patients say doctors should know and do: A qualitative study. *J. Homosex* **2017**, *64*, 1368–1389. [CrossRef] [PubMed]
20.  Ansara, Y.G. Challenging cisgenderism in the ageing and aged care sector: Meeting the needs of older people of trans and/or non-binary experience. *Australas J. Ageing* **2015**, *34*, 14–18. [CrossRef] [PubMed]
21.  Hunt, J.; Bristowe, K.; Chidyamatare, S.; Harding, R. 'They will be afraid of you': LGBTI people and sex workers' experience of accessing healthcare in Zimbabwe—An in-depth qualitative study. *BMJ Glob. Health* **2017**, *2*, e000168. [CrossRef] [PubMed]
22.  Hunt, J.; Bristowe, K.; Chidyamatare, S.; Harding, R. 'So isolation comes in, discrimination and you find many people dying quietly without any family support': Accessing palliative care for key populations—An in-depth qualitative study. *Palliat. Med.* **2019**, *33*, 685–692. [CrossRef] [PubMed]
23.  Eyssel, J.; Köhler, A.; Dekker, A.; Sehner, S.; Nieder, T.O. Needs and concerns of transgender individuals regarding interdisciplinary transgender healthcare: A non-clinical online survey. *PLoS ONE* **2017**, *12*, e0183014. [CrossRef] [PubMed]
24.  Goldhammer, H.; Maston, E.D.; Kissock, L.A.; Davis, J.A.; Keuroghlian, A.S. National findings from an LGBTI healthcare organizational needs assessment. *LGBTI Health* **2018**, *5*, 461–468. [CrossRef] [PubMed]
25.  Gonzales, G.; Quinones, N.; Attanasio, L. Health and access to care among reproductive-age women by sexual orientation and pregnancy status. *Womens Health Issues* **2019**, *29*, 8–16. [CrossRef] [PubMed]
26.  Green, K.E.; Feinstein, B.A. Substance use in lesbian, gay, and bisexual populations: An update on empirical research and implications for treatment. *Psychol Addict. Behav* **2012**, *26*, 265–278. [CrossRef] [PubMed]
27.  Loos, F.; Köhler, A.; Eyssel, J.; Nieder, T.O. Subjektive Indikatoren des Behandlungserfolges und Diskriminierungserfahrungen in der trans* Gesundheitsversorgung. Qualitative Ergebnisse einer Online-Befragung [Subjective indicators of treatment success and experiences of discrimination in interdisciplinary trans* healthcare: Qualitative results from an online survey]. *Zeitschr. Sexualforsch.* **2016**, *29*, 205–223.
28.  Meyer, I.H. Prejudice, social stress, and mental health in lesbian, gay and bisexual populations: Conceptual issues and research evidence. *Psychol. Bull.* **2003**, *129*, 674–697. [CrossRef]
29.  Plöderl, M.; Tremblay, P. Mental health of sexual minorities. A systematic review. *Int. Rev. Psychiatry* **2015**, *27*, 367–385. [CrossRef]
30.  Zeeman, L.; Sherriff, N.; Browne, K.; McGlynn, N.; Mirandola, M.; Gios, L.; Davis, R.; Sanchez-Lambert, J.; Aujean, S.; Pinto, N.; et al. A review of lesbian, gay, bisexual, trans and intersex (LGBTI) health and healthcare inequalities. *Eur. J. Public Health* **2018**. [CrossRef]
31.  Coleman, E.; Bockting, W.; Botzer, M.; Cohen-Kettenis, P.; De Cuypere, G.; Feldman, J.; Fraser, L.; Green, J.; Knudson, G.; Meyer, W.J.; et al. Standards of care for the health of transsexual, transgender, and gender-nonconforming people, Version 7. *Int. J. Transgend.* **2012**, *13*, 165–232. [CrossRef]
32.  Deutsche Gesellschaft für Sexualforschung. Geschlechtsinkongruenz, Geschlechtsdysphorie und Trans-Gesundheit: S3-Leitlinie Zur Diagnostik, Beratung und Behandlung [Gender Incongruence, Gender Dysphoria and Trans Health: S3-Guideline on Diagnostics, Counselling and Treatment]. Available online: https://www.awmf.org/leitlinien/detail/ll/138-001.html (accessed on 30 May 2019).
33.  Nieder, T.; Strauß, B. S3-Leitlinie zur Diagnostik, Beratung und Behandlung im Kontext von Geschlechtsinkongruenz, Geschlechtsdysphorie und Trans-Gesundheit [S3-Guideline on diagnosis, counselling and treatment in the context of gender incongruence, gender dysphoria and trans health]. *Zeitschr. Sexualforsch.* **2019**, *32*, 70–79.

34. Bundesärztekammer. Stellungnahme der Bundesärztekammer: Versorgung von Kindern, Jugendlichen und Erwachsenen mit Varianten/Störungen der Geschlechtsentwicklung [Statement of the German Medical Association: Care of children, adolescents and adults with Disorders of Sex Develpment, DSD]. *Dtsch. Arztebl.* **2015**. [CrossRef]

35. Cools, M.; Nordenström, A.; Robeva, R.; Hall, J.; Westerveld, P.; Flück, C.; Köhler, B.; Berra, M.; Springer, A.; Schweizer, K.; et al. Caring for individuals with a difference of sex development (DSD): A consensus statement. *Nat. Rev. Endocrinol.* **2018**, *14*, 415–429. [CrossRef] [PubMed]

36. Lee, P.A.; Nordenström, A.; Houk, C.P.; Ahmed, S.F.; Auchus, R.; Baratz, A.; Baratz Dalke, K.; Liao, L.M.; Lin-Su, K.; Looijenga, L.H.J., 3rd; et al. Global disorders of sex development update since 2006: Perceptions, approach and care. *Horm. Res. Paediatr.* **2016**, *85*, 158–180. [CrossRef] [PubMed]

37. Deutsche Gesellschaft für Urologie (DGU) e.V.; Deutsche Gesellschaft für Kinderchirurgie (DGKCH) e.V.; Deutsche Gesellschaft für Kinderendokrinologie und-Diabetologie (DGKED) e.V. (Eds.) S2k-Leitlinie. Varianten der Geschlechtsentwicklung [S2k-Guideline. Variations of Sex Development]. 2016. Available online: http://www.awmf.org/uploads/tx_szleitlinien/174-001l_S2k_Geschlechtsentwicklung-Varianten_2016-08_01.pdf (accessed on 30 May 2019).

38. Malouf, M.A.; Wisniewski, A.B. Differences of sex development/intersex populations. In *Lesbian, Gay, Bisexual, and Transgender Healthcare. A Clinical Guide to Preventive, Primary, and Specialist Care*; Eckstrand, K.L., Ehrenfeld, J.M., Eds.; Springer: Cham, Switzerland; Heidelberg, Germany; New York, NY, USA; Dordrecht, The Netherlands; London, UK, 2016; pp. 405–420.

39. McIntosh, C.A. Interdisciplinary care for transgender patients. In *Lesbian, Gay, Bisexual, and Transgender Healthcare. A Clinical Guide to Preventive, Primary, and Specialist Care*; Eckstrand, K.L., Ehrenfeld, J.M., Eds.; Springer: Cham, Switzerland; Heidelberg, Germany; New York, NY, USA; Dordrecht, The Netherlands; London, UK, 2016; pp. 339–349.

40. Lampalzer, U.; Behrendt, P.; Dekker, A.; Briken, P.; Nieder, T.O. Was benötigen LSBTI-Menschen angesichts ihrer Sexual- und Geschlechtsbiografien für eine bessere Gesundheitsversorgung? Eine qualitative Untersuchung in einer deutschen Großstadt [What Do LGBTI People Need for Better Health Care with Regard to their Sexual and Gender Biographies? A Qualitative Study in a German Metropolis]. *Zeitschr. Sexualforsch.* **2019**, *32*, 17–26.

41. Lampalzer, U.; Behrendt, P.; Dekker, A.; Briken, P.; Nieder, T.O. LSBTI* und Gesundheit: Partizipative Forschung und Versorgung im Zusammenspiel von Sexualwissenschaft, Psychologie und Medizin. In *Sexuelle und Geschlechtliche Vielfalt. Interdisziplinäre Perspektiven aus Wissenschaft und Praxis*; Timmermanns, S., Böhm, M., Eds.; Beltz Juventa: Weinheim, Germany, 2019; pp. 256–273.

42. Lampalzer, U.; Behrendt, P.; Köster, E.M.; Dekker, A.; Briken, P.; Nieder, T.O. *Abschlussbericht zum Projekt Herausforderungen und Probleme in der Gesundheitsversorgung und -förderung für Frauen, "Männer und LSBTI-Menschen in Hamburg" gefördert von der Behörde für Wissenschaft, Forschung und Gleichstellung der Freien und Hansestadt Hamburg*; UKE, Behörde für Wissenschaft, Forschung und Gleichstellung der Freien und Hansestadt Hamburg: Hamburg, Germany, 2018; Unpublished work.

43. Freie und Hansestadt Hamburg. Aktionsplan für Akzeptanz Geschlechtlicher und Sexueller Vielfalt. Available online: https://www.hamburg.de/contentblob/8080476/1a25022ddb800a8d89fd5616b2b5a654/data/d-broschuere-aktionsplan-fuer-akzeptanz-geschlechtlicher-und-sexueller-vielfalt-.pdf (accessed on 20 August 2019).

44. Eckstrand, K.L.; Ehrenfeld, J.M. (Eds.) *Lesbian, Gay, Bisexual, and Transgender Healthcare. A Clinical Guide to Preventive, Primary, and Specialist Care*; Springer: Cham/Heidelberg, Germany; New York, NY, USA; Dordrecht, The Netherlands; London, UK, 2016.

45. Smalley, K.B.; Warren, J.C.; Barefoot, K.N. *LGBT Health, Meeting the Needs of Gender and Sexual Minorities*; Springer: New York, NY, USA, 2018.

46. Cropley, A.J. *Qualitative Research Methods: A Practice-Oriented Introduction for Students of Psychology and Education*, 2nd ed.; Zinātne: Riga, Latvia, 2019.

47. Northridge, M.E.; McGrath, B.P.; Krueger, S.Q. Using Community-Based Participatory Research to Understand and Eliminate Social Disparities in Health for Lesbian, Gay, Bisexual, and Transgender Populations. In *The Health of Sexual Minorities. Public Health Perspectives on Lesbian, Gay, Bisexual and Transgender Populations*; Meyer, I.H., Northridge, M.E., Eds.; Springer: Boston, MA, USA, 2007; pp. 455–470.

48. Denzin, N.K. *The Research Act in Sociology*; Aldine: Chicago, IL, USA, 1970.

49. Mayring, P. Qualitative Inhaltsanalyse. In *Grundlagen und Techniken*, 11th ed.; Beltz: Weinheim, Germany, 2010.

50. Wolf, G.; Meyer, E. Sexuelle Orientierung und Geschlechtsidentität—(k)ein Thema in der Psychotherapie? [Sexual orientation and gender identity – a topic in psychotherapy or not?]. *Psychotherapeutenjournal* **2017**, *16*, 130–135.

51. Burkhalter, J.E. Smoking in the LGBT community. In *Cancer and the LGBT Community. Unique Perspectives from Risk to Survivorship*; Boehmer, U., Elk, R., Eds.; Springer: Heidelberg, Germany, 2015; pp. 63–80.

52. Berger, I.; Mooney-Somers, J. Smoking cessation programs for lesbian, gay, bisexual, transgender, and intersex people: A content-based systematic review. *Nicotine Tob. Res.* **2017**, *19*, 1408–1417. [CrossRef]

53. Lawrence, A.A. Transgender health concerns. In *The Health of Sexual Minorities: Public Health Perspectives on Lesbian, Gay, Bisexual, and Transgender Populations*; Meyer, I.H., Northridge, M.E., Eds.; Springer Science + Business Media: New York, NY, USA, 2007; pp. 473–505.

54. Weber, G.; Dodge, A. Substance use among gender and sexual minority youth and adults. In *LGBT Health. Meeting the Needs of Gender and Sexual Minorities*; Smalley, K.B., Warren, J.C., Barefoot, K.N., Eds.; Springer: New York, NY, USA, 2018; pp. 199–213.

55. Cohn, T.J.; Casazza, S.P.; Cottrell, E.M. The mental health of gender and sexual minority groups in context. In *LGBT Health. Meeting the Needs of Gender and Sexual Minorities*; Smalley, K.B., Warren, J.C., Barefoot, K.N., Eds.; Springer: New York, NY, USA, 2018; pp. 161–179.

56. Ott, A.; Garcia Nuñez, D. Der Substanzkonsum von trans* Personen aus der Minoritätenstressperspektive [Substance Use of Transgender and Gender Non-Conforming People from a Minority Stress Perspective]. *Suchttherapie* **2018**, *19*, 193–198.

57. Plöderl, M.; Kravolec, K.; Fartacek, C.; Fartacek, R. Homosexualität als Risikofaktor für Depression und Suizidalität bei Männern [Homosexuality as a risk factor for depression and suicidal behaviour in men]. *Blickpkt. Mann* **2009**, *7*, 28–37.

58. Plöderl, M.; Wagenmakers, E.J.; Tremblay, P.; Ramsay, R.; Kralovec, K.; Fartacek, C.; Fartacek, R. Suicide risk and sexual orientation: A Critical Review. *Arch. Sex. Behav.* **2013**, *42*, 715–727. [CrossRef]

59. Takács, J. *Social Exclusion of Young Lesbian, Gay, Bisexual and Transgender (LGBT) People in Europe*; ILGA-Europe & IGLYO: Brussels, Belgium; Amsterdam, The Netherlands, 2006.

60. Wolf, G. Trans* und Substanzgebrauch: Bedingungen und Behandlungsempfehlungen [Trans* People and Substance Abuse: Conditions and Recommendations for Treatment]. *Suchttherapie* **2018**, *19*, 186–192.

61. Wilson, C.; Cariola, L.A. LGBTQI+ youth and mental health: A systematic review of qualitative research. *Adolesc. Res. Rev.* **2019**. [CrossRef]

62. Elk, R.; Boehmer, U. The challenges remain: Needed next steps in alleviating the burden of cancer in the LGBT community. In *Cancer and the LGBT Community. Unique Perspectives from Risk to Survivorship*; Boehmer, U., Elk, R., Eds.; Springer: Heidelberg, Germany, 2015; pp. 313–328.

63. Fallinn-Bennett, K.; Henderson, S.L.; Nguyen, G.T.; Hyderi, A. Primary care, prevention, and coordination of care. In *Lesbian, Gay, Bisexual, and Transgender Healthcare. A Clinical Guide to Preventive, Primary, and Specialist Care*; Eckstrand, K.L., Ehrenfeld, J.M., Eds.; Springer: Cham/Heidelberg, Germany; New York, NY, USA; Dordrecht, The Netherlands; London, UK, 2016; pp. 95–114.

64. Kathrins, M.; Kolon, T.F. Malignancy in disorders of sex development. *Transl. Androl. Urol.* **2016**, *5*, 794–798. [CrossRef] [PubMed]

65. O'Hanlan, K.A.; Isler, C.M. Health care of lesbians and bisexual women. In *The Health of Sexual Minorities*; Meyer, I.H., Northridge, M.E., Eds.; Springer: Boston, MA, USA, 2007; pp. 506–522.

66. Centers for Disease Control and Prevention. HIV Among Gay and Bisexual Men. Available online: https://www.thebodypro.com/article/hiv-among-gay-and-bisexual-men (accessed on 25 June 2019).

67. Horvath, K.J.; Yared, N.; Lammert, S.; Lifson, A.; Kulasingam, S. HIV and other sexually transmitted infections within the gender and sexual minority community. In *LGBT Health. Meeting the Needs of Gender and Sexual Minorities*; Smalley, K.B., Warren, J.C., Barefoot, K.N., Eds.; Springer: New York, NY, USA, 2018; pp. 215–243.

68. Reisner, S.L.; Poteat, T.; Keatley, J.; Cabral, M.; Mothopeng, T.; Dunham, E.; Holland, C.E.; Max, R.; Baral, S.D. Global health burden and needs of transgender populations: A systematic review. *Lancet* **2016**, *388*, 412–436. [CrossRef]

69. Centers for Disease Control and Prevention. Start Talking. Stop HIV. Available online: https://www.cdc.gov/actagainstaids/campaigns/starttalking/index.html (accessed on 5 July 2019).

70. Braun, H.M.; Garcia-Grossman, I.R.; Quiñones-Rivera, A.; Deutsch, M.B. Outcome and Impact Evaluation of a Transgender Health Course for Health Profession Students. *LGBT Health* **2017**, *4*, 55–61. [CrossRef] [PubMed]

71. Craig, S.L.; Austin, A. The AFFIRM open pilot feasibility study: A brief affirmative cognitive behavioral coping skills group intervention for sexual and gender minority youth. *Child. Youth Serv. Rev.* **2016**, *64*, 136–144. [CrossRef]

72. Braun, H.M.; Ramirez, D.; Zahner, G.J.; Gillis-Buck, E.M.; Sheriff, H.; Ferrone, M. The LGBTQI health forum: An innovative interprofessional initiative to support curriculum reform. *Med. Educ. Online* **2017**. [CrossRef] [PubMed]

73. Costa, A.B.; Pase, P.F.; de Camargo, E.S.; Guaranha, C.; Caetano, A.H.; Kveller, D.; da Rosa Filho, H.T.; Catelan, R.F.; Koller, S.H.; Nardi, H.C. Effectiveness of a multidimensional web-based intervention program to change Brazilian health practitioners' attitudes toward the lesbian, gay, bisexual and transgender population. *J. Health Psychol.* **2016**, *21*, 356–368. [CrossRef] [PubMed]

74. Yingling, C.T.; Cotler, K.; Hughes, T.L. Building nurses' capacity to address health inequities: Incorporating lesbian, gay, bisexual and transgender health content in a family nurse practitioner programme. *J. Clin. Nurs.* **2017**, *26*, 2807–2817. [CrossRef] [PubMed]

75. Johnson, M.J.; Nemeth, L.S. Addressing health disparities of lesbian and bisexual women: A grounded theory study. *Womens Health Issues* **2014**, *24*, 635–640. [CrossRef]

76. Steele, L.S.; Tinmouth, J.M.; Lu, A. Regular health care use by lesbians: A path analysis of predictive factors. *Fam. Pr.* **2006**, *23*, 631–636. [CrossRef]

77. Warren, J.C.; Smalley, K.B.; Barefoot, K.N. Bisexual health. In *LGBT Health. Meeting the Needs of Gender and Sexual Minorities*; Smalley, K.B., Warren, J.C., Barefoot, K.N., Eds.; Springer: New York, NY, USA, 2018; pp. 293–305.

78. Baldwin, A.; Dodge, B.; Schick, V.; Herbenick, D.; Sanders, S.; Dhoot, R.; Fortenberry, D. Health and identity-related interactions between lesbian, bisexual, queer and pansexuel women and their healthcare providers. *Cult. Health Sex.* **2017**, *19*, 1181–1196. [CrossRef] [PubMed]

79. Bjorkman, M.; Malterud, K. Lesbian women's experiences with health care: A qualitative study. *Scand J. Prim. Health Care* **2009**, *27*, 238–243. [CrossRef] [PubMed]

80. Pufall, E.L.; Kall, M.; Shahmanesh, M.; Nardone, A.; Gilson, R.; Delpech, V.; Ward, H.; Positive Voices Study Group. Sexualized drug use ('chemsex') and high-risk sexual behaviours in HIV-positive men who have sex with men. *HIV Med.* **2018**, *19*, 261–270. [CrossRef]

81. Fuchs, W.; Ghattas, D.C.; Reinert, D.; Widmann, C. *Studie zur Lebenssituation von Transsexuellen in Nordrhein-Westfalen [Study on the life situation of transsexuals in North Rhine-Westphalia]*; Lesben- und Schwulenverband Landesverband Nordrhein-Westfalen e.V.: Köln, Germany, 2012.

82. Krell, C.; Oldemeier, K. *Coming-out—Und dann?! [Coming-out - And then?]*; Deutsches Jugendinstitut e.V.: München, Germany, 2015.

83. Safer, J.C.; Coleman, E.; Feldman, J.; Garofalo, R.; Hembree, W.; Radix, A.; Sevelius, J. Barriers to healthcare for transgender individuals. *Curr. Opin. Endocrinol. Diabetes Obes.* **2016**, *23*, 168–171. [CrossRef] [PubMed]

84. Schweizer, K.; Lampalzer, U.; Handford, C.; Briken, P. *Kurzzeitbefragung zu Strukturen und Angeboten zur Beratung und Unterstützung bei Variationen der körperlichen Geschlechtsmerkmale. Begleitmaterial zur Interministeriellen Arbeitsgruppe Inter- & Transsexualität [Short-term survey on structures and services for counselling and support in variations of sex characteristics. Supplementary material for the Interministerial Working Group on Inter- & Transsexuality]*; Bundesministerium für Familie, Senioren, Frauen und Jugend: Berlin, Germany, 2016.

85. De Blok, C.J.M.; Wiepjes, C.M.; Nota, N.N.; van Engelen, K.; Adank, M.A.; Dreijerink, K.M.A.; Barbé, E.; Konings, I.R.H.M.; den Heijer, M. Breast cancer risk in transgender people receiving hormone treatment: Nationwide cohort study in the Netherlands. *BMJ* **2019**, *365*, l1652. [CrossRef] [PubMed]

86. Braun, H.; Nash, R.; Tangpricha, V.; Brockman, J.; Ward, K.; Goodman, M. Cancer in transgender people: Evidence and methodological considerations. *Epidemiol. Rev.* **2017**, *39*, 93–107. [CrossRef]

87. Döhnert, U.; Wünsch, L.; Hiort, O. Gonadectomy in complete androgen insensitivity syndrome: Why and when? *Sex. Dev.* **2017**, *11*, 171–174. [CrossRef]

88. Pleskacova, J.; Hersmus, R.; Oosterhuis, J.W.; Setyawati, B.A.; Faradz, S.M.; Cools, M.; Wolffenbuttel, K.P.; Lebel, J.; Drop, S.L.; Looijenga, L.H. Tumor risk in disorders of sex development. *Sex. Dev.* **2010**. [CrossRef]

89. Dhejne, C.; Van Vlerken, R.; Heylens, G.; Arcelus, J. Mental health and gender dysphoria: A review of the literature. *Int. Rev. Psychiatry* **2016**, *28*, 44–57. [CrossRef]

90. Nieder, T.O.; Güldenring, A.; Köhler, A.; Briken, P. Trans*-Gesundheitsversorgung. Zwischen Entpsychopathologisierung und bedarfsgerechter Behandlung begleitender psychischer Störungen [Trans healthcare: Between depsychopathologization and a needs-based treatment of accompanying mental disorders]. *Nervenarzt* **2017**, *88*, 466–471. [CrossRef] [PubMed]

91. Van Lisdonk, J. *Living with Intersex/DSD. An Exploratory Study of the Social Situation of Persons with Intersex/DSD*; Netherlands Institute for Social Research: The Hague, The Netherlands, 2014.

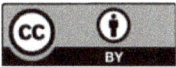

© 2019 by the authors. Licensee MDPI, Basel, Switzerland. This article is an open access article distributed under the terms and conditions of the Creative Commons Attribution (CC BY) license (http://creativecommons.org/licenses/by/4.0/).

International Journal of
*Environmental Research and Public Health*

MDPI

*Article*

# Effect of Same-Sex Marriage Referendums on the Suicidal Ideation Rate among Nonheterosexual People in Taiwan

I-Hsuan Lin [1], Nai-Ying Ko [2,3], Yu-Te Huang [4], Mu-Hong Chen [5,6], Wei-Hsin Lu [7,8,*] and Cheng-Fang Yen [9,10,*]

1   Department of Psychiatry, Yuan's General Hospital, Kaohsiung 80249, Taiwan; ihreneelin@gmail.com
2   Departments of Nursing, College of Medicine, National Cheng Kung University and Hospital,
    Tainan 70101, Taiwan; nyko@mail.ncku.edu.tw
3   Center of Infection Control, National Cheng Kung University Hospital, Tainan 70101, Taiwan
4   Department of Social Work and Social Administration, The University of Hong Kong,
    Hong Kong RM543, Hong Kong; Yuhuang@hku.hk
5   Department of Psychiatry, Taipei Veterans General Hospital, Taipei 11217, Taiwan; kremer7119@gmail.com
6   Division of Psychiatry, School of Medicine, National Yang-Ming University, Taipei 11221, Taiwan
7   Department of Psychiatry, Ditmanson Medical Foundation Chia-Yi Christian
    Hospital, Chia-Yi City 60002, Taiwan
8   Department of Senior Citizen Service Management, Chia Nan University of Pharmacy and Science,
    Tainan 60002, Taiwan
9   Department of Psychiatry, School of Medicine, College of Medicine, Kaohsiung Medical University,
    Kaohsiung 80708, Taiwan
10  Department of Psychiatry, Kaohsiung Medical University Hospital, Kaohsiung 80708, Taiwan
*   Correspondence: wiiseen@gmail.com (W.-H.L.); chfaye@cc.kmu.edu.tw (C.-F.Y.)

Received: 29 August 2019; Accepted: 16 September 2019; Published: 17 September 2019

**Abstract:** Taiwan held voter-initiated referendums to determine same-sex marriage legalization on 24 November 2018. This study aims to compare suicidal ideation rates in heterosexual and nonheterosexual participants of a first-wave survey (Wave 1, 23 months before the same-sex marriage referendums) and a second-wave survey (Wave 2, one week after the same-sex marriage referendums) in Taiwan and to examine the influence of gender, age, and sexual orientation on the change in suicidal ideation rates in nonheterosexual participants. In total, 3286 participants in Wave 1 and 1370 participants in Wave 2 were recruited through a Facebook advertisement. Each participant completed an online questionnaire assessing suicidal ideation. The proportions of heterosexual and nonheterosexual participants with suicidal ideation were compared between the Wave 1 and Wave 2 surveys. Suicidal ideation rates between participants in the Wave 1 and Wave 2 surveys were further compared by stratifying nonheterosexual participants according to gender, age, and sexual orientation. Nonheterosexual participants in the Wave 2 survey had a higher suicidal ideation rate than those in the Wave 1 survey, whereas no difference was observed in suicidal ideation rates between heterosexual participants in Wave 2 and Wave 1. Nonheterosexual participants who were female, younger, gay, lesbian, and bisexual in Wave 2 had a higher suicidal ideation rate than those in Wave 1. The suicidal ideation rate significantly increased in nonheterosexual participants experiencing the same-sex marriage referendums in Taiwan. Whether civil rights of sexual minority individuals can be determined through referendums should be evaluated.

**Keywords:** age; gender; same-sex marriage; sexual orientation; suicidality

## 1. Introduction

### 1.1. Suicide in Sexual Minorities

Suicide is a critical health issue among sexual minority individuals. A meta-analysis found that sexual minority youth reported significantly higher rates of suicidality than did their heterosexual counterparts [1]. A meta-analysis pooling 19 studies found that the prevalence of lifetime suicidal ideation in men who have sex with men was 34.97%, which is far higher than that in the general population [2]. Another meta-analysis pooling 30 studies found that sexual minority adults had nearly three- to five-times higher risks of suicidal attempts than did heterosexual individuals [3]. Research has found that most suicidal attempts are preceded by suicidal ideation [4,5]. Therefore, suicidal ideation warrants careful evaluation and intervention to prevent eventual suicide completion.

### 1.2. Same-Sex Marriage Bans: A Structural-Level Discrimination toward a Sexual Minority

According to the ecological systems theory [6], suicidality may result from complex interactions between sexual minority individuals and their environments. One of the individual–environmental interacting factors that may increase the suicidal risk of sexual minority individuals is stigma based on sexual orientation [7]. According to minority stress theory [8], socially-stigmatized individuals may experience chronic stress due to their minority statuses and consequently develop mental health problems. Sexual minority individuals may internalize sexuality-related oppression and experience stress caused by hiding and managing a socially-stigmatized identity, both of which further compromise their mental health [9]. In addition to perceived discrimination [10], the expectation of being discriminated against by others [11], internalized stigma [12], and structural stigma [13] has been identified as a contributor to mental health problems in sexual minority individuals. Same-sex marriage bans are one type of structural-level discrimination that differentially targets sexual minority individuals due to social exclusion and compromises their mental health [14,15]. Lesbian, gay, and bisexual (LGB), but not heterosexual, individuals living in states in the United States (U.S.) that passed constitutional amendments banning same-sex marriage experienced significant increases in mood disorder, generalized anxiety disorder, alcohol use disorder, and psychiatric comorbidity; the increase in psychiatric disorders was not found among LGB individuals living in states without these constitutional amendments [14]. LGB individuals reported that constitutional amendments banning same-sex marriage make them feel indignant about discrimination, as well as fearful, anxious, and hopeless about protecting their relationships and families [15]. These results demonstrated the harmful discriminating effects of passing same-sex marriage bans on the mental health of sexual minority individuals.

### 1.3. Same-Sex Marriage Campaign and Referendums in Taiwan

Sexual minority rights campaigners in Taiwan have strived for same-sex marriage legalization since the end of the 1980s. However, people in Taiwan traditionally regard homosexuality as a challenge to the family obligations mandated in Confucianism, and in particular, they require their offspring to continue the family bloodline. Moreover, the Civil Code's stipulation "an agreement to marry shall be made by the male and the female parties in their own concord" renders same-sex marriage difficult to legalize [16]. In the past two decades, overall, an attitude of social tolerance toward homosexuality has become widespread in Taiwan, which is mainly accounted for by improvement in education and liberal values related to gender roles [17]. The 2012 Taiwan Social Change Survey showed that for the first time, supporters of same-sex marriage outnumber those who oppose it [18]. The most encouraging progress of same-sex marriage legalization in Taiwan is that in May 2017, the Council of Grand Justices announced that the current Civil Code that barred same-sex marriage is a violation of the human right to equality and is unconstitutional, and the council directed that same-sex marriage should be legalized within two years. With such progress, sexual minority rights campaigners in Taiwan rejoiced at the prospect of same-sex marriage.

However, the progress of same-sex marriage has drawn substantial opposition, mainly from Christian groups, in Taiwan. In response to the ruling of the Council of Grand Justices on same-sex marriage, the group against same-sex marriage drafted two referendums to argue that legal reform should be made outside changes to the Civil Code, including Case No. 10: "Do you agree that marriage defined in the Civil Code should be restricted to the union between one man and one woman?" and Case No. 12: "Do you agree to the protection of the rights of same-sex couples in co-habitation on a permanent basis in ways other than changing of the Civil Code?". By contrast, the group lobbying for marriage equality drafted a referendum (Case No. 14: "Do you agree to the protection of same-sex marital rights with marriage as defined in the Civil Code?") to argue that separate legislation amounts to a form of discrimination. The results of the vote on 24 November 2018, indicated that Case No. 10 and Case No. 12 received overwhelming support, with 70.12% and 57.60% of voters in favor, respectively. By contrast, only 30.27% of voters supported Case No. 14. The results of voting suggested that the two referendums drafted by the group against same-sex marriage received considerably stronger support than the one by the group supporting marriage equality.

Research has shown that Asian countries exhibit considerably less tolerance for homosexuality than do European and North American countries [19]. Taiwan is the first Asian country to deliberate on same-sex marriage legalization through voter-initiated referendums. Nevertheless, the results of the referendums on 24 November 2018, definitely discouraged sexual minority individuals and minority rights campaigners. Given that voter-initiated referendums occur with some regularity and affect numerous minority groups [20], the effects of the same-sex marriage ban referendums on the mental health of sexual minority individuals in Taiwan warrants further study. The result of such a study may provide empirical evidence to understand the impacts of voter-initiated referendums on mental health in minority groups whose rights are restricted or rejected, as well as to inspect whether civil rights of any individual can be determined through referendums.

### 1.4. Aims and Hypotheses of this Study

The Investigation on the Attitude Toward Same-Sex Marriage in Taiwan is a two-wave online survey of people's attitude toward same-sex marriage and the mental health status of sexual minority individuals in Taiwan. The first wave (Wave 1) was conducted from 1–31 January 2017, 23 months before the same-sex marriage referendums. The second wave (Wave 2) was conducted from 1–31 December 2018, one week after the same-sex marriage referendums. The two aims and corresponding hypotheses of the present study are described below.

### 1.5. Aim I: To Compare the Suicidal Ideation Rate in Nonheterosexual and Heterosexual Participants between the Wave 1 and Wave 2 Surveys

The negative results of the same-sex marriage referendums directly discriminated and devaluated nonheterosexual people. Moreover, the groups opposing same-sex marriage spent a large amount of money to malign the image of sexual minority individuals through propaganda on mass media and social media. Research has found that greater exposure to same-sex marriage campaign advertisements is associated with high stress in sexual minority individuals, and negative advertisements evoke the feeling of sadness among them [20]. The same-sex marriage referendum process and result may also cause the exposure of sexual minority individuals to hostile interactions with neighbors, colleagues, and family members [21]. By contrast, heterosexual individuals are spared from developing mental health problems related to same-sex marriage bans [14]. Therefore, in the present study, we hypothesized that the suicidal ideation rate in nonheterosexual participants increased from the Wave 1 to Wave 2 surveys, whereas no significant difference was observed in suicidal ideation rates among heterosexual participants between the Wave 1 and Wave 2 surveys.

*1.6. Aim II: To Examine the Effects of Gender, Age, and Sexual Orientation on Differences in Suicidal Ideation Rates among Nonheterosexual Participants between the Wave 1 and Wave 2 Surveys*

Research has demonstrated the positive effects of formal same-sex relationships on psychological well-being in younger, but not in older, lesbians and gay men [22]. Research has also found that civil union legalization is the most beneficial for racial or ethnic minority women and women with lower levels of education [23]. Whether same-sex marriage referendums exert various psychological effects on nonheterosexual individuals with various genders, ages, and sexual orientations warrants further study. We hypothesized that differences existed in suicidal ideation rates among nonheterosexual participants of various genders, ages, and sexual orientations.

## 2. Methods

### 2.1. Participants

The method of recruiting participants is described elsewhere [24]. In brief, participants aged at least 20 years were recruited into the two-wave online survey through a Facebook advertisement. The Facebook advertisement included a headline, main text, pop-up banner, and weblink to the study questionnaire website. The advertisement appeared in the News Feed of Facebook, which is a streaming list of updates from the user's connections and advertisers. News feed advertisements are more effective in terms of recruitment metrics for studies [25]. We targeted the advertisement to Facebook users by location (Taiwan) and language (Chinese). The de-duplication protocol used in the present study to identify multiple submissions and preserve data integrity included cross-validation of the eligibility of key variables and examination of discrepancies in key data, as well as checking for unusually fast completion time (<10 minutes) [26]. Moreover, each Internet Protocol address could be registered to complete the online questionnaire once only.

Participants were not given any incentives for participation. All subjects gave their informed consent for inclusion before they participated in the study. The study was conducted in accordance with the Declaration of Helsinki, and the protocol was approved by the Ethics Committee of Kaohsiung Medical University Hospital (KMUHIRB-EXEMPT(II)-20160065). The study design involved respondents' online response to the recruitment advertisement and questionnaire anonymously, which allowed the respondents to decide freely whether to join or not, and their personal information was kept secure. Owing to the anonymity of participants, we could not determine how many participants responded to both surveys. Therefore, the data of the two waves of the survey was analyzed independently. The IRB thus agreed that this study did not require obtaining informed consent from the respondents.

### 2.2. Measures

#### 2.2.1. Suicidal Ideation

We used the question "Do you have any suicide ideation?" on the Revised 5-item Brief Symptom Rating Scale to inquire participants' suicidal ideation during the past week. Participants were asked to rate the severity of suicidal ideation on a 5-point scale: 0, not at all; 1, a little bit; 2, moderately; 3, quite a bit; and 4, extremely [27]. Participants who rated ≥2 on the item were classified as having significant suicidal ideation.

#### 2.2.2. Demographic Variables

Data on participants' gender (female, male, and transgender), age, and sexual orientation (heterosexual, bisexual, homosexual, pansexual, asexual, and unsure) were collected. According to sexual orientation, participants were classified into heterosexual and nonheterosexual (including bisexual, homosexual, and others) groups. According to age, participants were classified into the age groups of 20–29, 30–39, and ≥40 years.

## 2.3. Procedure and Statistical Analysis

The proportions of gender, age, and suicidal ideation were compared between the Wave 1 and Wave 2 surveys in heterosexual and nonheterosexual groups by using the $x^2$ test. Because of multiple comparisons, a $p$-value of <018 (0.05/3) was considered statistically significant for all tests. The proportions of nonheterosexual participants with suicidal ideation were compared between Wave 1 and Wave 2 surveys in various gender (female, male, and transgender), age (20–29, 30–39, and ≥40 years), and sexual orientation groups (homosexual, bisexual, and others) by using the $x^2$ test. Because of multiple comparisons, a $p$-value of <006 (0.05/9) was considered statistically significant for all tests.

## 3. Results

A total of 3423 and 1395 Facebook users completed the online questionnaire in Wave 1 and Wave 2, respectively. Among them, 137 and 25 were excluded from analysis because they were underage (<20 years) or had an erroneous value for age (>100 years) in Wave 1 and Wave 2, respectively. The final data of 3286 participants (1456 heterosexual and 1830 nonheterosexual individuals) in Wave 1 and 1370 participants (540 heterosexual and 830 nonheterosexual individuals) in Wave 2 was analyzed. Table 1 shows the results of a comparison of demographic characteristics between participants in the Wave 1 and Wave 2 surveys. In nonheterosexual groups, higher numbers of transgender individuals were found in the Wave 2 (3.9%) than in Wave 1 (1.9%) survey ($x^2$ = 9.488, $p$ = 0.009). Higher numbers of heterosexual participants aged 20–29 years (44.0% vs. 29.1%) and lower numbers of heterosexual participants aged ≥40 years (19.2% vs. 35.2%) were found in the Wave 1 survey than in the Wave 2 survey ($x^2$ = 64.554, $p$ < 0.001).

### 3.1. Change in Suicidal Ideation Rates between Heterosexual and Nonheterosexual Participants

Table 1 also shows the results of a comparison of suicidal ideation rates between participants in the Wave 1 and Wave 2 surveys. Nonheterosexual participants in the Wave 2 survey (24.6%) had a higher suicidal ideation rate than nonheterosexual participants in the Wave 1 survey (15.4%) ($x^2$ = 32.145, $p$ < 001), whereas no difference was observed in suicidal ideation rates between heterosexual participants in Wave 1 (6.3%) and Wave 2 (5.2%) surveys ($x^2$ = 877, $p$ = 349).

**Table 1.** Comparison of demographic characteristics and suicidal ideation rates in heterosexual and nonheterosexual participants between the Wave 1 and Wave 2 surveys.

| Variables | Heterosexual | | | | Non-Heterosexual | | | |
|---|---|---|---|---|---|---|---|---|
| | Wave 1 (n = 1456) n (%) | Wave 2 (n = 540) n (%) | $x^2$ | $p$ | Wave 1 (n = 1830) n (%) | Wave 2 (n = 830) n (%) | $x^2$ | $p$ |
| Gender | | | | | | | | |
| Female | 1132 (77.8) | 416 (77.0) | 3.202 | 0.202 | 917 (50.1) | 412 (49.6) | 9.488 | 0.009 |
| Male | 311 (21.4) | 123 (22.8) | | | 879 (48.0) | 386 (46.5) | | |
| Transgender | 13 (0.9) | 1 (0.2) | | | 34 (1.9) | 32 (3.9) | | |
| Age (years) | | | | | | | | |
| 20–29 | 640 (44.0) | 157 (29.1) | 64.554 | <0.001 | 1075 (58.7) | 472 (56.9) | 2.207 | 0.332 |
| 30–39 | 536 (36.8) | 193 (35.7) | | | 611 (33.4) | 279 (33.6) | | |
| 40 or older | 280 (19.2) | 190 (35.2) | | | 144 (7.9) | 79 (9.5) | | |
| Suicidal ideation | | | | | | | | |
| No | 1380 (94.8) | 506 (93.7) | 0.877 | 0.349 | 1548 (84.6) | 626 (75.4) | 32.145 | <0.001 |
| Yes | 76 (5.2) | 34 (6.3) | | | 282 (15.4) | 204 (24.6) | | |

### 3.2. Changes in Suicidal Ideation Rates in Nonheterosexual Participants of Various Genders, Ages, and Sexual Orientations

Table 2 shows the results of a comparison of suicidal ideation rates in nonheterosexual participants of various genders, ages, and sexual orientations between the Wave 1 and Wave 2 surveys. Nonheterosexual women exhibited a significant increase in suicidal ideation rates from the Wave 1 to Wave 2 surveys (14.0% vs. 36.4%, $\chi^2$ = 26.125, $p$ < 0.001). Suicidal ideation rates in nonheterosexual men tended to increase from the Wave 1 to Wave 2 surveys (16.8% vs. 23.3%, $\chi^2$ = 7.371, $p$ = 0.007), but the difference was not statistically significant. No significant increase in suicidal ideation rates was detected in nonheterosexual transgender individuals from the Wave 1 to Wave 2 surveys (17.6% vs. 28.1%, $\chi^2$ = 1.031, $p$ = 0.310).

Nonheterosexual participants aged 20–29 years (17.0% vs. 27.3%, $\chi^2$ = 21.642, $p$ < 0.001) and aged 30–39 years (13.7% vs. 22.6%, $\chi^2$ = 10.837, $p$ = 0.001) exhibited higher suicidal ideation rates in the Wave 2 survey than in the Wave 1 survey. No difference was observed in the suicidal ideation rate in older nonheterosexual participants (aged ≥40 years) between Wave 1 and Wave 2 (10.4% vs. 15.2%, $\chi^2$ = 1.092, $p$ = 0.296).

Gay and lesbian (16.6% vs. 26.4%, $\chi^2$ = 21.838, $p$ < 0.001) and bisexual participants (11.1% vs. 23.2%, $\chi^2$ = 15.408, $p$ < 0.001) exhibited higher suicidal ideation rates in the Wave 2 survey than in the Wave 1 survey. No difference was observed in the suicidal ideation rate in the participants with pansexual, asexual, and unsure sexual orientations between Wave 1 and Wave 2 (17.1% vs. 18.1%, $\chi^2$ = 0.052, $p$ = 0.820).

**Table 2.** Comparison of suicidal ideation rates in nonheterosexual participants between the Wave 1 and Wave 2 surveys: gender, age, and sexual orientation effects.

| Variables | Suicidal idea | | $\chi^2$ | $p$ |
| --- | --- | --- | --- | --- |
| | Yes $n$ (%) | No $n$ (%) | | |
| Gender | | | | |
| Female | | | | |
| Wave 1 ($n$ = 917) | 128 (14.0) | 789 (86.0) | 26.125 | <0.001 |
| Wave 2 ($n$ = 412) | 105 (36.4) | 307 (74.5) | | |
| Male | | | | |
| Wave 1 ($n$ = 879) | 148 (16.8) | 731 (83.2) | 7.371 | 0.007 |
| Wave 2 ($n$ = 386) | 90 (23.3) | 296 (76.7) | | |
| Transgender | | | | |
| Wave 1 ($n$ = 34) | 6 (17.6) | 28 (82.4) | 1.031 | 0.310 |
| Wave 2 ($n$ = 32) | 9 (28.1) | 23 (71.9) | | |
| Age (years) | | | | |
| 20-29 | | | | |
| Wave 1 ($n$ = 1075) | 183 (17.0) | 892 (83.0) | 21.642 | <0.001 |
| Wave 2 ($n$ = 472) | 129 (27.3) | 343 (72.7) | | |
| 30-39 | | | | |
| Wave 1 ($n$ = 611) | 84 (13.7) | 527 (86.3) | 10.837 | 0.001 |
| Wave 2 ($n$ = 279) | 63 (22.6) | 216 (77.4) | | |
| 40 or older | | | | |
| Wave 1 ($n$ = 144) | 15 (10.4) | 129 (89.6) | 1.092 | 0.296 |
| Wave 2 ($n$ = 79) | 12 (15.2) | 67 (84.8) | | |
| Sexual orientation | | | | |
| Homosexual | | | | |
| Wave 1 ($n$ = 1166) | 194 (16.6) | 972 (83.4) | 21.838 | <0.001 |
| Wave 2 ($n$ = 531) | 140 (26.4) | 391 (73.6) | | |
| Bisexual | | | | |
| Wave 1 ($n$ = 424) | 47 (11.1) | 377 (88.9) | 15.408 | <0.001 |
| Wave 2 ($n$ = 194) | 45 (23.2) | 149 (76.8) | | |
| Others (pansexual, asexual and unsure) | | | | |
| Wave 1 ($n$ = 240) | 41 (17.1) | 199 (82.9) | 0.052 | 0.820 |
| Wave 2 ($n$ = 105) | 19 (18.1) | 86 (81.9) | | |

## 4. Discussion

The results of the present study revealed that nonheterosexual participants in the Wave 2 survey had a higher suicidal ideation rate than those in the Wave 1 survey, whereas no difference was found in suicidal ideation rates in heterosexual participants between Wave 2 and Wave 1. Nonheterosexual participants who were female, younger (aged 20–39 years), gay, lesbian, and bisexual in Wave 2 had a higher suicidal ideation rate than those in Wave 1.

### 4.1. Suicidal Ideation in LGB Participants Experiencing Same-Sex Marriage Referendums

The present study found that the suicidal ideation rate in nonheterosexual participants significantly increased from Wave 1 (conducted 23 months before the same-sex marriage referendums) to Wave 2 (conducted one week after the same-sex marriage referendums), whereas the suicidal ideation rate did not significantly change in heterosexual participants. The same-sex marriage referendums might specifically influence the suicidal ideation rate among sexual minority individuals in Taiwan in two ways: the campaigns against same-same marriage before the referendums and the negative results of the referendums. First, the groups opposing same-sex marriage in Taiwan spread a considerable amount of incorrect information and rumors to malign same-sex marriage and sexual minority individuals through social media and public media, as they proposed the referendums against same-sex marriage. For example, they claimed that the legalization of same-sex marriage would lead to the widespread outbreak of the contagion of human immunodeficiency virus infection, depopulation in Taiwan, and the deterioration of traditional family values. These misleading portrayals and negative stereotypes spread in the media demoralized sexual minority individuals and directly disturbed their emotional regulation. Research in the U.S. found that exposure to negative same-sex marriage campaign advertisements evoked the feeling of sadness among lesbian, gay, bisexual, and/or transgender individuals [20]. Research in Australia found that more frequent exposure to negative media messages about same-sex marriage was associated with greater psychological distress [28]. Moreover, LGB individuals might internalize distorted images and point of views into their self-appraisals and feel ashamed of their LGB identity [29].

Second, although the 2012 Taiwan Social Change Survey found that supporters of same-sex marriage outnumbered those opposing it [18], the large amount of false information broadcast by anti-LGB campaigners certainly influenced the values of people in Taiwan to a certain extent. Research has shown that public campaigns debating anti-gay policies, such as same-sex marriage, may foster a negative social climate for sexual minority individuals [30]. After the proposal of referendums in Taiwan, sexual minority individuals had to interact with neighbors, colleagues, and family members who adopted the viewpoints broadcast by the groups opposing same-sex marriage for half a year. According to the social identity threat theories of stigma [31], cues from the social environment that are appraised as potentially harmful to one's stigmatized social identity engender a threat, which in turn creates involuntary stress responses. Stigma-related stress deteriorates victims' emotion dysregulation and cognitive processes and further confers the risk of psychopathology [32]. A previous study had a similar result that LGB people reported comparatively worse life satisfaction, mental health, and overall health in constituencies with higher rates of voters saying "no" to the same-sex plebiscite [33].

Third, the result that a certain group of voters favored that sexual minority individuals only have the right to cohabit but not marry according to the Civil Code definitely discriminated between sexual minority individuals and heterosexual individuals. Creating laws ruling that sexual minority individuals do not have the same rights as heterosexual individuals reinforced the marginalized and socially-devalued statuses of sexual minority individuals [21,30]. The European Social Survey determined that sexuality-based discrimination has significant negative effects on the self-related health and subjective well-being of victims [34]. The results of the present study support that referendums on the civil rights of sexual minority individuals represent a source of stress for this sexual minority and may have significant negative effects on the mental health of sexual minority individuals and increases their suicide risk. Whether the civil rights of sexual minority individuals can be determined through voter-initiated referendums should be comprehensively evaluated. Mental health professionals must develop prevention and intervention strategies for suicide risk in LGB individuals experiencing referendums that decide their civil rights.

*4.2. Gender Differences in the Change in Suicidal Ideation Rates*

The present study found that nonheterosexual women had significantly exhibited higher suicidal ideation rates in the Wave 2 survey than in the Wave 1 survey ($p < 0.001$), whereas suicidal ideation rates in nonheterosexual men tended to increase, but not significantly ($p = 0.007$). This gender difference might be partially attributed to the double stigma that many lesbians experience as both lesbians and women [35]. Taiwanese society considers women subordinate to men. In the past decade, women's reproductive health, empowerment, and labor market have improved significantly [36]. However, the gender gap in social status remains nonuniform. For example, the gender pay gap still exists in Taiwan, with women earning 85.4% of the average hourly income of men [36]. Moreover, a longitudinal study in Australia found that nonheterosexual women were more disadvantaged in health and wellbeing than nonheterosexual men [37]. As a structural stigma, the result of the referendums may interact with individual disadvantages, including sexual minority and underprivileged gender, which may cause lesbian individuals to become vulnerable to the frustration caused by failure in changing the Civil Code for same-sex marriage legalization. The result indicated the importance of considering gender differences in psychological reactions to major events related to sexual minority rights.

In the present study, suicidal ideation rates did not significantly increase in nonheterosexual transgender individuals from the Wave 1 to Wave 2 surveys. The small number of nonheterosexual transgender participants in the present study limited the possibility of drawing a conclusion on the effect of the same-sex marriage referendums on the mental health of nonheterosexual transgender individuals. Subgroups of nonheterosexual individuals may have had various experiences during the period of the same-sex marriage referendums. The questions of whether nonheterosexual transgender individuals feel marginalized in the debates and whether they consequently feel uninvolved in the same-sex marriage movement warrant further study.

*4.3. Age Differences in the Change in Suicidal Ideation Rates*

The present study found that nonheterosexual participants aged 20–29 years exhibited the most significant increase in the suicidal ideation rate, followed by those aged 30–39 years, from the Wave 1 to Wave 2 surveys, whereas no difference was observed in the suicidal ideation rate in those aged ≥40 years ($p = 0.296$). Research has demonstrated that young people have a more tolerant attitude toward homosexuality than older people in Taiwan [17]. Younger nonheterosexual participants may have an overly optimistic expectation of legalizing same-sex marriage based on the atmosphere they perceived from their peers, whereas older nonheterosexual participants may have a pessimistic expectation based on the social stigma prevailing in Taiwan for a long time. Various expectations may result in various levels of shock and disappointment in response to the results of the referendums and further caused the difference in changes in suicidal ideation rates in various age groups of nonheterosexual participants. Moreover, nonheterosexual participants in early adulthood may still strive to establish their sexual identity and self-worth. The result of the referendums may disappoint their establishment of sexual identity and compromise their psychological well-being. The result indicated the importance of considering age when developing prevention and intervention programs for suicidality in nonheterosexual individuals experiencing the legalization of policies hostile to any sexual minority.

*4.4. Sexual Orientation Differences in the Change in Suicidal Ideation Rates*

The present study found that gay, lesbian, and bisexual, but not pansexual, asexual, and unsure, participants had increased suicidal ideation rates from the Wave 1 to Wave 2 surveys. No epidemiological study has examined the proportions of pansexual, asexual, and unsure individuals in Taiwan. In total,

7.3% and 7.7% of participants in the Wave 1 and Wave 2 surveys, respectively, labeled their sexual orientation as pansexual, asexual, or unsure; these proportions were lower than those of individuals who labeled themselves as homosexual (35.5% in Wave 1 and 38.8% in Wave 2) and bisexual (12.9% in Wave 1 and 14.2% in Wave 2). Individuals whose sexual orientations are pansexual, asexual, or unsure are minor groups in the sexual minority. Their experiences in the debates of same-sex marriage require additional studies to deepen the understanding of various sexual minority groups.

*4.5. Limitations*

The present study has some limitations. First, although recruiting participants through Facebook can deliver large numbers of participants quickly, cheaply, and with minimal effort compared with mail and phone recruitment, access to Facebook is not universal to people of all ages. A 2018 analysis found that 68.4% of active Facebook users in Taiwan were aged between 18 and 44 [38]. Moreover, people are not equally motivated to use Facebook [39]. Although the female:male ratio of Facebook uses in Taiwan is about 1:1 [38], no data shows the distribution of sexual orientation in Facebook users in Taiwan. Therefore, whether young lesbians are more likely to participate in Facebook as a way of creating a social community and more likely to express suicidal ideation warrants further study.

Second, the distributions of heterosexual and nonheterosexual participants in the current study were not congruent with those in the general population. The number of female heterosexual respondents was higher than that of male heterosexual respondents in both waves of the survey.

Third, the Wave 2 survey was conducted one week after the referendums. The nonheterosexual participants might be in a state of great anger and disappointment. Studies with relatively long follow-up periods are needed to examine the longer term change in suicidal ideation.

Fourth, participants' suicidal ideation might develop in various biological, cognitive, and emotional contexts. The present study did not clarify the mechanisms for the increased suicidal ideation rate in nonheterosexual participants. The results of previous studies may provide possible explanations for the mechanisms through which voter referendums affect the mental health of sexual minority individuals in the U.S. [20,29,40]. However, whether these mechanisms proposed based on the U.S. sociocultural background can well explain the increased suicidal ideation rate in nonheterosexual participants in Taiwan warrants further study.

## 5. Conclusions

The suicidal ideation rate significantly increased in nonheterosexual individuals affected by the same-sex marriage referendums in Taiwan. Nonheterosexual participants who were female, younger, gay, lesbian, and bisexual were particularly vulnerable to the effects of the same-sex marriage referendums and had an increased suicidal ideation rate. The result indicated that the same-sex marriage ban referendums had a negative effect on the mental health of sexual minority individuals in Taiwan. The results also indicated the importance of considering gender, age, and sexual orientation differences in psychological reactions to major events related to sexual minorities. In addition to the inspection of whether civil rights of sexual minority individuals can be determined through referendums, factors that can protect sexual minority individuals from the hurt of structural stigma such as same-sex marriage bans warrant study. For example, research found that perceiving a greater immediate social network can buffer the effect of exposure to negative media messages about same-sex marriage on psychological distress [28]. Perceived poor social support also mediates a large portion of the effects of structural stigma on LGB outcomes [33].

**Author Contributions:** N.-Y.K. and C.-F.Y. conceived of, designed, and performed the study; Y.-T.H. and M.-H.C. analyzed the data; I.-H.L., W.-H.L., and C.-F.Y. wrote the paper.

**Funding:** This research was partially funded by the Ministry of Science and Technology, Taiwan, Grant Number MOST 107-2314-B-037-102-MY3 and by the Kaohsiung Medical University Hospital, Grant Number KMUH107-7R69.

**Conflicts of Interest:** The authors declare no conflict of interest. The founding sponsors had no role in the design of the study; in the collection, analyses, or interpretation of the data; in the writing of the manuscript; nor in the decision to publish the results.

## References

1. Marshal, M.P.; Dietz, L.J.; Friedman, M.S.; Stall, R.; Smith, H.A.; McGinley, J.; Thoma, B.C.; Murray, P.J.; D'Augelli, A.; Brent, D.A. Suicidality and depression disparities between sexual minority and heterosexual youth: A meta-analytic review. *J. Adolesc. Health* **2011**, *49*, 115–123. [CrossRef] [PubMed]
2. Luo, Z.; Feng, T.; Fu, H.; Yang, T. Lifetime prevalence of suicidal ideation among men who have sex with men: A meta-analysis. *BMC Psychiatry* **2017**, *17*, 406. [CrossRef] [PubMed]
3. Hottes, T.S.; Bogaert, L.; Rhodes, A.E.; Brennan, D.J.; Gesink, D. Lifetime prevalence of suicide attempts among sexual minority adults by study sampling strategies: A systematic review and meta-analysis. *Am. J. Public Health* **2016**, *106*, e1–e12. [CrossRef] [PubMed]
4. Deykin, E.Y.; Buka, S.L. Suicidal ideation and attempts among chemically dependent adolescents. *Am. J. Public Health* **1994**, *84*, 634–639. [CrossRef] [PubMed]
5. Klimes-Dougan, B.; Free, K.; Ronsaville, D.; Stilwell, J.; Welsh, C.J.; Radke-Yarrow, M. Suicidal ideation and attempts: A longitudinal investigation of children of depressed and well mothers. *J. Am. Acad. Child Adolesc. Psychiatry* **1999**, *38*, 651–659. [CrossRef] [PubMed]
6. Bronfenbrenner, U. *The Ecology of Human Development*; Harvard University Press: Cambridge, MA, USA, 1979.
7. Hatzenbuehler, M.L. The social environment and suicide attempts in lesbian, gay, and bisexual youth. *Pediatrics* **2011**, *127*, 896–903. [CrossRef]
8. Meyer, I.H. Prejudice, social stress, and mental health in lesbian, gay, and bisexual populations: Conceptual issues and research evidence. *Psychol. Bull.* **2003**, *129*, 674–697. [CrossRef] [PubMed]
9. Almeida, J.; Johnson, R.M.; Corliss, H.L.; Molnar, B.E.; Azrael, D. Emotional distress among LGBT youth: The influence of perceived discrimination based on sexual orientation. *J. Youth Adolesc.* **2009**, *38*, 1001–1014. [CrossRef]
10. Mays, V.M.; Cochran, S.D. Mental health correlates of perceived discrimination among lesbian, gay, and bisexual adults in the United States. *Am. J. Public Health* **2001**, *91*, 1869–1876. [CrossRef]
11. McCabe, S.E.; Bostwick, W.B.; Hughes, T.L.; West, B.T.; Boyd, C.J. The relationship between discrimination and substance use disorders among lesbian, gay, and bisexual adults in the United States. *Am. J. Public Health* **2010**, *100*, 1946–1952. [CrossRef]
12. Tatum, A.K. The interaction of same-sex marriage access with sexual minority identity on mental health and subjective wellbeing. *J. Homosex.* **2017**, *64*, 638–653. [CrossRef] [PubMed]
13. Hatzenbuehler, M.L. Structural stigma and the health of lesbian, gay, and bisexual populations. *Curr. Dir. Psychol. Sci.* **2014**, *23*, 127–132. [CrossRef]
14. Hatzenbuehler, M.L.; McLaughlin, K.A.; Keyes, K.M.; Hasin, D.S. The impact of institutional discrimination on psychiatric disorders in lesbian, gay, and bisexual populations: A prospective study. *Am. J. Public Health* **2010**, *100*, 452–459. [CrossRef] [PubMed]
15. Rostosky, S.S.; Riggle, E.D.B.; Horne, S.G.; Miller, A.D. Lesbian, gay, and bisexual individuals' psychological reactions to amendments denying access to civil marriage. *Am. J. Orthopsychiatry* **2010**, *80*, 302–310. [CrossRef] [PubMed]
16. Hsu, C.Y.; Yen, C.F. Taiwan: Pioneer of the health and well-being of sexual minorities in Asia. *Arch. Sex Behav.* **2017**, *46*, 1577–1579. [CrossRef] [PubMed]
17. Cheng, Y.A.; Wu, F.C.F.; Adamczyk, A. Changing attitudes toward homosexuality in Taiwan, 1995–2012. *Chin. Social Rev.* **2016**, *48*, 317–345. [CrossRef]
18. Chang, Y.H.; Tu, S.H.; Liao, P.S. *Taiwan Social Change Survey 2012, Phase 6, Wave 3*; Institute of Sociology, Academia Sinica: Taipei City, Taiwan, 2013.
19. World Value Survey Association. World Value Survey Wave 6: 2010–2014; WVSA. 2014. Available online: http://www.worldvaluessurvey.org/WVSOnline.jsp (accessed on 20 August 2019).
20. Flores, A.R.; Hatzenbuehler, M.L.; Gates, G.J. Identifying psychological responses of stigmatized groups to referendums. *Proc. Natl. Acad. Sci. USA* **2018**, *115*, 3816–3821. [CrossRef] [PubMed]

21. Rostosky, S.S.; Riggle, E.D.B.; Horne, S.G.; Miller, A.D. Marriage amendments and psychological distress in lesbian, gay, and bisexual (LGB) adults. *J. Couns. Psychol.* **2009**, *56*, 56–66. [CrossRef]
22. Bariola, E.; Lyons, A.; Leonard, W. The mental health benefits of relationship formalisation among lesbians and gay men in same-sex relationships. *Aust. N. Z. J. Public Health* **2015**, *39*, 530–535. [CrossRef]
23. Everett, B.G.; Hatzenbuehler, M.L.; Hughes, T.L. The impact of civil union legislation on minority stress, depression, and hazardous drinking in a diverse sample of sexual-minority women: A quasi-natural experiment. *Soc. Sci. Med.* **2016**, *169*, 180–190. [CrossRef]
24. Huang, Y.T.; Chen, M.H.; Hu, H.F.; Ko, N.Y.; Yen, C.F. Role of mental health in the attitude toward same-sex marriage among people in Taiwan. *J. Formos. Med. Assoc.* **2019**. [CrossRef]
25. Ramo, D.E.; Rodriguez, T.M.; Chavez, K.; Sommer, M.J.; Prochaska, J.J. Facebook recruitment of young adult smokers for a cessation trial: Methods, metrics, and lessons learned. *Internet Interv.* **2014**, *1*, 58–64. [CrossRef] [PubMed]
26. Bowen, A.M.; Daniel, C.M.; Williams, M.L.; Baird, G.L. Identifying multiple submissions in Internet research: Preserving data integrity. *AIDS Behav.* **2008**, *12*, 964–973. [CrossRef] [PubMed]
27. Wu, C.Y.; Lee, J.I.; Lee, M.B.; Liao, S.C.; Chang, C.M.; Chen, H.C.; Lung, F.W. Predictive validity of a five-item symptom checklist to screen psychiatric morbidity and suicide ideation in general population and psychiatric settings. *J. Formos. Med. Assoc.* **2016**, *115*, 395–403. [CrossRef] [PubMed]
28. Verrelli, S.; White, F.A.; Harvey, L.J.; Pulciani, M.R. Minority stress, social support, and the mental health of lesbian, gay, and bisexual Australians during the Australian Marriage Law Postal Survey. *Aust. Psychol.* **2019**, *54*, 336–346. [CrossRef]
29. Russell, G.M.; Richards, J.A. Stressor and resilience factors for lesbians, gay men, and bisexuals confronting anti-gay politics. *Am. J. Community Psychol.* **2003**, *31*, 313–328. [CrossRef]
30. Russell, G.M. *Voted Out: The Psychological Consequences of Anti-Gay Politics*; New York University: New York, NY, USA, 2000.
31. Major, B.; O'Brien, L.T. The social psychology of stigma. *Annu. Rev. Psychol.* **2005**, *56*, 393–421. [CrossRef]
32. Hatzenbuehler, M.L. How does sexual minority stigma "get under the skin"? A psychological mediation framework. *Psychol. Bull.* **2009**, *135*, 707–730. [CrossRef]
33. Perales, F.; Todd, A. Structural stigma and the health and wellbeing of Australian LGB populations: Exploiting geographic variation in the results of the 2017 same-sex marriage plebiscite. *Soc. Sci. Med.* **2018**, *208*, 190–199. [CrossRef]
34. Van der Star, A.; Bränström, R. Acceptance of sexual minorities, discrimination, social capital and health and well-being: A cross-European study among members of same-sex and opposite-sex couples. *BMC Public Health* **2015**, *15*, 812. [CrossRef]
35. Connolly, C.M. A feminist perspective of resilience in lesbian couples. *J. Fem. Fam. Ther.* **2006**, *18*, 137–162. [CrossRef]
36. Foundation of Women's Rights Promotion and Development: SDGs for Women, Women for SDGs: Actions from Taiwan 2019. Available online: http://www.globalgender.org/upload/media/status/Web%20_%20Women%20for%20SDGs%20-%20Actions%20from%20Taiwan%202019%20Feb..pdf (accessed on 20 August 2019).
37. Perales, F. The health and wellbeing of Australian lesbian, gay and bisexual people: A systematic assessment using a longitudinal national sample. *Aust. N.Z. J. Public Health* **2019**, *43*, 281–287. [CrossRef] [PubMed]
38. Analysis of Sex and Age Distributions of Facebook Active Users in Taiwan. Available online: https://www.marketersgo.com/marketing/201804/2017-social-media-analysis-report/ (accessed on 13 September 2019).
39. Bobkowski, P.; Smith, J. Social media divide: Characteristics of emerging adults who do not use social network websites. *Media Cult. Soc.* **2013**, *35*, 771–781. [CrossRef]
40. Maisel, N.C.; Fingerhut, A.W. California's ban on same-sex marriage: The campaign and its effects on gay, lesbian, and bisexual individuals. *J. Soc. Issues* **2011**, *67*, 242–263. [CrossRef]

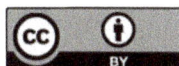

© 2019 by the authors. Licensee MDPI, Basel, Switzerland. This article is an open access article distributed under the terms and conditions of the Creative Commons Attribution (CC BY) license (http://creativecommons.org/licenses/by/4.0/).

International Journal of
*Environmental Research and Public Health*

MDPI

*Article*

# Sexually Transmitted Infections and Associated Factors in Homosexuals and Bisexuals in Granada (Spain) during the Period 2000–2015

Isabel Llavero-Molino [1], María Teresa Sánchez-Ocón [2], María Ángeles Pérez-Morente [3],*, Beatriz Espadafor-López [4], Adelina Martín-Salvador [5], Encarnación Martínez-García [6] and César Hueso-Montoro [6]

1    Hospital La Axarquía, Andalusian Health System, 29740 Vélez-Málaga, Spain
2    University Hospital Virgen de las Nieves, Andalusian Health System, 18014 Granada, Spain
3    Faculty of Health Sciences, University of Jaén, 23071 Jaén, Spain
4    Sexually Transmitted Infection Clinic, Andalusian Health System, 18012 Granada, Spain
5    Faculty of Health Sciences, University of Granada, 52005 Melilla, Spain
6    Faculty of Health Sciences, University of Granada, 18016 Granada, Spain
*    Correspondence: mmorente@ujaen.es

Received: 18 July 2019; Accepted: 13 August 2019; Published: 16 August 2019

**Abstract:** Sexually transmitted infections (STIs) are a major public health issue. Previous research shows the vulnerability of the homosexual and bisexual population, as well as the influence of economic, political, and cultural determinants. The aim of this study was to describe the socio-demographic healthcare profile and the main risk factors associated with STIs in homosexuals and bisexuals seen at the STI clinic in Granada (Spain) during the years 2000–2015. Infection prevalences were compared between the economic crisis period (2008–2014) and the rest of the years analysed. A cross-sectional observational and analytical study was conducted by reviewing 261 clinical records of individuals with suspected or present infection. Univariate, bivariate, and multivariate analyses were performed. 91.2% of the individuals were men, and 8.8% were women, with the mean age being 28.61 (SD = 9.35, Range = 17–74) years old. The prevailing sexual orientation identity was homosexual. 94.2% were single. The main reason for consultation was HIV. Differences in prevalence were found between crisis and non-crisis years (OR = 3.91; 95% CI = 1.73–9.19). In conclusion, their profile was that of a young, single man suspecting possible HIV infection. STI prevalence was significantly higher in the years of economic recession in comparison to the rest of the years.

**Keywords:** sexually transmitted diseases; risk factors; sexual and gender minorities

## 1. Introduction

Sexually Transmitted Infections (STIs) are a major public health issue, both due to their morbidity rates and the complications and sequelae associated with them. Recent studies have noted the existence of certain groups that are particularly vulnerable to STIs, such as immigrants, adolescents, sex workers, men who have sex with men (MSM), and bisexuals [1,2]. MSM are a special interest group because of the increase in the prevalence of HIV and other STIs in recent decades [3].

The latest data published by the European Centre for Disease Prevention and Control (ECDC) for the years 2016 (syphilis) and 2017 (congenital syphilis, gonorrhoea, chlamydia trachomatis, and lymphogranuloma venereum) report an increase in these infections in different population groups. More specifically, in the case of syphilis, 66% of the new cases reported, in which the transmission category is provided, were in MSM [4]. Almost all of the reported cases of lymphogranuloma venereum were in MSM [5]. 10% of the reported cases of chlamydia infections were in MSM [6]. 47% of the cases of gonorrhoea infection were in MSM [7]. Finally, with respect to HIV, transmission in MSM was the most frequent, accounting for 54.3% of all reported cases [8].

The number of new HIV diagnoses in MSM continues to rise in the United States. In 2016, these diagnoses accounted for 82% of new diagnoses, with the age group at highest risk of new diagnosis being those between 13 and 24 years old, this group having experienced an increase of 24% in the number of new diagnoses since 2010 [9]. Syphilis cases also show a steady increase since 2008 in MSM, according to a study conducted in 20 U.S. cities [10].

Certain properties of an individual's sexual behaviour, such as levels of promiscuity, early first sexual intercourse, number of sexual partners, and correctness of condom usage, determine the level of vulnerability in this group [11,12]. In addition, the following stand out: the use of alcohol and drugs, the use of the Internet and other new technologies to easily find and meet sexual partners, the optimism caused by the emergence of antiretroviral treatments, and the lack of effectiveness of prevention programmes [13–19].

The economic, cultural, and political situation has repercussions inth e area of public health and, more specifically, in the incidence of STIs. Spain endured an economic crisis between 2008 and 2014, in which some STIs, such as syphilis and gonorrhoea, which were considered virtually eradicated, resurfaced. In addition, the incidence of other infections, such as HIV, hepatitis, and Human Papillomavirus (HPV), also increased, when HPV control appeared to have been achieved [20].

Based on the above, the general objective of this study was to analyse the socio-demographic characteristics, and healthcare received, as well as the main risk behaviours in relation to STIs in the homosexual and bisexual population seen at the STI clinic in Granada during the years 2000–2015. During this period, some years have been characterised by a strong economic recession (2008–2014). Given the importance of this recession as a social determinant, the specific objective was thus to analyse the differences in the prevalence of these infections between this period and the rest of the years included in the study.

## 2. Materials and Methods

A cross-sectional observational analytic study was conducted by reviewing the medical records at the Sexually Transmitted Infection Clinic in Granada. A total of 261 cases of homosexual and bisexual individuals were analysed. These cases had been extracted from a larger sample of 1536 clinical records that were collected as part of a study which had been carried out by the research team since 2012.

For the selection of these clinical records, records of adult individuals without cognitive impairment who visited the clinic for suspicious reasons or the presence of an STI were considered. Individuals were identified as potential participants when a condition which suggested a possible future diagnosis was met, as stated in the record: symptoms, control, contact follow-up, and HIV.

The sample size was calculated to detect differences in a binary variable (in this case, presence, or absence of STI), seeking to detect differences of 20% in two years, with a statistical power of 80%, provided that the test was performed with an error of $\alpha = 5\%$. The number of clinical records needed per year was 97. In order to select the records, the first and last record numbers were taken from the archive of each year's new records. Subsequently, an annual sample was extracted using systematic random sampling. The study period covers 15 years (2000 to 2015).

The variables collected were the following: socio-demographic (age, sex, nationality, occupation, employment status, level of education, marital status, sexual orientation identity); clinical care received (reason for visit, previous visit, number of subsequent visits, and number of new subsequent episodes); risk indicators (regular partner, period of time since last sexual contact without a condom, number of partners in the last month, number of partners in the last year, contact with a sex worker, regular partner having symptoms, drug use, frequency of drug use, previous STIs, and age of first sexual intercourse).

The following variables, registered in the clinical records as nominal variables, were transformed into ordinal variables for the ease of analysis: the period since last sexual contact without a condom; the number of partners in the last month; and number of partners in the last year. Similarly, the following variables were coded as binary for bivariate analysis: the level of education; marital status; and the reason for the visit.

STI diagnosis was included as the dependent variable and coded as binary (yes/no), following the pattern established by other studies in this line of research [21]. This variable was compared to the rest of the variables described above, which were considered to be independent variables for this analysis. Finally, in order to meet the specific objective, the records were grouped into two time periods: 2000–2007 and 2015, which correspond to the years of absence of the crisis or economic recession, and 2008–2014, which correspond to the years of recession, according to data from the Spanish Ministry of Economy and Business [22].

The data were gathered in a data collection sheet created specifically for this purpose and then transferred to a computerised database. In order to address the general objective of the study, the univariate analysis was carried out first. For quantitative variables, descriptive statistics were computed (mean, median, interquartile range, 95% confidence interval). For qualitative variables, absolute frequencies and percentages were calculated. Subsequently, bivariate analyses were carried out to compare the dependent variable with the independent variables. The Mann-Whitney *U*-test was used if the independent variable was quantitative. This non-parametric test was chosen due to the absence of normality of the analysed variables. This was verified by the Kolmogorov-Smirnov and Shapiro-Wilk tests, as well as by the ordinal nature of some study variables and the small sample size obtained in some comparison groups. For qualitative independent variables, the Chi-squared test ($\chi^2$) or the generalisation of Fisher's exact test was used where applicable.

In order to address the specific objective of the study, the frequency and percentage of STI diagnoses in the crisis and non-crisis periods were first calculated. It was then determined whether there were significant differences in STI prevalence between the two periods using the Chi-squared test. Finally, a multiple logistic regression was performed to control for potential confounding factors, taking the presence or absence of STIs as the dependent variable and the crisis/non-crisis period as an independent variable. These factors were identified after comparing the samples from both study periods on the basis of the variables described above. The tests already described were used for the bivariate analyses. In order to measure the strength of the association, the odds ratio was calculated with its corresponding 95% CI. Once the regression model was generated, the fitting conditions were checked the: collinearity between variables was explored by calculating the Variance Inflation Factor (VIF); the linearity of the dependent variable was checked against the quantitative variables included in the model; calibration was determined by means of the Hosmer–Lemeshow test for goodness of fit; and discrimination was determined according to the value of the area under the ROC curve.

Univariate and bivariate analyses were conducted using the Statistical Package for the Social Sciences (SPSS) program, version 22, (IBM, New York, USA, for Windows). Multiple logistic regression was performed with the R Commander software, version 3.2.2, Free Software Foundation's GNU General Public License, Project R-UCA in Spanish. The statistical significance threshold was set at $p < 0.05$.

Before this study was carried out, approval was obtained from the Biomedical Research Ethics Committee of the province of Granada and from the Management Directorate of the Granada-Metropolitano Health District, which is responsible for the STI clinic where the research was carried out. Patient data were handled with the utmost confidentiality and in compliance with the Spanish Organic Law 15/1999, of the 13th of December, on Personal Data Protection, and the Spanish Organic Law 3/2018, of the 5th of December, on Personal Data Protection and guarantee of digital rights.

## 3. Results

Figure 1 shows the progression of the number of records analysed in the sample that corresponded to homosexual and bisexual individuals.

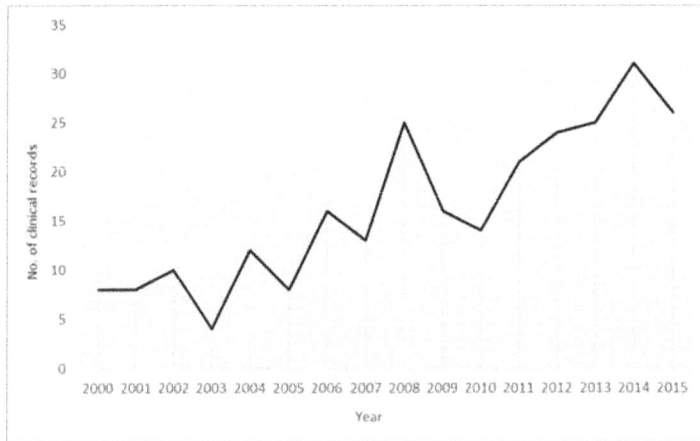

**Figure 1.** Progression of clinical records of the homosexual and bisexual population (2000–2015).

Table 1 displays the characteristics of the sample in relation to the socio-demographic variables, healthcare received, and risk indicators.

**Table 1.** Sample characteristics.

| Socio-Demographic Data | | | | |
|---|---|---|---|---|
| | **Mean** | **95% CI** | **Me** | **IQR** |
| Age (*n* = 261) | 28.61 | 24.47–29.75 | 26.00 | 10 |
| | | *n* | | % |
| Sex (*n* = 261) | | | | |
| Male | | 238 | | 91.2% |
| Female | | 23 | | 8.8% |
| Nationality (*n* = 258) | | | | |
| Spanish | | 230 | | 89.1% |
| Non-Spanish | | 28 | | 10.9% |
| Occupation (*n* = 250) | | | | |
| Other occupations/Unpaid occupation | | 126 | | 50.4% |
| Student | | 124 | | 49.6% |
| Employment status (*n* = 244) | | | | |
| Employed | | 91 | | 37.3% |
| Unemployed | | 25 | | 10.2% |
| Retired | | 4 | | 1.6% |
| Student | | 124 | | 50.8% |
| Level of education (*n* = 253) | | | | |
| No education | | 1 | | 0.4% |
| Primary/Elementary/Basic education | | 13 | | 5.1% |
| Secondary education | | 46 | | 18.2% |
| Vocational training | | 33 | | 13.0% |
| Higher education | | 160 | | 63.2% |

**Table 1.** *Cont.*

| Marital status (n = 258) | | |
|---|---|---|
| Single | 243 | 94.2% |
| Married/Common-law marriage | 9 | 3.5% |
| Separated/Divorced | 6 | 2.3% |
| **Sexual orientation identity (n = 261)** | | |
| Bisexual | 57 | 21.8% |
| Homosexual | 204 | 78.2% |
| **Clinical care received** | | |
| | *n* | % |
| Reason for visit (n = 261) | | |
| Symptoms | 75 | 28.7% |
| Control | 14 | 5.4% |
| Contact follow-up | 2 | 0.8% |
| HIV | 170 | 65.1% |
| Previous visit (n = 211) | | |
| Yes | 52 | 24.6% |
| No | 159 | 75.4% |

| | Mean | 95% CI | Me | IQR |
|---|---|---|---|---|
| No. of subsequent visits (n = 260) | 1.19 | 1.06–1.33 | 1.00 | 0 |
| No. of new subsequent episodes (n = 259) | 0.69 | 0.54–0.84 | 0.000 | 1 |

| **Risk indicators** | | |
|---|---|---|
| | *n* | % |
| Has regular partner (n = 244) | | |
| Yes | 123 | 50.4% |
| No | 121 | 49.6% |
| Contact with sex worker (n = 126) | | |
| Yes | 8 | 6.3% |
| No | 118 | 93.7% |
| Regular partner has symptoms (n = 76) | | |
| Yes | 39 | 51.3% |
| No | 37 | 48.7% |
| Uses drugs (n = 165) | | |
| Yes | 50 | 30.3% |
| No | 115 | 69.7% |
| Frequency of drug use (n = 47) | | |
| Usually | 14 | 29.8% |
| Sporadically | 31 | 66.0% |
| Not currently | 2 | 4.3% |
| Previous Sexually Transmitted Infections (STIs) (n = 217) | | |
| Yes | 54 | 24.9% |
| No | 163 | 75.1% |

| | Mean | 95% CI | Me | IQR |
|---|---|---|---|---|
| Period since last sexual contact without a condom (n = 184) | 2.62 | 2.49–2.75 | 3.00 | 1 |
| No. of partners in the last month (n = 244) | 1.59 | 1.48–1.71 | 1.00 | 1 |
| No. of partners in the last year (n = 241) | 3.13 | 2.95–3.32 | 3.00 | 2 |
| Age of first sexual intercourse (n = 172) | 17.76 | 17.29–18.22 | 17 | 3 |

n = sample size; 95% CI = 95% Confidence Interval; Me = Median; IQR = Interquartile Range; Period of time since last sexual contact without a condom: 1 = never, 2 = less than one month, 3 = one to six months, 4 = six to 12 months, 5 = more than 12 months; No. of partners in the last month: 1 = 0–1, 2 = 2, 3 = 3–5, 4 = more than 5; No. of partners in the last year: 1 = 0–1, 2 = 2, 3 = 3–5, 4 = 6–10, 5 = 11–20, 6 = more than 20.

STI diagnosis was recorded in 132 cases, with a negative diagnosis in 50 of them (37.9%) and a positive diagnosis in 82 of them (62.1%).

No statistically significant differences were found in this variable when compared to the rest of the variables (Tables 2–4).

**Table 2.** STI diagnosis vs. Socio-demographic characteristics.

| Variables | Negative STI Diagnosis | | | | | Positive STI Diagnosis | | | | | $p$ |
|---|---|---|---|---|---|---|---|---|---|---|---|
| | $n$ | Mean | Me | 95% CI | IQR | $n$ | Mean | Me | 95% CI | IQR | |
| Age ($n = 132$) | 50 | 31.38 | 28 | 27.84–34.92 | 14 | 82 | 28.40 | 26 | 26.48–30.33 | 10 | ns |
| | $n$ | | | % | | $n$ | | | % | | $p$ |
| Sex ($n = 132$) | | | | | | | | | | | |
| Male | 44 | | | 37.0% | | 75 | | | 63.0% | | ns |
| Female | 6 | | | 46.2% | | 7 | | | 53.8% | | |
| Nationality ($n = 132$) | | | | | | | | | | | |
| Spanish | 46 | | | 38.3% | | 74 | | | 61.7% | | ns |
| Non-Spanish | 4 | | | 33.3% | | 8 | | | 66.7% | | |
| Occupation ($n = 126$) | | | | | | | | | | | |
| Other occupations/Unpaid occupation | 24 | | | 33.8% | | 47 | | | 66.2% | | ns |
| Student | 22 | | | 40.0% | | 33 | | | 60.0% | | |
| Employment status ($n = 124$) | | | | | | | | | | | |
| Employed | 19 | | | 38.0% | | 31 | | | 62.0% | | ns |
| Unemployed | 4 | | | 25.0% | | 12 | | | 75.0% | | |
| Retired | 2 | | | 66.7% | | 1 | | | 33.3% | | |
| Student | 22 | | | 40.0% | | 33 | | | 60.0% | | |
| Level of education ($n = 126$) | | | | | | | | | | | |
| Higher education | 33 | | | 37.9% | | 54 | | | 62.1% | | ns |
| Others | 15 | | | 38.5% | | 24 | | | 61.5% | | |
| Marital status ($n = 131$) | | | | | | | | | | | |
| Single | 44 | | | 36.4% | | 77 | | | 63.6% | | ns |
| Others | 5 | | | 50.0% | | 5 | | | 50.0% | | |
| Sexual orientation identity ($n = 132$) | | | | | | | | | | | |
| Bisexual | 16 | | | 50.0% | | 16 | | | 50.0% | | ns |
| Homosexual | 34 | | | 34.0% | | 66 | | | 66.0% | | |

$n$ = sample size; 95% CI = 95% Confidence Interval; Me = Median; IQR = Interquartile Range; $p$ = $p$-Value; ns = not significant.

**Table 3.** STI diagnosis vs. Healthcare received.

| Variables | Negative STI Diagnosis | | | | | Positive STI Diagnosis | | | | | $p$ |
|---|---|---|---|---|---|---|---|---|---|---|---|
| | $n$ | | | % | | $n$ | | | % | | |
| Reason for visit ($n = 32$) | | | | | | | | | | | |
| Others | 33 | | | 39.8% | | 50 | | | 60.2% | | ns |
| HIV | 17 | | | 34.7% | | 32 | | | 65.3% | | |
| Previous visit ($n = 110$) | | | | | | | | | | | |
| Yes | 10 | | | 24.4% | | 31 | | | 75.6% | | ns |
| No | 28 | | | 40.6% | | 41 | | | 59.4% | | |
| | $n$ | Mean | Me | 95% CI | IQR | $n$ | Mean | Me | 95% CI | IQR | $p$ |
| No. of subsequent visits ($n = 131$) | 49 | 0.92 | 1.00 | 0.63–1.20 | 1 | 82 | 1.38 | 1.00 | 1.07–1.69 | 2 | ns |
| No. of new subsequent episodes ($n = 131$) | 49 | 0.57 | 0.00 | 0.32–0.83 | 1 | 82 | 1.09 | 0.00 | 0.77–1.40 | 2 | ns |

$n$ = sample size; $p$ = $p$-Value; Me = Median; 95% CI = 95% Confidence Interval; IQR = Interquartile Range; ns = not significant.

**Table 4.** STI diagnosis vs. Risk indicators.

| Variables | Negative STI Diagnosis | | Positive STI Diagnosis | | *p* |
|---|---|---|---|---|---|
| | *n* | % | *n* | % | |
| Regular Partner (*n* = 122) | | | | | |
| Yes | 26 | 43.3% | 34 | 56.7% | *ns* |
| No | 21 | 33.9% | 41 | 66.1% | |
| Contact with sex worker (*n* = 66) | | | | | |
| Yes | 2 | 40.0% | 3 | 60.0% | *ns* |
| No | 21 | 34.4% | 40 | 65.6% | |
| Regular partner having symptoms (*n* = 36) | | | | | |
| Yes | 9 | 56.25% | 7 | 43.75% | *ns* |
| No | 6 | 30.0% | 14 | 70.0% | |
| Uses drugs (*n* = 74) | | | | | |
| Yes | 7 | 33.3% | 14 | 66.7% | *ns* |
| No | 25 | 47.2% | 28 | 52.8% | |
| Frequency of drug use (*n* = 18) | | | | | |
| Usually | 2 | 33.3% | 4 | 66.7% | *ns* |
| Sporadically | 5 | 41.7% | 7 | 58.3% | |
| Previous STIs (*n* = 109) | | | | | |
| Yes | 10 | 33.3% | 20 | 66.7% | *ns* |
| No | 32 | 40.5% | 47 | 59.5% | |

| | *n* | Mean | Me | 95% CI | IQR | *n* | Mean | Me | 95% CI | IQR | *p* |
|---|---|---|---|---|---|---|---|---|---|---|---|
| Period since last sexual contact without a condom (*n* = 88) | 35 | 2.71 | 3.00 | 2.36–3.07 | 1 | 5347 | 2.34 | 2.00 | 2.15–2.53 | 1 | *ns* |
| No. of partners in the last month (*n* = 122) | 47 | 1.70 | 2.00 | 1.47–1.94 | 1 | 75 | 1.72 | 1.00 | 1.50–1.94 | 1 | *ns* |
| No. of partners in the last year (*n* = 120) | 45 | 3.40 | 4 | 2.99–3.81 | 1 | 75 | 3.05 | 3 | 2.72–3.38 | 2 | *ns* |
| Age of first sexual intercourse (*n* = 78) | 33 | 18.39 | 18.0 | 17.05–19.74 | 5 | 45 | 17.40 | 17.0 | 16.42–18.38 | 2 | *ns* |

*n* = sample size; *p* = *p*-Value; Me = Median; 95% CI = 95% Confidence Interval; IQR = Interquartile Range; ns = not significant; Period of time since last sexual contact without a condom: 1 = never, 2 = less than one month, 3 = one to six months, 4 = six to 12 months, 5 = more than 12 months; No. of partners in the last month: 1 = 0–1, 2 = 2, 3 = 3–5, 4 = more than 5; No. of partners in the last year: 1 = 0–1, 2 = 2, 3 = 3–5, 4 = 6–10, 5 = 11–20, 6 = more than 20.

When analysing the presence of STIs between the crisis and non-crisis periods, it was found that, during the non-crisis period, 50% of diagnoses were positive and 50% of diagnoses were negative (*n* = 33 in a sample of 66). In contrast, in the crisis period, the percentages were 74.24% (*n* = 49) for positive diagnoses, and 23.75% (*n* = 17) for negative diagnoses, also in a sample of 66 cases. There was an increase in the number of STIs diagnosed during the crisis period versus the non-crisis period, with this difference being statistically significant (*p* = 0.004) (Figure 2).

In order to analyse whether the statistical association observed could be conditioned by a possible confounding factor related to any of the variables described above, we compared potential confounds (socio-demographic variables and risk indicators) in the sample between both time periods.

The results showed that, in both periods, the populations were homogeneous in all of the variables compared, except for nationality (*p* = 0.002) and number of partners in the last month (*p* < 0.001), in which statistically significant differences were found.

After fitting this association with these two factors using logistic regression (Table 5), a statistically significant association was still observed (*p* = 0.001) with an odds ratio value (crisis/non-crisis period) of 3.91 (95% CI: 1.73–9.19).

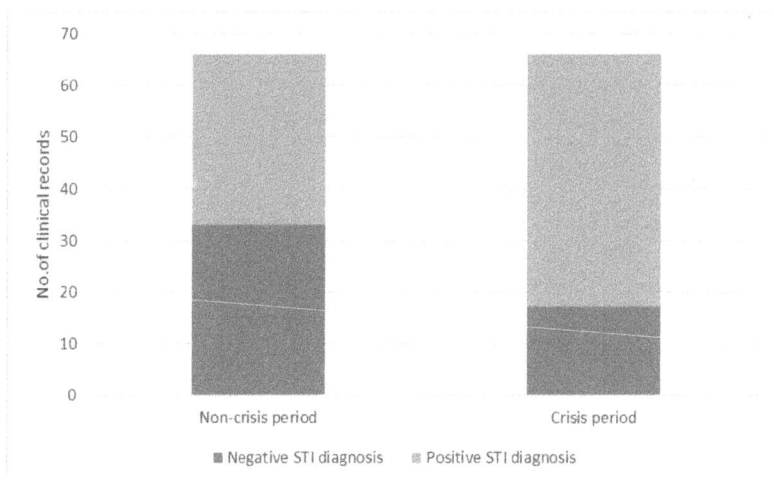

**Figure 2.** Sexually Transmitted Infections (STIs) diagnosis vs. Crisis/Non-crisis period.

**Table 5.** Logistic regression for STI diagnosis vs. Crisis.

| Variables | Crude OR | Adjusted OR (95% CI) | *p* | VIF |
|---|---|---|---|---|
| *Crisis* | | | | |
| Yes | 2.88 (1.40–6.10) | 3.91 (1.73–9.19) | 0.001 | 1.16 |
| No | Ref. | Ref. | | |
| *Nationality* | | | | |
| Non-Spanish | 1.24 (0.37–4.87) | 1.35 (0.32–6.07) | 0.680 | 1.11 |
| Spanish | Ref. | Ref. | | |
| *No. of partners in the last month* | 1.02 (0.68–1.55) | 1.27 (0.80–2.09) | 0.317 | 1.19 |

OR = Odds Ratio; 95% CI = 95% Confidence Interval; VIF = Variance Inflation Factor; Calibration using the Hosmer–Lemeshow goodness-of-fit test: $\chi^2 = 1.5644$, df = 8, $p = 0.991$; Discrimination according to the ROC curve: area under the ROC curve with a value of 0.67 (95% IC = 0.57–0.75).

## 4. Discussion

### 4.1. Main Findings

With regards to the number of homosexual and bisexual individuals who have visited the study clinic, the progressive increase in cases throughout the study period is noteworthy. This increase may be linked to the progressive reduction of stigma and social discrimination against these minority groups, which might lead to the increased self-determination of their sexual behaviour or sexual orientation and the public manifestation thereof. In spite of being in the midst of a process of change in the attitudes of the general population towards these communities, it should be pointed out that there is still a discriminatory attitude that perpetuates their vulnerability even more. Previous studies have highlighted the existing association between stigma and discrimination against these groups, including low self-esteem, depression, and substance use. All of this is conducive to risky sexual practice [13].

In the study period, in the analysed individuals who received their serological test results, a greater prevalence was observed in positive STI diagnoses in comparison to negative STI diagnoses. This finding is in consonance with a recent study in which 365 MSM were monitored, resulting in 253 individuals being diagnosed with one or more STIs during the first two years, with an incidence rate of 90.4 per 100 individuals per year. Other studies suggest that the issue of STIs in the MSM population has been increasing in recent decades, largely due to the risky behaviours adopted by this population [13], while mentioning improvements in biomedical HIV interventions as one of the factors influencing the adoption of risky behaviours [23].

In terms of healthcare indicators, the reason for visit relating to suspected HIV infection was the most common, followed by STI symptoms. It is noteworthy that three-quarters of the sample reported no previous STIs and that the majority of the individuals did not make a previous visit due to suspected STIs. This illustrates the role of these specialised clinics as referral centres for addressing this health issue in this population group [11].

Drug use is a risk factor reported by other investigations which indicate that risky practices are often related to drug use and to certain places of sexual contact, such as private parties, clubs, and saunas [24]. The results found in the present study are not significant in this sense, but a trend can certainly be observed in this respect.

Another risk indicator analysed was the period since the last sexual contact without a condom, with data pointing to inconsistent and infrequent condom use. With respect to the number of partners in the last month and in the last year, the data extrapolated from the clinical records yield a value of between 1–2 partners in the last month and 5–10 in the last year. Both inconsistent condom use and having a large number of sexual partners have been described by other studies as predictors of STI risk, mainly in the adolescent population [24,25].

The age of first sexual intercourse was around the age of 17 years. Other authors [12,26] point to the beginning of sexual relations at even earlier ages, around 15 years old. It is well known that an early onset in this type of relation promotes the occurrence of risky sexual behaviours, as well as an increased risk of contracting STIs [11].

Finally, regarding the specific objective, it should be noted that there was an increase in the prevalence of STIs during the crisis period in comparison to the non-crisis period. This finding is consistent with a previous study by the authors [27] which, unlike the present research, was conducted on the general population and covered a shorter period. In line with the contributions of other authors [28,29], the negative effect of financial crises on infectious conditions is particularly noteworthy. Greece, one of the European countries that has suffered most from the financial crisis, is a prime example of this, where several studies [30,31] have revealed an increase in prevalence of several infectious conditions, including HIV, pointing to budget cuts and the dismantling of a third of all EU prevention programmes between 2009–2010 as possible causes [31]. Interestingly, one of the studies published on the economic crisis and communicable diseases in Europe [32] highlights how STIs and vulnerable groups, such as immigrants, drug users, homeless people, and MSM would be affected.

## 4.2. Limitations

Among the limitations of the present study, first of all, is the fact that the results cannot be extrapolated to the general population of homosexuals and bisexuals since this study was carried out in a single clinic. Of the total number of records collected for the research project, of which this study forms a part, the sample of homosexual and bisexual individuals accounted for 17%. According to a survey carried out in several European countries, 14% of Spanish people between the ages of 14 and 29 would identify themselves as lesbian, gay, bisexual or transgender (LGBT) [33]. Taking into account that the age of the individuals in the records analysed was around 26 and 29 years old, it is fairly safe to conclude that the representation obtained is equivalent to that observed in the general population. However, it should be kept in mind that the distribution by sex differs from the aforementioned survey, with men being more represented than women. It should also be taken into consideration that our sample focuses mainly on men who identify as homosexual or bisexual, whereas the scientific literature consulted refers to MSM, who may view themselves as heterosexual, while still including homosexual and bisexual men.

In addition, being a specialised clinic, the subjects who visit it are attributed to risky behaviour for merely visiting it. In this sense, an underreporting of certain behaviours due to the effect of social desirability cannot be ruled out either, as the clinical records are completed by means of a personal interview.

The percentage of values missing in some of the variables should be taken into account. In some cases, this absence responds to the lack of completion of the clinical record, which could not be controlled in this study. In other cases; however, these were values that were not suitable for collection due to the profile of the individual studied. For this reason, it was preferred to carry out an analysis of the complete cases per variable, showing the sample size analysed in each variable.

Another limitation has to do with the type of design used. In spite of analysing a wide time series, since it is a cross-sectional study, the associations found can only be considered to be causal hypotheses.

### 4.3. Implications for Practice and Research

The results of this research would reinforce the idea of the need to develop education programmes for the prevention of STIs, especially in vulnerable groups, such as homosexual and bisexual populations, that inform and provide tools on what these infections imply and promote the adoption of attitudes, strategies, and personal behaviours that enable these populations to protect themselves from STIs. Emphasis should be placed on prioritising their initiation in these health education programmes from an early age before the first risky behaviours begin. In addition, health policy actions are needed to strengthen specialised STI care and work on prevention through the Internet [23].

In line with the above, one aspect that has not been dealt with in this research, but which will be the subject of future studies, has to do with the use of new technologies through the Internet to search for sexual partners. Increased use of these technologies, especially among younger people, has been demonstrated in other studies reviewed, which reported that young MSM currently meet their first sexual partners through the Internet [34]. Other studies conclude that this practise should be considered to be a risk factor for contracting STIs and HIV [19,35].

The study involved a low number of female individuals. It is, therefore, necessary to conduct future studies that include more women or that are exclusively developed on a female population.

In addition, further longitudinal studies should be carried out to establish more solid causal relationships than those observed in this research, as well as qualitative studies to determine the reasons associated with risky sexual practices from the perspective of homosexual and bisexual individuals.

### 5. Conclusions

As a conclusion, during the period 2000–2015, the profile of the individuals who visited the sexually transmitted infection clinic were mostly young homosexual men of Spanish nationality whose predominant marital status was single. The main reasons for the visit were the suspicion of HIV infection and STI symptoms, with a positive STI diagnosis prevailing when a serological test was performed. No statistically significant differences were found in STI diagnoses when other factors were compared, such as socio-demographic factors, factors relating to the healthcare received, and risk indicators. Differences in STI prevalence were found between crisis and non-crisis periods, with increased STI prevalence during the crisis period.

**Author Contributions:** Conceptualization—I.L.-M., M.Á.P.-M. and C.H.-M.; Data curation—I.L.-M., M.T.S.-O., M.Á.P.-M. and B.E.-L.; Methodology—I.L.-M., M.Á.P.-M., A.M.-S., E.M.-G. and C.H.-M.; Software—C.H.-M.; Supervision—M.Á.P.-M. and C.H.-M.; Writing—Original draft—I.L.-M., M.Á.P.-M. and C.H.-M.; Writing—Review & editing—I.L.-M., M.T.S.-O., M.Á.P.-M., B.E.-L., A.M.-S., E.M.-G. and C.H.-M.

**Funding:** This research received no external funding.

**Acknowledgments:** The authors would like to thank all members of the STI clinic team in the province of Granada, as well as nurses from the Esperanza Cano Romero and María Visitación Mingorance Ruiz, for their help in collecting the data.

**Conflicts of Interest:** The authors declare no conflict of interest.

## References

1. Johnston, L.G.; Alami, K.; El Rhilani, M.H.; Karkouri, M.; Mellouk, O.; Abadie, A.; Rafif, N.; Ouarsas, L.; Bennani, A.; Omari, B.E. HIV, syphilis and sexual risk behaviours among men who have sex with men in Agadir and Marrakesh, Morocco. *Sex. Transm. Infect.* **2013**, *89* (Suppl. 3), 45–48. [CrossRef] [PubMed]

2. Godoy, P. La vigilancia y el control de las infecciones de transmisión sexual: Todavía un problema pendiente. *Gac. Sanit.* **2011**, *25*, 263–266. [CrossRef] [PubMed]

3. De Mosteyrín, S.F.; del Val Acebrón, M.; de Mosteyrín, T.F.; Guerrero, M.L.F. Prácticas y percepción del riesgo en hombres con infección por el virus de la inmunodeficiencia humana que tienen sexo con otros hombres. *Enferm. Infecc. Microbiol. Clin.* **2014**, *32*, 219–224. [CrossRef] [PubMed]

4. European Centre for Disease Prevention and Control. Syphilis. In *ECDC Annual Epidemiological Report for 2016*; ECDC: Stockholm, Sweden, 2018.

5. European Centre for Disease Prevention and Control. Lymphogranuloma venereum. In *ECDC Annual Epidemiological Report for 2017*; ECDC: Stockholm, Sweden, 2019.

6. European Centre for Disease Prevention and Control. Chlamydia infection. In *ECDC Annual Epidemiological Report for 2017*; ECDC: Stockholm, Sweden, 2019.

7. European Centre for Disease Prevention and Control. Gonorrhoea. In *ECDC. Annual Epidemiological Report for 2017*; ECDC: Stockholm, Sweden, 2019.

8. Ministerio de Sanidad, Consumo y Bienestar Social. Vigilancia Epidemiológica del VIH y SIDA en España 2017. Available online: https://www.mscbs.gob.es/ciudadanos/enfLesiones/enfTransmisibles/sida/vigilancia/doc/InformeVIH_SIDA_2018_21112018.pdf (accessed on 10 April 2019).

9. Center for Disease Control and Prevention; National Center for HIV/AIDS, Viral Hepatitis, STD, and TB Prevention Division of HIV/AIDS. HIV Surveillance—Men Who Have Sex with Men (MSM) through 2017. Available online: https://www.cdc.gov/hiv/pdf/library/slidesets/cdc-hiv-surveillance-slides-msm-2017.pdf (accessed on 31 July 2019).

10. An, Q.; Wejnert, C.; Bernstein, K.; Paz-Bailey, G. Syphilis screening and diagnosis among men who have sex with men, 2008–2014, 20 U.S. cities. *J. Acquir. Immune Defic. Syndr.* **2017**, *75* (Suppl. 3), S363–S369. [CrossRef] [PubMed]

11. De Munain, J.L. Epidemiología y control actual de las infecciones de transmisión sexual. Papel de las unidades de ITS. *Enferm. Infecc. Microbiol. Clin.* **2019**, *37*, 45–49. [CrossRef] [PubMed]

12. Teva, I.; Bermúdez, M.; Buela-Casal, G. Variables sociodemográficas y conductas de riesgo en la infección por el VIH y las enfermedades de transmisión sexual en adolescentes: España, 2007. *Rev. Esp. Salud Publ.* **2009**, *83*, 30–320. [CrossRef]

13. Folch, C.; Fernández-Dávila, P.; Ferrer, L.; Soriano, R.; Díez, M.; Casabona, J. Conductas sexuales de alto riesgo en hombres que tienen relaciones sexuales con hombres según tipo de pareja sexual. *Enferm. Infecc. Microbiol. Clin.* **2014**, *32*, 341–349. [CrossRef] [PubMed]

14. Operario, D.; Choi, K.; Chu, P.L.; McFarland, W.; Secura, G.M.; Behel, S.; MacKellar, D.; Valleroy, L. Prevalence and correlates of substance use among young Asian Pacific Islander men who have sex with men. *Prev. Sci.* **2006**, *7*, 19. [CrossRef] [PubMed]

15. Folch, C.; Esteve, A.; Zaragoza, K.; Muñoz, R.; Casabona, J. Correlates of intensive alcohol and drug use in men who have sex with men in Catalonia, Spain. *Eur. J. Public Health* **2009**, *20*, 139–145. [CrossRef] [PubMed]

16. Folch, C.; Marks, G.; Esteve, A.; Zaragoza, K.; Muñoz, R.; Casabona, J. Factors associated with unprotected sexual intercourse with steady male, casual male, and female partners among men who have sex with men in Barcelona, Spain. *AIDS Educ. Prev.* **2006**, *18*, 227–242. [CrossRef]

17. Coll, J.; Fumaz, C.R. Drogas recreativas y sexo en hombres que tienen sexo con hombres: Chemsex. Riesgos, problemas de salud asociados a su consumo, factores emocionales y estrategias de intervención. *Rev. Enf. Emerg.* **2016**, *15*, 77–84.

18. Fernández-Dávila, P.; Zaragoza Lorca, K. Internet y riesgo sexual en hombres que tienen sexo con hombres. *Gac. Sanit.* **2009**, *23*, 380–387. [CrossRef] [PubMed]

19. Jacques Aviñó, C.; García de Olalla, P.; Díez, E.; Martín, S.; Caylà, J.A. Explicaciones de las prácticas sexuales de riesgo en hombres que tienen sexo con hombres. *Gac. Sanit.* **2015**, *29*, 252–257. [CrossRef] [PubMed]

20. Vázquez, F. El incremento de las infecciones de transmisión sexual en el siglo XXI: Nuevos retos y aparición de nuevas patologías. *Enferm. Infecc. Microbiol. Clin.* **2011**, *29*, 77–78. [CrossRef] [PubMed]

21. Horn, K.; Swartz, J.A. A comparative analysis of lifetime medical conditions and infectious diseases by sexual identity, attraction, and concordance among women: Results from a National US survey. *Int. J. Environ. Res. Public Health* **2019**, *16*, 1399. [CrossRef]
22. Ministerio de Economía y Competitividad. La Economía Española Cierra 2013 con un Crecimiento del 0,2%, una Décima Superior al Trimestre Previo. Available online: http://www.mineco.gob.es/stfls/mineco/prensa/ficheros/noticias/2014/140227_NP_rpCN4T13.pdf (accessed on 28 May 2019).
23. Chow, E.P.F.; Grulich, A.E.; Fairley, C.K. Epidemiology and prevention of sexually transmitted infections in men who have sex with men at risk of HIV. *Lancet HIV* **2019**, *6*, e396–e405. [CrossRef]
24. Calatrava, M.; López-Del Burgo, C.; de Irala, J. Factores de riesgo relacionados con la salud sexual en los jóvenes europeos. *Med. Clin.* **2012**, *138*, 534–540. [CrossRef]
25. Câmara, S.G.; Sarriera, J.C.; Carlotto, M.S. Predictores de conductas sexuales de riesgo entre adolescentes. *Rev. Interam. Psicol.* **2007**, *41*, 161–166.
26. Castro, A.; Bermúdez, M.; Madrid, J.; Buela-Casal, G. Variables psicosociales que influyen en el debut sexual de adolescentes en España. *Rev. Interam. Psicol.* **2011**, *43*, 83–94.
27. Pérez-Morente, M.A.; Sánchez-Ocón, M.T.; Martínez-García, E.; Martín-Salvador, A.; Hueso-Montoro, C.; García-García, I. Differences in sexually transmitted infections between the precrisis period (2000–2007) and the crisis period (2008–2014) in Granada, Spain. *J. Clin. Med.* **2019**, *8*, 277. [CrossRef]
28. Suhrcke, M.; Stuckler, D.; Suk, J.E.; Desai, M.; Senek, M.; McKee, M.; Tsolova, S.; Basu, S.; Abubakar, I.; Hunter, P.; et al. The impact of economic crises on communicable disease transmission and control: A systematic review of the evidence. *PLoS ONE* **2011**, *6*, e20724. [CrossRef] [PubMed]
29. Llácer, A.; Fernández-Cuenca, R.; Martínez-Navarro, F. Crisis económica y patología infecciosa. Informe sespas 2014. *Gac. Sanit.* **2014**, *28*, 97–103. [CrossRef] [PubMed]
30. Mckee, M.; Karanikolos, M.; Belcher, P.; Stuckler, D. Austerity: A failed experiment on the people of Europe. *Clin. Med.* **2012**, *12*, 346–350. [CrossRef] [PubMed]
31. Kentikelenis, A.; Karanikolos, M.; Papanicolas, I.; Basu, S.; Mckee, M.; Stuckler, D. Health effects of financial crisis: Omens of a Greek tragedy. *Lancet* **2011**, *378*, 1457–1458. [CrossRef]
32. Rechel, B.; Suhrcke, M.; Tsolova, S.; Suk, J.E.; Desai, M.; McKee, M.; Stuckler, D.; Abubakar, I.; Hunter, P.; Senek, M.; et al. Economic crisis and communicable disease control in Europe: A scoping study among national experts. *Health Policy* **2011**, *103*, 168–175. [CrossRef] [PubMed]
33. Dalia Research. Counting the LGBT Population: 6% of Europeans Identify as LGBT. 2019. Available online: https://daliaresearch.com/counting-the-lgbt-population-6-of-europeans-identify-as-lgbt (accessed on 20 May 2019).
34. Bolding, G.; Davis, M.; Hart, G.; Sherr, L.; Elford, J. Where young MSM meet their first sexual partner: The role of the Internet. *AIDS Behav.* **2007**, *11*, 522–556. [CrossRef] [PubMed]
35. Blackwell, C.W. Men who have sex with men and recruit bareback sex partners on the internet: Implications for STI and HIV prevention and client education. *Am. J. Mens Health* **2008**, *2*, 306–313. [CrossRef] [PubMed]

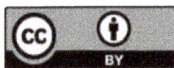

© 2019 by the authors. Licensee MDPI, Basel, Switzerland. This article is an open access article distributed under the terms and conditions of the Creative Commons Attribution (CC BY) license (http://creativecommons.org/licenses/by/4.0/).

International Journal of
*Environmental Research
and Public Health*

MDPI

*Review*

# A Systematic Review of Sexual Minority Women's Experiences of Health Care in the UK

Catherine Meads [1], Ros Hunt [1,*], Adam Martin [2] and Justin Varney [3]

[1]  Faculty of Health, Education, Medicine and Social Care, Anglia Ruskin University, Cambridge CB1 1PT, UK
[2]  Academic Unit of Health Economics, Leeds Institute of Health Sciences, University of Leeds,
     Leeds LS2 9JT, UK
[3]  Director of Public Health, Birmingham City Council, Birmingham City Council'10 Woodcock Street,
     Birmingham B7 4BL, UK
*   Correspondence: ros.hunt@virgin.net

Received: 23 July 2019; Accepted: 17 August 2019; Published: 21 August 2019

**Abstract:** Sexual minority women (SMW) experience worse health and disproportionate behavioural risks to health than heterosexual women. This mixed-methods systematic review evaluated recent studies on health experiences of UK SMW, published 2010–2018. Analysis was through narrative thematic description and synthesis. Identified were 23,103 citations, 26 studies included, of which 22 provided qualitative and nine quantitative results. SMW had worse health experiences that might impact negatively on access, service uptake and health outcomes. Findings highlighted significant barriers facing SMW, including heteronormative assumptions, perceptions and experiences of negative responses to coming out, ignorance and prejudice from healthcare professionals, and barriers to raising concerns or complaints. Little information was available about bisexual and trans women's issues. Findings highlighted the need for explicit and consistent education for healthcare professionals on SMW issues, and stronger application of non-discrimination policies in clinical settings.

**Keywords:** sexual minority women; SMW; lesbian; bisexual; trans; health inequalities; heterosexism

## 1. Background

Sexual minority women (SMW) include women defining themselves by sexual identity (lesbians, bisexual women), behaviour (women who have sex with women, women who have sex with men and women) or relationship status (women who are married to or cohabit with other women).

Although there is a limited evidence base [1–4], in general, SMW experience worse mental health [5], worse physical health [6,7] and higher risk factors for physical ill-health [8–11] than their heterosexual counterparts. Due to lack of outcome-focused research [12], it is unclear whether difficulties with healthcare access are driving worse physical and mental health.

There have been several international systematic reviews on SMW's experiences of healthcare in specific settings. A systematic review of lesbian disclosure to primary care providers [13] included 30 studies (one from UK). It found that a wide variety of attributes of lesbians, healthcare providers and setting affected disclosure. Safety was important for disclosure as was relevancy, health status, how likely a person was to be out overall, and relationship status. The review highlighted the importance of enquiring about sexual orientation rather than presuming heterosexuality. Socio-demographic factors such as age, ethnicity and education did not have clear links with disclosure.

A meta-ethnographic systematic review of lesbian's experiences of childbirth [14] included 13 studies (four from UK). They identified four main themes: encountering and managing overt and covert prejudice, acknowledging the confidence that can be created when professionals present knowledge about lesbian lifestyle and even small gestures of appropriate support, disclosure of sexual orientation being important but risky unless the patient was in charge of the context or situation, and the need for acceptance of the lesbian family by recognising both mothers.

A systematic review of sexual minority people's needs and experiences for end of life and palliative care [15] included 12 studies (one from UK); most of the information for women was related to cancer. The evidence consistently showed the need for all of the health professionals involved in end of life care to be better educated to explore sexual preferences of their patients, avoid heterosexist assumptions, and recognise the importance of partners in decision-making. Health professionals also need to recognise the importance of supportive groups where sexual minority people feel safe to reveal their sexuality, feel accepted and be understood by the support group.

Reasons why sexual minority people may not feel comfortable about revealing their sexual orientation include heteronormativity or overt homophobia. Heteronormativity is the assumption that people are heterosexual. This can result in attitudes and behaviours that exclude people who are not heterosexual (for example assuming a woman of reproductive age who is having regular sexual activity may become pregnant unless contraception is used). Homophobia in a healthcare related setting can manifest as inappropriate refusal to provide care, providing sub-optimal care or inappropriate words or behaviour whilst providing care.

There have been no recent systematic reviews covering the experiences of SMW in a breadth of settings nor specifically from the UK. This systematic review includes all recent evidence on SMW's experiences of UK healthcare in a variety of settings. It focuses on UK research only as experience of healthcare is likely to be very different in other countries because of differences in healthcare delivery and different perceptions of homosexuality and bisexuality. This is a mixed-methods systematic review using both qualitative and quantitative methods on the same topic because neither alone can provide the richness of information available. Mixed methods systematic reviews can provide triangulation of results and increased value compared to either method on its own, and increase the relevance of the findings for decision makers [16].

## 2. Methods

A protocol for the whole project investigating all aspects of health and experience of healthcare in SMW was registered with the Prospero database (No. CRD42016050299). This part of the project investigated experiences of UK healthcare in any setting by SMW (lesbians, bisexual women, women who have sex with women (WSW) and women who have sex with men and women (WSMW), same sex married or cohabiting women or other non-defined non-heterosexual women). Trans women were included if they also identified as SMW. Self-report or objectively measured health experiences were included, from any published or unpublished research (i.e., grey literature reports available on LGBT organisation websites) dated from 2010 onwards.

### 2.1. Searches

Searches were conducted in June 2018 and included results from previous searches for related projects. Databases (platforms) searched were CAB abstracts (Ovid), Cinahl (Elsevier), Cochrane CENTRAL (Cochrane Library), Embase (OVID), Medline (Elsevier), PsycInfo (OVID), Social Policy and Practice (OVID), and Science Citation Index (Web of Science). EPPI-Reviewer 4, Endnote and Microsoft Excel were used to sift citations. Search terms included relevant Medical Subject Heading (MESH) terms and text words for sexual minority identity, behaviour and relationship status.

In addition to database searches, reviews and summaries of lesbian, gay, bisexual and trans (LGB&T) health were examined for additional evidence to ensure all relevant studies were included. Hand search of several relevant journals was conducted (Journal of Homosexuality (2017–June 2018), LGBT Health (2017–June 2018) Journal of LGBT Health Research (all issues), Journal of Lesbian Studies (2014–2018) and Journal of Gay and Lesbian Mental Health (2014–2018)) as different journals are indexed in different databases and entry time varies.

Previous projects by the first author (CM) were sifted for relevant research and, from a previous project, a list of active LGBT health researchers and their publications were reviewed. Web pages of several researchers and organisations who had published health research in SMW were searched. The UK National LGB&T Partnership monthly newsletter from February to August 2018 was sifted to find recent unpublished research. UK national survey websites were examined for relevant information on SMW health (for example, Health Survey for England, Integrated Household Survey, Scottish Health Survey, Welsh Health Survey).

*2.2. Study Selection, Data Extraction, Quality Assessment*

Full text copies of studies that may match the inclusion criteria were obtained. Two reviewers (CM and RH) checked study eligibility. For quantitative data one reviewer independently extracted data from studies into tables (CM) and these were checked by another reviewer (AM), with disagreements resolved through discussion. For qualitative studies relevant results were copied from the included studies into a separate document for reorganisation by descriptive themes. Characteristics and results of included studies were described. (See Table 1 for characteristics of included studies and Table 2 for quantitative results). The Critical Appraisal Skills Programme (CASP) qualitative studies checklist was used to assess quality of interview and focus group studies (Table 3). The question on the CASP qualitative checklist not having yes/cannot tell/no responses was omitted (i.e., question 10 on the value of the research). The CASP checklist for cohort studies was used to assess quality of the quantitative studies in order to give consistency in quality assessment strategy across studies (see Table 4). Questions on this checklist not having yes/cannot tell/no responses were omitted (i.e., study results and their precision, and implications of the results) as these are reported in the results section where appropriate. Studies providing both qualitative and quantitative results were assessed with both checklists. The Confidence in the Evidence from Reviews of Qualitative Research (CERQual) approach [17] was used to summarise our confidence in the systematic review findings across the included studies (Table 5). The review finding headings in the text of the results section correspond to the CERQual assessments in Table 5.

*2.3. Synthesis Methods*

Synthesis of the quantitative results was through narrative description and tabulation. Meta-analysis was not appropriate due to heterogeneity of study designs and outcomes measured. Synthesis of qualitative studies was through thematic synthesis. One researcher (CM) extracted all quotes and author's analyses from the included studies, coded them and organised them into descriptive themes. A second researcher (RH) independently coded the quotes and author's analyses and organised them into another set of descriptive themes. Both researchers together then used the two sets of descriptive themes they had developed to establish analytical themes. These were then reanalysed by the second researcher, who selected illustrative quotations from the original studies to be reported alongside analytical themes. CERQual analysis was then used to develop the finally reported themes. Both researchers had experience analysing qualitative research, one through conducting systematic reviews (CM) and one from conducting primary qualitative research (RH). Neither (CM) nor (RH) had been involved in the conduct of any of the included studies. Combining the qualitative and quantitative results was undertaken in the discussion section, in order to give meaning to the body of evidence as a whole.

**Table 1.** Characteristics of included studies.

| Study Author, Year | Study Design Method | Population, Setting | Number of Participants (Total Number in Study) | Recruitment | Sexual Orientation Ascertainment | Outcomes of Interest | Funding Publication Status |
|---|---|---|---|---|---|---|---|
| Almack et al. 2010 | Four focus groups | LGB community | 5 SMW (n = 15 total) | Unclear | Self-report | End of life care issues | Fully published, Funded by Burdett Trust for Nursing and Help the Aged (now Age UK) |
| Balding 2014 | Health-Related Behaviour Survey | School year 10—aged 14–15 | 1916 Cambridgeshire girls, of which 92 LGBT (n = 3918 total) | Through schools | Self-report LGB | GP practice issues | Grey literature report. Schools Health Education Unit. |
| Bristowe et al. 2018 | Semi-structured interviews | LGB community with advanced illnesses or their carers | 18 SMW (n = 40 total) | Through palliative care teams (three hospital, three hospice), and nationally through social/print media and LGBT community networks | Self-report LGB | Experience of receiving care when facing advanced illness | Fully published. Marie Curie Research Grant Scheme |
| Carter et al. 2013 | Individual and small group interviews | SMW in community | 5 SMW (n = 5 total) | Unclear | Self-report | Cervical screening issues | Fully published, funding unclear |
| Cherguit et al. 2013 | Semi-structured interviews | SMW in community | 10 lesbian mothers (n = 10 total) | Via a donor conception charity then snowball. | Self-report lesbian | Midwifery and delivery issues | Fully published, not funded |
| Elliot et al. 2014 | English General Practice Patient Survey 2009/10 | Women in community attending GPs | 1,021,541 women of which 0.6% lesbian, 0.5% bisexual. 86.1% heterosexual (n = 2,169,718 total) | Through GP surgeries | Self-report LGB using ONS categories | GP practice issues | Fully published, funded by UK Govt. Department of Health |
| Evans and Barker 2010 | Survey (open-ended questions) | Community | 47 women of which 44 SMW (n = 62 total) | Adverts including in Diva magazine | Self-report | Issues around mental health counselling | Fully published, funder unclear |
| Fenge 2014 | Semi-structured interviews at home or workplace. | Community | 1 lesbian (n = 4 total) | Snowball sample | Self-report | Bereavement experiences | Fully published, funding unclear |
| Fish 2010 | Semi-structured interviews | SMW in the community with breast cancer or had partner with breast cancer | 17 SMW (n = 17 total) | Flyers via networks, websites, email lists, LB women's groups, cancer care services and Age Concern | Self-report | Breast cancer care experiences and issues | Grey literature, funded by National Cancer Action Team |

**Table 1.** *Cont.*

| Study Author, Year | Study Design Method | Population, Setting | Number of Participants (Total Number in Study) | Recruitment | Sexual Orientation Ascertainment | Outcomes of Interest | Funding Publication Status |
|---|---|---|---|---|---|---|---|
| Fish and Bewley 2010 | Survey (open ended questions) | SMW in the community | 5909 lesbian and bisexual women ($n$ = 5909 total) | Promotional materials in gay and mainstream media and other distribution channels. | Self-report sexual minority | Nature of healthcare experiences, recommendations for improving services and any other healthcare experiences | Fully published, funded by Lloyds TSB Charitable Foundation |
| Fish and Williamson 2016 | Semi-structured interviews | LGB people in the community diagnosed with cancer in previous 5 years | 6 lesbians ($n$ = 15 total) | Radio interviews, LGBT press articles, 50 local mainstream media cancer groups, LGBT community-based groups, social media | Self-report LGB | Experiences of cancer care | Fully published, funded by Hope Against Cancer charity |
| Formby 2011 (and Formby 2011b) | Survey and focus groups | SMW in the community | 54 SMW ($n$ = 54 total) | Online and through local press, LGBT networks and commercial gay scene | Self-report | Sexual health services | Fully published, funder unclear |
| GEO 2018 | Survey (online only) | LGBTI aged 16 or over | N women not given but approx. 45,402 (42%) ($n$ = 108,100 total) | Via stakeholders, Pride events, national media, GEO, government social media, television interviews and online video | Self-report | Experiences of health services | Grey literature, funded by UK government |
| Guasp 2011 | Survey | Older LGB and heterosexual, community | N women unclear, n SMW unclear. ($n$ = 2086 total) | Through YouGov panel supplemented with social media campaign | Unclear | Future care (other results not presented by gender) | Grey literature report. Funded by Stonewall |
| Humphreys et al. 2016 | Survey and 3 focus groups | SMW in the community | 101 women ($n$ = 101 total) | Through National LGB&T Partnership social media | Self-report | Healthcare experiences | Grey literature, funding unclear |
| Ingham et al. 2016 | Semi-structured interviews | Older women in community | 8 women who had lost a same-sex partner ($n$ = 8 total) | Adverts to relevant charities, support groups and services | Self-report partnership status | Bereavement experiences | Fully published, funding unclear |
| Knocker 2012 | Interviews | Older lesbians in community or sheltered housing | 4 lesbians ($n$ = 8 total) | Unclear | Self-report | Experiences of health and social care | Grey literature report, funded by Joseph Rowntree Foundation |
| Lee et al. 2011 | Unstructured interviews | Lesbian mothers | 8 lesbians ($n$ = 8 total) | Snowballing from first participant | Self-report | Positive and negative experiences of maternity care | Fully published, not funded |

157

**Table 1.** *Cont.*

| Study Author, Year | Study Design Method | Population, Setting | Number of Participants (Total Number in Study) | Recruitment | Sexual Orientation Ascertainment | Outcomes of Interest | Funding Publication Status |
|---|---|---|---|---|---|---|---|
| Light and Ormandy 2011 | Survey and 6 focus groups | Community | Survey 611 LGB women (n = 611 total), 60 in focus groups | Online survey, via Manchester Pride and Manchester Lesbian and Gay Foundation | Self-report | Cervical screening service experiences | Grey literature report, funded by NHS Cervical Screening Programme |
| Macredie 2010 | Survey, with open and closed questions | LGBT in community | 114 LB women (n = 212 total) | Convenience sample, including from pubs and clubs | Self-report lesbian/gay women or bisexual women | Fertility, screening (most results not split by gender) | Grey literature report. Commissioned by NHS Bradford and Airedale |
| McDermott et al. 2016 | Survey and interviews | LGBT people in the community aged 16–25 years who had experienced self-harm or suicidal feelings, and mental health services staff | Survey 336 women (n = 789 total), interviews number of women unclear (n = 29 total) | LGBT organisations and social networks, LGBT mental health organisations | Self-report LGB or queer | Experiences of mental health services | Grey literature, funded by Department of Health Policy Research Programme |
| Price 2010 (and Price 2012) | Semi-structured interviews | LGB carers of people with dementia | 11 SMW (n = 21 total) | Through Alzheimers' Society then online fora, conference, advertising, word of mouth | Unclear | Experiences of dementia services | Fully published, funding unclear |
| River 2011 | Survey (open and closed questions) | LGBT people aged over 50 | 144 SMW n = 283 total) | Through Polari Group mailing list, specialist websites, emails to community lists and social and campaigning groups in London | Self-report LGB | Experiences of GP services | Grey literature, funded by Age Concern England |
| Urwin and Whittaker 2016 | English General Practice Patient Survey 20012/14 | Women in community attending GPs | 1,138,653 women of which 0.6% lesbian, 0.4% bisexual. 91.9% heterosexual (n = 2,807,320 total) | Through GP surgeries | Self-report LGB using ONS categories | GP practice use | Fully published, not funded |
| Westwood 2016 (and Westwood 2016b) | Semi-structured interviews | Older LGB in community or sheltered housing | 36 SMW (n = 60 total) | Convenience sample via online adverts social networks, word of mouth, | Self-report various self-labels | Housing and residential care provision, concerns around dementia care | Fully published, funding unclear |
| Willis et al. 2011 | Two focus groups and semi-structured interviews | Care stakeholders including carers | 2 lesbian carers (n = 10 total) | Multiple channels including electronic fliers, Facebook, LGBT organisations | Self-report | Carers' experiences | Fully published, University of Birmingham seedcorn funding |

Abbreviations: GP—general practice; LB—lesbian and bisexual women; LGB—lesbian, gay and bisexual; LGBT—lesbian, gay, bisexual and transgender; ONS—Office for National Statistics.

Table 2. Quantitative results.

| Study | | Lesbian | Bisexual | Mixed | Heterosexual/Comparator | Statistical Significance | Notes |
|---|---|---|---|---|---|---|---|
| Balding 2014 | Visited GP within previous 6 months | NG | NG | 84% (77/92) | 76% (146/1916) | NG | Comparator is Cambridgeshire girls |
| | Felt uncomfortable or very uncomfortable talking to doctor or other surgery staff on last visit | NG | NG | 34% (31/92) | 26% (50/1916) | NG | |
| Elliott et al. 2014 | Trust and confidence in doctor = not at all | 5.3% (95% CI 4.7–5.9) | 5.3% (95% CI 4.6–6.0) | NG | 3.9% (95% CI 3.8–3.9) | $p < 0.001$ both | Precise numbers for each question varied, numbers by sexual orientation not given. Adjusted percentages controlled for age, race/ethnicity, self-rated health, deprivation quintiles |
| | Doctor communication any item = poor or very poor | 11.7% (95% CI 10.8–12.5) | 12.8% (95% CI 11.9–13.7) | NG | 9.3% (95% CI 9.2–9.4) | $p < 0.001$ both | |
| | Nurse communication any item = poor or very poor | 7.8% (95% CI 7.1–8.4) | 6.7% (95% CI 5.9–7.5) | NG | 4.5% (95% CI 4.5–4.6) | $p < 0.001$ both | |
| | Overall satisfaction = fairly or very dissatisfied | 4.9% (95% CI 4.3–5.5) | 4.2% (95% CI 3.6–4.8) | NG | 3.9% (95% CI 3.8–3.9) | $p < 0.001$ and $p = 0.31$ | |
| GEO 2018 | Did not discuss or disclose sexual orientation because afraid of a negative reaction | NG | NG | 15.6% (cis) | NG | NG | Results given separately for cis and trans women. No heterosexual comparator for cis SMW. Nine percent of trans women were heterosexual, but results not given separately for SMW transwomen (or versus heterosexual transwomen) |
| | Did not discuss or disclose sexual orientation because had a bad experience in past | NG | NG | 5.8% (cis) | NG | NG | |
| | Did not discuss or disclose sexual orientation because afraid of being outed | NG | NG | 5.4% (cis) | NG | NG | |
| | Unsuccessful in accessing mental health services | NG | NG | 9% (cis) | NG | NG | |
| | Rated access to mental health services 'not at all easy' | NG | NG | 27.4% (cis) | NG | NG | |
| | Experience of mental health services mainly or completely negative | NG | NG | 22.2% (cis) | NG | NG | |
| | Accessing sexual health services not easy | 31% | NG | 12.1% (cis) | NG | NG | |
| | Had to wait too long to access sexual health services | NG | NG | 11.5% (cis) | NG | NG | |
| | Was not able to go at a convenient time | NG | NG | 8.9% (cis) | NG | NG | |
| | Worried, anxious or embarrassed about going to sexual health services | NG | NG | 7.1% (cis) | NG | NG | |
| | Sexual health services were not close | NG | NG | | NG | NG | |

**Table 2.** *Cont.*

| Study | Lesbian | Bisexual | Mixed | Heterosexual/ Comparator | Statistical Significance | Notes |
|---|---|---|---|---|---|---|
| GEO 2018 — Did not know where to go to access sexual health services | NG | NG | 5.9% (cis) | NG | NG | Results given separately for cis and trans women. No heterosexual comparator for cis SMW. Nine percent of trans women were heterosexual, but results not given separately for SMW transwomen (or versus heterosexual transwomen) |
| GEO 2018 — GP was not supportive | NG | NG | 4.2% (cis) | NG | NG | |
| GEO 2018 — GP did not know where to refer for sexual health services | NG | NG | 2.3% (cis) | NG | NG | |
| GEO 2018 — Experience of sexual health services mainly or completely negative | NG | NG | 17.3% (cis) | NG | NG | |
| Guasp 2011 — Experienced discrimination, hostility or poor treatment because of their sexual orientation when using GP services | NG | NG | 17% | NG | NG | Numbers unclear, 40% of these incidents within previous 5 years |
| Guasp 2011 — Been excluded from a consultation or decision-making process with regard to their partner's health or care needs | NG | NG | 14% | 6% | NG | Numbers unclear |
| Guasp 2011 — Hidden the existence of a partner when accessing services like health, housing and social care | NG | NG | 12% | <1% | NG | Numbers unclear |
| Humphreys et al. 2016 — Negative experience of GP/Primary care | NG | NG | 47% (24/51) | NG | NG | Denominator numbers unclear |
| Humphreys et al. 2016 — Negative experience of hospital | NG | NG | 66% (18/27) | NG | NG | |
| Humphreys et al. 2016 — Negative experience in a mental health setting | NG | NG | 66% (4/6) | NG | NG | |
| Humphreys et al. 2016 — Negative experience in sexual health clinic | NG | NG | 57% (8/14) | NG | NG | |
| Light and Ormandy 2011 — Refused or discouraged from having a cervical screen by a health professional because of their sexual orientation | NG | NG | 14% (70/500) | NG | NG | |
| Light and Ormandy 2011 — Refused a cervical screen or advised it was not necessary | NG | NG | 6% (7/114) | NG | NG | |
| Macredie 2010 — Found screening staff to be helpful but lacking in knowledge of lesbian and bisexual women | NG | NG | 57% (33/62) | NG | NG | Of those screened |
| Macredie 2010 — Found screening staff to be unhelpful and lacking in knowledge of lesbian and bisexual women | NG | NG | 12% (7/62) | NG | NG | |
| River 2011 — Bad experiences of General Practice | NG | NG | 31% (45/144) | NG | NG | |
| Urwin and Whittaker 2016 — Odds ratio of visiting a family practitioner for any reason | 0.803 (0.755–0.854) | 0.887 (0.817–0.963) | NG | Referent | $p < 0.001$ and $p = 0.004$ | Adjusted for patient and GP practice characteristics |

Abbreviations: GEO—Government Equalities Office; 95% CI—95% confidence interval; cis—cisgender; GP—general practitioner; NG—not given.

**Table 3.** Critical Appraisal Skills Programme (CASP) quality assessment of qualitative studies.

| No | Study | 1 | 2 | 3 | 4 | 5 | 6 | 7 | 8 | 9 | 10 |
|----|-------|---|---|---|---|---|---|---|---|---|----|
| 1 | Almack et al. 2010 | Y | Y | Y | Y | Y | CT | CT | Y | Y | Y |
| 2 | Bristowe et al. 2018 | Y | Y | Y | Y | Y | CT | CT | Y | Y | Y |
| 3 | Carter et al. 2013 | Y | Y | Y | Y | Y | CT | CT | CT | Y | Y |
| 4 | Cherguit et al. 2012 | Y | Y | Y | Y | Y | Y | Y | Y | Y | Y |
| 5 | Evans and Barker 2010 | Y | Y | Y | Y | Y | Y | Y | Y | Y | Y |
| 6 | Fenge 2014 | Y | Y | Y | Y | Y | N | Y | Y | Y | Y |
| 7 | Fish 2010 | Y | Y | Y | Y | Y | CT | Y | N | Y | Y |
| 8 | Fish and Bewley 2010 | Y | Y | Y | Y | Y | CT | Y | Y | Y | Y |
| 9 | Fish and Williamson 2016 | Y | Y | Y | Y | Y | Y | Y | Y | Y | Y |
| 10 | Formby 2011 | Y | Y | Y | Y | Y | N | Y | CT | Y | Y |
| 11 | Guasp 2011 | Y | Y | Y | Y | Y | N | Y | CT | Y | Y |
| 12 | Humphreys et al. 2016 | Y | Y | CT | Y | Y | CT | CT | N | Y | Y |
| 13 | Ingham et al. 2016 | Y | Y | Y | Y | Y | Y | CT | Y | Y | Y |
| 14 | Knocker 2012 | Y | Y | Y | CT | Y | N | CT | N | Y | Y |
| 15 | Lee et al. 2011 | Y | Y | Y | Y | Y | Y | Y | Y | Y | Y |
| 16 | Light and Ormandy 2011 | Y | Y | Y | Y | Y | CT | Y | Y | Y | Y |
| 17 | Macredie 2010 | Y | Y | Y | CT | Y | CT | CT | N | Y | N |
| 18 | McDermott et al. 2016 | Y | Y | Y | Y | Y | CT | Y | Y | Y | Y |
| 19 | Price 2015 | Y | Y | Y | Y | Y | CT | Y | Y | Y | Y |
| 20 | River 2011 | Y | Y | Y | Y | Y | N | Y | CT | Y | CT |
| 21 | Westwood 2016 | Y | Y | Y | Y | Y | CT | Y | CT | Y | Y |
| 22 | Willis et al. 2011 | Y | Y | Y | Y | Y | CT | CT | Y | Y | Y |

Checklist questions were: 1. Was there a clear statement of the aims of the research? 2. Is a qualitative methodology appropriate? 3. Was the research design appropriate to address the aims of the research? 4. Was the recruitment strategy appropriate to the aims of the research? 5. Was the data collected in a way that addressed the research issue? 6. Has the relationship between researcher and participants been adequately considered? 7. Have ethical issues been taken into consideration? 8. Was the data analysis sufficiently rigorous? 9. Is there a clear statement of findings? 10. How valuable is the research? Abbreviations: Y—yes; CT—cannot tell; N—no; N/A—not applicable.

**Table 4.** CASP quality assessment of quantitative studies.

| | Study | 1 | 2 | 3 | 4 | 5a | 5b | 6a | 6b | 9 | 10 | 11 |
|---|-------|---|---|---|---|----|----|----|----|---|----|----|
| 1 | Balding 2014 | y | y | y | ct | ct | ct | n/a | n/a | y | y | n/a |
| 2 | Elliott et al. 2014 | y | y | y | y | y | y | n/a | n/a | y | y | y |
| 3 | GEO 2018 | y | y | y | y | y | ct | n/a | n/a | y | y | y |
| 4 | Guasp 2011 | y | y | y | y | ct | n | n/a | n/a | y | y | y |
| 5 | Humphreys et al. 2016 | y | ct | ct | y | ct | n | n/a | n/a | n | ct | y |
| 6 | Light and Ormandy 2011 | y | y | ct | y | ct | n | n/a | n/a | y | y | y |
| 7 | Macredie 2010 | y | ct | ct | y | ct | n | n/a | n/a | y | y | y |
| 8 | River 2011 | y | y | ct | y | ct | n | n/a | n/a | y | y | y |
| 9 | Urwin and Whittaker 2016 | y | y | y | y | y | y | n/a | n/a | y | y | y |

Checklist questions were: 1. Did the study address a clearly focused issue? 2. Was the cohort recruited in an acceptable way? 3. Was the exposure (SMW status) accurately measured to minimise bias? 4. Was the outcome accurately measured to minimise bias? 5a. Have the authors identified all important confounding factors? 5b) Have they taken account of the confounding factors in the design and/or analysis? 6a. Was the follow up of subjects complete enough? 6b. Was the follow up of subjects long enough? 9. Do you believe the results? 10. Can the results be applied to the local population? 11. Do the results of this study fit with other available evidence? Abbreviations: y—yes; ct—cannot tell; n—no; n/a—not applicable.

**Table 5.** CERQual qualitative evidence profile.

| | Summary of Review Findings | Qualitative Studies Contributing* | Methodological Limitations | Relevance | Coherence | Adequacy | Assessment of Confidence in the Evidence | Explanation of CERQual Assessment |
|---|---|---|---|---|---|---|---|---|
| 1 | Unhelpful health ambience. Women reported that the environment did not include them | 3,5–7, 10,12,14,17,19,20 | Minor methodological concerns due to sample size of some studies and some data coding and analysis undertaken by only one researcher | Very minor concerns. Some studies are extremely local, but the studies together present a coherent picture | Very minor concerns as data consistent within and across studies | Very minor concerns despite low number of participants in some studies. Studies together provide rich data | High | This finding was graded as high as together these 10 studies present a coherent picture of women's experience. Larger studies confirm findings of smaller studies. Rich data supports findings. |
| 2 | Assumed Heterosexuality /Heteronormativity | 2,4–12,17,20 | Very minor methodological considerations due to lack of clarity concerning researcher role and potential bias in design and analysis of most studies. | Very minor concerns. Some studies very local or in big cities, | Very minor concerns. Findings are consistent within and across studies | Minor concerns due to small sample size of some studies. Larger studies provide very rich data and confirm findings of smaller studies. | High | This finding was graded as high despite very minor concerns in a minority of studies as together these studies provide rich data from a wide variety of settings. The 12 studies included provide a consistent picture regardless of service setting and service user group |
| 3 | Being Out or not | 1,3–14,16,19,20 | Very minor methodological considerations due to lack of clarity concerning researcher role and potential bias in design and analysis of most studies. | Very minor concerns. All demonstrate relevance to overall topic | Very minor concerns. Consistency across studies demonstrated. Data support findings | Studies together provide rich data across a variety of health and social care settings | High | This finding was graded as high despite some studies having a small number of participants as there was consistency of findings regardless of setting, geographical location and service user group. Sixteen studies contributed to this finding and rich data were evidenced |
| 4 | Responses to Being Out | 4,5,7–9,12,15–17,22 | Very minor methodological considerations due to lack of clarity concerning researcher role and potential bias in design and analysis of most studies. | Very minor concerns. All demonstrate relevance to overall topic | Very minor concerns. Data consistent within and across studies | Minor concerns due to sample size in some studies which offered little data about women's experience, | High | This finding was graded as high despite minor concerns as ten studies contributed to this theme and larger studies provided consistent, rich data which supported the findings of smaller studies |
| 5 | Ignorance | 3,5,8,10,12,15–17,22 | Very minor methodological considerations due to lack of clarity concerning researcher role and potential bias in design and analysis of most studies. | Very minor concerns. All demonstrate relevance to overall topic | Very minor concerns. Data consistent within and across studies | Minor concerns as some studies were aiming to improve particular services. | High | This finding was graded as high as nine studies contributing to this theme provided rich data to support findings. Consistency and relevance across the studies assures the findings. |

**Table 5.** *Cont.*

| | Summary of Review Findings | Qualitative Studies Contributing* | Methodological Limitations | Relevance | Coherence | Adequacy | Assessment of Confidence in the Evidence | Explanation of CERQual Assessment |
|---|---|---|---|---|---|---|---|---|
| 6 | Impact on SMW | 2,3,7,10–13,15,16,20 | Very minor methodological considerations due to lack of clarity concerning researcher role and potential bias in design and analysis of most studies. | Minor concerns. All demonstrate relevance to overall topic | Very minor concerns. Data consistent within and across studies | Moderate concerns as half of these studies were categorised as 'grey' literature and half had small numbers of participants | Moderate-High | This finding was graded as moderate to high as a half of the studies were categorised as grey literature and half had relatively small numbers of participants. Despite this, data were consistent across studies. |
| 7. | Challenging/ Complaining | 4,7–9,12,16,20 | Very minor methodological considerations due to lack of clarity concerning researcher role and potential bias in design and analysis of most studies. | Minor concerns | Very minor concerns. Data consistent within and across studies | Minor concerns, as this theme was not the focus of studies in most cases and the data were moderately rich | Moderate | This finding was graded as moderate. The data were consistent but lacked richness. |

* Numbers here refer to the studies in Table 3 – CASP assessment of qualitative studies, rather than the reference list.

## 3. Results

A total of 23,103 citations were identified, 22,763 from the first searches and 340 from the second searches (see Figure 1). Full texts of 692 papers were screened for potential relevancy. There were 26 studies included, described in 29 papers, of which 22 provided qualitative results and nine provided quantitative results (studies providing both quantitative and qualitative results were [18–22]. The main reasons for exclusion were that results were not given separately for women and that the papers were not on experiences of UK healthcare. For a full list of references to included studies please see Supplementary Material.

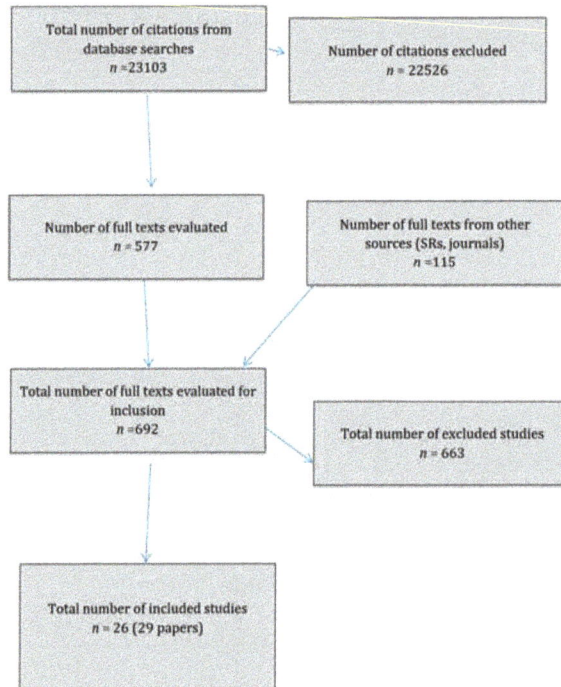

**Figure 1.** PRISMA* flow diagram. *Preferred Reporting Items for Systematic Reviews and Meta-Analyses.

Characteristics of included studies are described in Table 1. Participants in the studies were from the general community and varied in ages from schoolchildren [23] to over 50 [22]. Some of the studies were very large [24] and some compared results from lesbians and bisexual women or SMW to heterosexual women [25] whereas others were small and some recruited lesbians only [26]. The service areas varied from describing experiences of general health services [19] to describing very specific services such as cancer care [27], sexual health services [28] or midwifery [29]. Nine studies provided quantitative results (Table 2) of which two also contributed qualitative results [20,22]. In total, 22 studies provided qualitative results.

*3.1. Qualitative Study Results*

### 3.1.1. Unhelpful Health Ambience

One theme which emerges strongly from the literature regardless of the types of health care provided is the physical context and ambience of the interaction. The patient journey was fraught with expectations of heteronormativity (assumption of heterosexuality) throughout, but initial impressions given by the images in waiting areas, leaflets, forms to be completed, and vocabulary used by staff members were likely to set the tone for any consultation. The visual and non-verbal environment created as a patient progresses through the system can be supportive and enabling, or it can reinforce that their identity is not recognised and give a perception of exclusion. Simple changes to promote visible inclusion of SMW makes a huge difference however the current reality was overwhelmingly that images, leaflets and language were identified by women as making assumptions of heterosexuality.

With respect to forms, for example, one patient felt that her legal relationship was devalued four years after the advent of civil partnership:

"The booking clerk asked me about my marital status. I said I'm civil partnered, she said what's that? I said this is my partner we are in a civil partnership. She said I'll put you down as single" [27] (p. 6).

Leaflets available in waiting areas, pictures on walls and information leaflets equally failed to depict diversity:

"They were all very heterosexual and there was absolutely no mention of a gay relationship or partners. So it didn't feel it was; it didn't feel it could be about me" [30] (p. 298).

Alternatively, leaflets were simply inappropriate; women reported having to 'translate' information to make it appropriate to their situations.

"We were given a print out of a document that would help a straight couple having problems having children, information included for example that 'you should be having sex regularly'. This clearly does not relate to our situation at all" [19] (p. 15).

Respondents to Fish [26] concerning cancer care similarly found the ambience in waiting rooms and support groups to be alien, and focused on aspects of life which they felt were not relevant to them.

For women seeking acceptance, appropriate leaflets and posters with the inclusion of diverse imagery and content would be signifiers that a service was LGB(T) friendly and safe, and contribute to a positive consultation experience. Several different lesbian respondents in River [22] commented on the desirability of indicating the service's openness by visual means such as posters depicting same sex couples, and commented that LGB specific leaflets would provide useful information for women who were not part of the LGB community and who had little other access to LGB specific health information. As Westwood [31] points out, heterosexuality is privileged by the absence of images and leaflets which include LGBT people. Findings such as these were confirmed by other researchers for example Carter et al. [32] in the context of maternity services and Cherguit et al. [29] in the context of co-mothering.

One respondent suggested that LGBT specific leaflets were actively removed from waiting areas. A lesbian respondent [22] saw the sudden disappearance of Broken Rainbow (domestic violence in same sex relationships support service) from the General Practitioner (GP) surgery as possible evidence that LGBT specific leaflets were thrown away or hidden.

Respondents were not entirely negative; many who were accessing fertility clinics praised the LGBT friendliness and one women particularly wanted to be a participant in Cherguit et al.'s [29] study in order to record her positive experience throughout the process.

Ambience is important as it sets the tone for the rest of the interaction with the service and impacts on what follows in terms of women's expectations of welcome or prejudice.

3.1.2. Assumed Heterosexuality/Heteronormativity

It could reasonably be assumed that a lack of LGBT friendly images and leaflets meant that staff did not have lesbian and bisexual women in mind when providing a service and this inevitably led to heterosexist assumptions in personal interactions. Respondents reported that language used by staff during consultations was experienced as exclusive [20,27,29], and required women to contradict assumptions in order to come out, creating a power dynamic, which some women reported as disabling [19,33]. Some women commented that it could be difficult to identify whether they were experiencing overt discrimination due to their sexual orientation, or simply poor practice which would have been similar, although differently expressed, regardless of their sexuality [29,33]

Assumptions of heterosexuality were likely to be influential in different ways. Firstly, women felt unwelcome and that the service, whatever it was, was not aimed at them [27,33,34]; in many instances this would then influence women's decisions as to whether or not to be open about their sexuality [20,33,35]. Secondly assumptions were made about what it was to be a lesbian or a woman who has sex with women [33]. As a result of these assumptions, relationships with professionals were considered to be less good than they might have been, women felt less able to discuss their sexual orientation and therefore the clinicians were unable to make holistic decisions about care and support; This in turn could have resulted in less good (medical) care being provided [19,20,27,32].

Basic expressions of heterosexism (overt or covert discrimination on the grounds of not being heterosexual) were reported by women in many studies. Typically, this included failure by staff to recognise the same sex partner as that, a partner.

"On the day, the locum firstly ignored my introduction as 'partner' and continued to call me 'friend' for the rest of the session" [19] (p. 16).

Even when the evidence of the partner was physically present, professionals apparently found it difficult to treat or speak to female partners in the same way as they would have treated or spoken to husbands or male partners. Again this is evidenced across many services, such as ante-natal classes:

"Kept saying 'right, mums over here, dads, I mean or partners', so she said 'dads, I mean partners!' about 74 times before she finally got her head around just saying partners" [29] (p. 1273).

Issues around the inclusion of same-sex partners in consultations were often mentioned regardless of the setting. A number of participants described instances where partners were negated or derogated [33]. The acceptance of same sex partners was particularly important as women wanted their partners recorded as next of kin and to be the person making decisions for them if required [27,33]. Many felt that their relationships were not recognised:

"(The receptionist) refused to put down my partner's name and partner/next of kin, kept saying 'I'll just put friend', I said, no, I want you to put partner and she looked at me all lips pursed and said, 'I'll just put friend.'" [19] (p. 16).

Heterosexist norms and systems were often applied routinely without adaption for non-heterosexual patients. For example, for lesbian patients, hair loss following chemotherapy meant that something as apparently simple as a wig fitting could become problematic. The only available hairstyles were long and very feminine and often inappropriate for some women's usual style [33].

Although negative experiences outweighed the positive, neutral or positive interactions were reported where same sex partners were accepted without comment by all staff [19,29]. It is perhaps concerning that professionals not reacting negatively to a woman with a same sex partner was worthy of positive comment from respondents. Commenting on the services received for end of life care in a hospital setting, one woman reported:

"I actually found that all the agencies that I had to deal with were totally professional and really helpful and supportive." [30] (p. 297).

3.1.3. Being "Out" or Not

Whether or not women chose to be open about their sexuality with health professionals was a complex topic with many factors impacting on the decision. Coming out to professionals potentially impacted the physical and psychological treatment women received. How health professionals responded to women declaring their sexuality contributed to women's overall experience of services received. In many cases this was influenced by the experiences of the service until the point of meeting the relevant health professional. Fear of prejudice or discrimination based either on previous experience or experience of friends meant that many women chose not to share information about their sexuality. Others chose to share information about their sexuality dependent on whether they thought that this would be medically relevant [20,32,33]. This could be problematic if women were seeking gynaecological treatment as they were unsure as to the relevance of their sexuality to the consultation [32]. If neither patient nor professional mention sexuality and so are unaware of possible health implications, then the potential for compounding the problem increases and the importance of this aspect of life in planning care is missed.

Some women expressed a wish to maintain control of who knew about their sexuality and made a new decision about coming out with respect to each professional they met. Confidentiality was of particular concern when confidentiality policies were unclear [27,32]. Other women requested that their sexuality be recorded on their patient notes so that they did not continually have to come out, although this was not always possible, as in one instance a woman was told it was not information that was recorded in the personal details [32]. The power dynamic of "coming out" is clearly important to SMW and the persistent levels of sexual orientation hate crime and workplace discrimination remind us that disclosure is not without risk [36].

A common theme, regardless of the area of health care, was the awkwardness of coming out. Carter et al.'s [32] research into lesbian and bisexual women's experiences of cervical screening comments that raising the topic could be difficult usually because of assumptions of heterosexuality, but other women in Humphreys and Worthington [19] identified lack of time in appointments as the influential factor. Additionally, women found that they were asked questions about contraception when the smear test was in progress, which was experienced as a particularly difficult time to discuss their sexual identity [20].

A common experience was that women felt that they were forced to be out; typically.

"I wouldn't mind, but I didn't really want to 'come out' to my nurse—she kept asking about contraception and sex—I had no choice but to tell her" [20] (p. 35).

For women who had not previously been open about a same sex relationship, there was the possibility of needing to change their usual practice at a time of ill-health or partner death and thus a time of vulnerability.

"The death of a partner becomes a very public thing so it's an issue and it forces you into a situation you weren't quite ready for" [30] (p. 295).

The result of not coming out might mean that women passively accepted the false assumptions being made about them; this could be uncomfortable, but for some women it provided a feeling of safety and was preferable as it avoided the potential for overt prejudice [32,35].

### 3.1.4. Responses to Being Out

Although many women experienced neutral or positive responses from their healthcare professional, a worrying number received negative responses.

"One couple-counsellor from the agency claimed she could not understand me. She said that I was attractive, had everything going for me, and didn't really understand what my problem was" [34] (p. 386).

Negative responses were frequently reported in the context of cervical screening:

"It was her face, I'll never forget it but she was physically repulsed, and that is how it felt, she was absolutely appalled" [20] (p. 34).

Women also reported the professional gasping [22], physically recoiling [20] or receiving a lecture during an ultrasound of the necessity for a child to have both a mother and a father [19].

On the other hand, there were many reports across all settings of supportive practitioners; these were particularly prominent in the research about women's experiences of being out in GP services [22].

Interestingly, women were occasionally uncertain whether a comment made was intended to be supportive or was homophobic. For example:

"When Jessica was born she said 'oh aren't you lucky you didn't have a boy because you wouldn't know how to deal with penis' and it's like 'what!' (laugh) you don't expect that from a doctor" [29] (p. 1273).

The experiences of this consultation, previous health interactions and general experience of discrimination all contribute to the way in which ambiguous comments are understood.

### 3.1.5. Ignorance

There were a worrying number of reports of medical ignorance with regards to SMW's health. Many, but not all, of these examples were concerned with whether women should be undergoing cervical screening as health professionals did not agree amongst themselves about whether a smear test was required. This comment was typical of respondents' experiences:

'Nurse and doctor have always said I don't need one—lesbians cannot get cervical cancer, so of course, I won't go through an embarrassing procedure I don't need' [20] (p. 32).

Additionally, medical staff appeared ignorant about SMW's sexual health in general. One woman who asked for dental dams rather than condoms was met with blankness, confusion and uncertainty [19]. On another occasion midwives seemed unable to differentiate between the two women in a couple, treating the one who was pregnant as if she had previously given birth when in fact it was her partner who had done so [26].

### 3.1.6. Impact on Sexual Minority Women

The inevitable result of negative experiences was that women either delayed or did not access health care. Carter et al. [32] noted that some participants avoided healthcare of any kind whilst others had not registered with a GP or changed their contact details. "Two (women in this study) avoided going to the GP when they had a problem which resulted in delayed treatment" [32] (p. 137).

For others the treatment might have been less good, for example following a mastectomy:

"The decision not to have reconstruction meant that the consultant did not perform the operation and this led to a reduction in the quality of her surgery" [27] (p. 15).

Likewise, in a counselling context, lack of knowledge was perceived to impact negatively [34].

In consultations, an atmosphere of discomfort and embarrassment, regardless of the vocabulary used could result in patients and partners feeling unable to take full advantage of the consultation and thus received a potentially less good service:

"If we'd had someone treating us that was maybe, was very relaxed about, you know, our sexuality, or whatever, I think it might have just made it a bit easier to ask questions" [27] (p. 5).

Finally, negative experiences added to feelings of being marginalised or different with the potential for associated loss of confidence and self-esteem:

"If you were feeling bad about yourself, you've got low self-esteem or, you know, had the experience of homophobic abuse, and then you went somewhere and you couldn't find the information you wanted, it kind of reinforces the difference" [27] (p. 17).

Affirming responses result in better consultations. Two women in the Humphreys and Worthington [18] study reported that they would ask more questions on the next visit, or feel confident to see the professional again with any future issues.

### 3.1.7. Challenging/Complaining

When experiencing what they considered to be discriminatory language or treatment, women considered complaining but rarely did so. One woman highlighted a variety of reasons for not complaining:

"There's also that thing of if you complain do you, you know, you get branded in some way (laugh) and it was, also its also a structural thing, so its not that anyone, you know, I couldn't say that person was homophobic and complain about them" [29] (p. 1273).

Another had no confidence that a complaint would be taken seriously and raised an important point:

"Looking back I should have complained about her, but didn't feel confident enough—what if the person I complained to was just as homophobic" [20] (p. 33).

Willis et al. [37] in their research with LGBT carers note that "Overt experiences of discrimination were considered not worth reporting because of the emotional resources required to challenge discriminatory treatment from health care professions" [37] (p. 1312). Complaining was often seen as an unavailable option as it might lead to less favourable treatment.

### 3.1.8. Bisexual and Trans Participants

Of the 22 studies included in this review, bisexual respondents were included in 19 studies and women who identified as trans were included in six studies. We have chosen to report bisexual and trans women's experiences separately to ensure that their specific experiences are represented. Most of the issues raised by bisexual and trans women were similar to issues raised by women who identified as gay, lesbian or queer, for example complaints about insensitivity including assumptions about the implications of their self-definition as bisexual or trans, but the issues impacted on them differently.

Some women pointed out that their bisexuality was invisible; women were sometimes disbelieved. One woman currently in a relationship with a woman was assumed to be a lesbian despite her otherwise respectful treatment and her insistence that she was bisexual [19]. Another woman describes feeling hurt when asked if she had 'switched sides' [19] and a woman accessing counselling felt that the counsellor actively denied her bisexuality and wanted her to realise that she was really straight [35]. If a woman had a woman partner at the time of the consultation, it was assumed that she was a lesbian and did not/had not had sex with men, an assumption that could be medically risky and denies the validity of bisexual identity.

There is very little research or acknowledgement of trans SMW and what limited research has been undertaken into trans women's experiences focuses on their gender identity rather than their sexual orientation. A vital issue for lesbian or bisexual transwomen was their gender status. For those who were ill or coming towards the end of their life, the urgency for being treated and dying as women was crucial:

"I'm not ready to die. I want my surgery first, and I was hanging on in there. It was important to me to be buried as a woman, not half and half, you know, with the physical side of it" [38] (p. 27).

Young people reported long waits for appointments at gender assignment clinics which impacted on their mental health:

"Yeah, it took a month ... it took a month for the ... for the referral to sort of like be processed by them and then their response was, 'We can't see you for six months,' which obviously, you know, started making me feel about the same again from before [suicidal]" [39] (p. 65).

Lack of respect for women's status took many forms, including failure to use the correct pronoun [38], this was sometimes then extended as clinicians struggled to process non-heterosexual identities of trans women. There were frequent reports of gender not being recognised:

"In 2008 I had knee surgery and woke up on a male ward—clearly they had looked at my face and overruled my notes" [19] (p. 16).

Women in this group were also questioned and treated inappropriately:

"Bearing in mind I had given him my history, he actually asked me about my periods" [19] (p. 16). And on another occasion:

"I was scheduled for a small bit of surgery and was asked to give a pregnancy test. I pointed out that I was not only a gay woman but also post-op male-to-female trans. The reply was 'Well, best to be sure'" [19] (p. 16).

Lack of awareness resulted in 'outing' women:

"I've been in resus where I didn't know if I was going to survive or not... just with curtains. And you can hear every conversation...Some doctors have said to me, 'How long have you been transgendered for?' And everybody has heard" [38] (p. 29).

A lack of realisation that following usual protocols would impact disproportionately on trans women was reported. In one instance, detained in a psychiatric hospital, in addition to taking no action to make her feel comfortable as a trans person, a woman was not allowed a razor, so her beard grew, to the inevitable detriment of her mental health [37].

### 3.2. Quantitative Comparative Results

Four included studies compared results for SMW and heterosexual women [18,23,25,40]. They tended to show SMW had worse experiences when accessing healthcare (see Table 2). For example Elliott et al. [25] published an evaluation of the English General Practice Patient Survey by gender and sexual orientation. The weighted percentages reporting no trust or confidence in the doctor was 5.3% (95% CI 4.7 to 5.9) in lesbians and 5.3% (95% CI 4.6 to 6.0) in bisexual women, compared to 3.9% (95% CI 3.8 to 3.9) in heterosexual women. Both differences were statistically significantly worse for SMW. There was also significantly worse doctor communication and nurse communication. More SMW were fairly or very dissatisfied with care than heterosexual women and for lesbians this was statistically significant.

Urwin and Whittaker [40] published another evaluation of the English General Practice Patient Survey, looking at inequalities of GP use by sexual orientation. They found that lesbians and bisexual women were less likely to visit the GP than heterosexual women in the previous 3 months (adjusted OR = 0.80 (95% CI 0.76 to 0.85 and OR = 0.89 (95% CI 0.82 to 0.96)) and this was not affected by the proportion of GPs who were women. On the other hand, a survey of schoolchildren in Cambridgeshire [23] found that 84% of sexual minority girls had been to the doctor's surgery in the previous 6 months compared to 76% of Cambridgeshire girls, and that 34% of sexual minority girls had felt uncomfortable or very uncomfortable talking to the doctor or other surgery staff compared to 26% of Cambridgeshire girls.

### 3.3. General Experience of Health from Non-Comparative Studies

A very large survey of LGBT experiences of everyday life in the UK [24] included 108,100 responses (see Table 2). Most of the chapter on health gave numerical results for men and women combined, but there were some results for SMW, but only for cisgender rather than both cisgender and trans women. The results showed widespread difficulties with accessing services, including for mental health and sexual health.

A survey commissioned by the LGBT Partnership [19] on SMW experiences of healthcare found that the majority were of GP/primary care (51%) but also included hospital (33%), sexual health clinic (14%), mental health (6%), fertility clinic (2%) and dentistry (1%). There were more negative experiences in mental health services and hospitals than sexual health clinics and GP/primary care services. The majority of the negative experiences reported took place in the previous year to the survey (i.e., 2014–2015). The main themes for the negative experiences were assumption of heterosexuality, clinicians being uncomfortable with minority sexual orientation, participants being given incorrect or incomplete information based on sexual orientation, bad treatment (possibly) not related to coming out, partner not being acknowledged, experience of overt homophobia or biphobia, or clinicians ignoring the patient disclosing their sexual orientation.

A survey of older LGBT people [22] found that 43% of SMW had had good experiences with their general practice and 31% reported bad experiences. These included overhearing homophobic comments, overt prejudice from a GP towards their partner with cancer, assumptions of heterosexuality by all staff including receptionists, lack of awareness of SMW's issues, partners being ignored, shock and embarrassment by health staff on disclosure, and inappropriate disclosure of sexual orientation to a third party.

Two UK studies were found on cervical screening attitudes and uptake in lesbians and bisexual women [20,32] and one provided quantitative results. Light et al. [20] conducted a multi-method evaluation of a project delivered by the then Lesbian and Gay Foundation (LGF - now LGBT Foundation) with SMW in the Northwest of England. From the survey, although 91% agreed that SMW should have cervical screening, only 70.5% of those eligible had accessed screening in the previous five years and 48% within the previous 3 years. There was clear evidence found that SMW had been misinformed by being told they did not need a cervical smear and 14% of those eligible had been actively refused or discouraged from having a smear test by a health professional as a direct result of their sexual orientation. When they did attend, many SMW were subjected to heteronormative assumptions. Following this survey, a public information campaign was run by LGF called 'Are you ready for your screen test?'. This was well received and accepted by lesbians and bisexual women in the North West and was evaluated by a second survey with 345 responses. The campaign resulted in an additional 22% of those aged 25 or more having gone for a cervical screen and a further 8% having booked a cervical smear appointment.

## 4. Discussion

### 4.1. Summary of Findings

This rigorously conducted and innovative mixed-methods systematic review included 26 studies, of which 22 provided qualitative results and nine provided quantitative results (two studies provided both quantitative and qualitative results [18–22]). All included studies were relevant to the delivery of UK healthcare services. A major strength of the findings is the demonstration of consistency across studies, including studies generated by small organisations and by the UK government, and the coherence of findings across qualitative and quantitative studies. This is systematic review is innovative in that there are very few mixed-methods systematic reviews and there have been no previous systematic reviews of SMW's experiences of UK healthcare. It is also one of very few to incorporate CERQual assessment of outcomes (Table 5).

In addition to the protections afforded by the Equality Act (2010), the National Health Service (NHS) constitution states that "Respect, dignity, compassion and care should be at the core of how patients... are treated". Although some women in specific services reported that this was the case, the majority of women included in these studies reported otherwise. Years of experience of prejudice means that women need positive signs/images that a service will be LGBT friendly. Negative expectations were confirmed by a plethora of experiences such as the ambience of the service and the attitude of reception staff, inappropriate protocols that needed to be followed, language used, assumptions made and apparent ignorance of SMW's health needs.

First impressions are important, thus images and leaflets in waiting areas set the tone of what could be expected. What might appear as a minor issue to others has a greater impact on those who have experiences of discrimination—images and the use of language are important in building up a trusting atmosphere. In many instances it is this pervasive heteronormativity that directly influences women's decisions on coming out or not to the professional they see, and therefore potentially limits their ability to receive holistic care. Systems that allowed appropriate registration of same-sex partners, and attitudes of reception staff prior to a consultation with the relevant professional, all contributed to women's assessment of whether they would be treated respectfully and their identities meaningfully recognised. Appropriate posters and leaflets are important, but if a service provides these, expectations are raised and the agencies would then need to ensure that a service that fulfils those expectations is provided. Inclusion and openness which is tokenistic is likely to have a detrimental outcome.

Health professionals were seemingly unable to adapt information given and procedures followed to SMW's specific situations; this was particularly obvious in fertility clinics and cervical screening. However, at times of reconstructing their self-image, for example as a cancer patient, it is unhelpful if a woman's physical style or style of dress and hair has to be amended to fit in with what NHS provision apparently considers to be the norm for women. Equally striking was the apparent ignorance of health professionals about SMW's health needs as clearly demonstrated by the inconsistent information provided about cervical screening. Extremely worrying here is the increased medical risk to women as evidenced by confusing a woman who is a first time mother with her partner who has given birth, or ignoring her history and refusing a bisexual woman a smear test as her current partner is a woman.

It is essential to remember that interactions with services tend to occur at a time of difficulty, illness, vulnerability or crisis. Coupled with fear of discrimination, this is not a time when women are likely to feel able to challenge or complain about poor treatment, unthinking assumptions about them and their lives or apparent active homophobia. SMW reported heteronormative assumptions leaving them with the choice of either going along with these assumptions or challenging them and thus risking negative reactions and potential breaches of confidentiality.

In order to form a trusting and open relationship with professionals, SMW need to feel respected for who they are. As is clear, the negation of partners, the use of inappropriate vocabulary and assumptions all militate against this. What SMW expect from the health professional is no different from what all patients expect and is promised in the NHS constitution. Health practitioners need to be aware that treating people equally and respectfully does not mean treating them the same, but making adjustments appropriate to their life situations. The assumed heterosexuality that SMW may encounter influences every aspect of their journey through services.

The impact of the experiences of marginalisation, labelling and direct discrimination cannot be underestimated. The way in which staff interacted with SMW might well be open to interpretation and many women expecting negative responses may thus interpret ambiguous responses negatively. It was also possible that the professionals in question were simply lacking in people skills so that all patients were treated equally poorly. It must be remembered that complaints voiced by many patients may impact differently on SMW; for example, meeting different doctors at every appointment in ongoing treatment means that women may constantly be deciding whether or not to come out, with the potential additional stress that this might entail.

One further comment is on the use of the term 'disclose' when women are considering whether or not to share their identity with professionals. In current English usage this term carries negative connotations, for example in 'disclosing' a criminal record. Such language is unlikely to encourage women to be open about who they are.

The quantitative comparative studies demonstrated that SMW experience worse interaction with UK health and social care in a wide variety of settings and services than heterosexual women. The non-comparative studies, including one extremely large survey by the UK Government Equalities Office [24], found very worrying trends in difficulty with accessing a wide variety of health and care services.

*4.2. Strengths and Weaknesses of the Systematic Review*

A major strength of this systematic review is the combining of findings from qualitative and quantitative research. Other strengths include extensive searches from a number of different sources. We assessed quality of individual studies using CASP questionnaires appropriate to the different study designs, to give an element of consistency in questions about bias assessment across qualitative and quantitative studies.

We used a wide definition of SMW including identity, behaviour and partnership. Although they are different concepts, (some women identify as lesbian whilst having sex with men, some women identify as heterosexual whilst having sex with women, and women can identify as lesbian or bisexual without being sexually active or being in a partnership) they are all representative of sexual minority status. The studies used self-report for the experience of healthcare and this may therefore result in responder bias, but it is unclear why responder bias might be stronger in SMW than heterosexual respondents. There is a potential conflict of interest where a charity or other small group seeks to demonstrate an issue in order to redress a wrong.

Several studies combined results for men and women and thus picking out issues specifically related to women was challenging. In the qualitative systematic review we used direct quotations rather than narratives from the papers where the author's analyses incorporated both men's and women's issues so that we could report the women's experiences. We used rigorous methods to synthesise the findings from a large number of studies to generate themes applicable to multiple health care delivery situations.

We also used CERQual [17] to generate evidence profiles of our findings to show how the relevance, coherence, adequacy and methodological limitations of individual studies impacted on our overall qualitative findings under each of the headings in the main text.

### 4.3. Comparison to Previous Research

There have been previous systematic reviews on UK LGB health but none focusing on SMW and on experience of healthcare. There have been no previous mixed-methods systematic reviews in this area incorporating CERQual assessment of outcomes. A wide-ranging systematic review on health, education, employment, housing and other topics, [3] written for the UK Government Equalities Office, included small sections on the use and experience of mental health services, satisfaction with health care and discrimination, and recommendations for policy, but did not distinguish between men's and women's health experiences. An extensive overview of health needs of lesbian and bisexual women [41] looked at experiences and expectations regarding healthcare providers also found negative experiences, lower satisfaction and fewer than half of SMW being out to their GPs. SMW frequently reported that healthcare providers assumed they were heterosexual, and that they were not given a chance to 'come out'. When women did come out this information was commonly ignored, and occasionally negative comments were made.

There is a clear gap in research into bisexual women and trans SMW's experiences, and this biases the perspectives to those of lesbian-identified women, especially in quantitative research where SMW are often combined for analysis due to limited sample size.

### 5. Implications and Recommendations for Practitioners

Many health care staff feel that they give person-centred care to all of their patients or clients including SMW, and therefore they do not need to know about their sexuality. A survey by the Stonewall Charity on the treatment of LGBT people within UK health and social care services [34] found a worrying amount of lack of knowledge and understanding of the issues, unfairness, negativity and some blatant discrimination by staff.

There is a need to incorporate SMW issues into guidelines for healthcare. A systematic review of primary care guidelines for LGB people [42] included 11 guidelines (two from UK). They found that the currently available guidelines for LGB care are philosophically and practically consistent, and synthesised recommendations could be readily applied to existing primary care systems with minimal change and no cost to practice systems, but staff training would be needed. The Lesbian, Gay, Bisexual and Trans Public Health Outcomes Framework Companion Document [11] sets out the evidence base related to each public health indicator, and makes clear recommendations for action at local, regional and national levels. Regarding healthcare it recommends that

"Commissioners should use the data available to them to assess whether mainstream services they have commissioned are accessible to and appropriate for LGBT people".

And also that

"Commissioners should ensure provision of specialist services, where appropriate, to address specific healthcare needs available in their local area."

There is a need for including issues around care for SMW in medical, nursing and allied professional training curricula. A recent review of UK issues around nursing care [43] concluded that, although a number of studies internationally had investigated LGBT nursing care and how it could be introduced into the nursing curriculum, there were no recent UK studies. There was little attention paid to LGBT patients' needs in many university nursing programmes, resulting in nurses being less than confident when nursing LGBT patients [43]. Concepts of homosexuality were difficult for nurses who were not being exposed to SMW, because SMW were not coming out in a nursing context. Experiences of lesbians should be made clear to staff to enable them to become familiar with the needs of this population and understand and modify the way they provide care. Health professionals also need to learn to abolish prejudice to enable them to deliver comprehensive and appropriate care.

## 6. Conclusions

There is very little research published on SMW health [1] and even less on experiences of healthcare. This mirrors the general trend of little investment in LGBT research [12]. There is clear and consistent evidence, despite limited research, that SMW face barriers to accessing and experiencing positive care. There is a strong need to enhance healthcare professionals' understanding of how to provide culturally competent care for LGBT people and to understand this group's health needs. Despite the fact that the NHS has a sexual orientation information standard guideline and training to support implementation, changing attitudes is not straightforward. It is unclear how long it will take for equality and diversity messages to filter through to front line healthcare staff resulting in practice change. While the current status quo continues, SMW continue to receive poor and inappropriate care in many situations.

**Supplementary Materials:** The following are available at http://www.mdpi.com/1660-4601/16/17/3032/s1, References to included studies.

**Author Contributions:** Conceptualization: J.V. and C.M., methodology: C.M. and R.H., methods: C.M., A.M. and R.H., formal analysis: C.M., A.M. and R.H., writing—original draft preparation: C.M. and R.H., writing—review and editing: all; project administration: C.M., funding acquisition: not applicable.

**Funding:** This research received no specific grant from any funding agency in the public, commercial, or not-for-profit sectors.

**Conflicts of Interest:** The authors declare that there is no conflict of interest.

## References

1. Blondeel, K.; Say, L.; Chou, D.; Toskin, I.; Khosla, R.; Scolaro, E.; Temmerman, M. Evidence and knowledge gaps on the disease burden in sexual and gender minorities: A review of systematic reviews. *Int. J. Equity Health* **2016**, *15*, 16. [CrossRef]

2. Edmondson, D.; Hodges, R.; Williams, H. *The Lesbian, Gay, Bisexual and Trans Public Health Outcomes Framework Companion Document*; updated; National LGB&T Partnership: London, UK, 2016.

3. Hudson-Sharp, N.; Metcalf, H. *Inequality among Lesbian, Gay Bisexual and Transgender Groups in the UK: A Review of Evidence*; National Institute of Economic and Social Research: London, UK, 2016.

4. Meads, C.; Pennant, M.; McManus, J.; Bayliss, S. *A Systematic Review of Lesbian, Gay, Bisexual and Transgender Health in the West Midlands Region of the UK Compared to Published UK Research*; University of Birmingham: Birmingham, UK, 2011; Available online: http://www.birmingham.ac.uk/Documents/collegemds/haps/projects/WMHTAC/REPreports/2009/LGBThealth030409finalversion.pdf (accessed on 26 January 2011).

5. Semlyen, J.; King, M.; Varney, J.; Hagger-Johnson, G. Sexual orientation and symptoms of common mental disorder or low wellbeing: Combined meta-analysis of 12 UK population health surveys. *BMC Psychiatry* **2016**, *16*, 67. [CrossRef] [PubMed]

6. Saunders, C.L.; Mendonca, S.; Lyratzopoulos, Y.; Abel, G.A.; Meads, C. Associations between sexual orientation, and overall and site-specific diagnosis of cancer: Evidence from two national patient surveys in England. *J. Clin. Oncol.* **2017**, *35*, 3654–3661. [CrossRef]

7. Robinson, C.; Galloway, K.Y.; Bewley, S.; Meads, C. Lesbian and bisexual women's gynaecological conditions: A systematic review. *BJOG* **2017**, *124*, 381–392. [CrossRef]

8. Hodson, K.; Meads, C.; Bewley, S. Lesbian and bisexual women's likelihood of becoming pregnant: A systematic review. *BJOG* **2017**, *124*, 393–402. [CrossRef]

9. Meads, C.; Moore, D. Breast cancer in lesbians and bisexual women: Systematic review of incidence, prevalence and risk studies. *BMC Public Health* **2013**, *13*, 1127. [CrossRef]

10. Shahab, L.; Brown, J.; Hagger-Johnson, G.; Michie, S.; Semlyen, J.; West, R.; Meads, C. Sexual orientation identity and tobacco and hazardous alcohol use: Findings from a cross-sectional English population survey. *BMJ Open* **2017**, *7*, e015058. [CrossRef] [PubMed]

11. Williams, H.; Varney, J.; Taylor, J.; Fish, J.; Durr, P.; Elan-Cane, C. *The Lesbian, Gay, Bisexual and Trans Public Health Outcomes Framework Companion Document*; Lesbian and Gay Foundation: Manchester, UK, 2013.

12. Coulter, R.W.; Kenst, K.S.; Bowen, D.J.; Scout. Research funded by the National Institutes of Health on the health of lesbian, gay, bisexual and transgender populations. *Am. J. Public Health* **2014**, *104*, e105–e112. [CrossRef]

13. St. Pierre, M. Under what conditions do lesbians disclose their sexual orientation to primary healthcare providers? A review of the literature. *J. Lesbian Stu.* **2012**, *16*, 199–219. [CrossRef]

14. Dahl, B.; Fylkesnes, A.M.; Sørlie, V.; Malterud, K. Lesbian women's experiences with healthcare providers in the birthing context: A meta-ethnography. *Midwifery* **2013**, *29*, 674–681. [CrossRef] [PubMed]

15. Harding, R.; Epiphaniou, E.; Chidgey-Clark, J. Needs, experiences, and preferences of sexual minorities for end-of-life care and palliative care: A systematic review. *J. Palliat. Med.* **2012**, *15*, 602–611. [CrossRef] [PubMed]

16. Harden, A. *Mixed-Methods Systematic Reviews: Integrating Quantitative and Qualitative Findings*; National Center for the Dissemination of disability Research (NCDDR): Washington, WA, USA, 2010.

17. Lewin, S.; Bohren, M.; Rashidian, A.; Munthe-Kaas, H.; Glenton, C.; Colvin, C.J.; Garside, R.; Noyes, J.; Booth, A.; Tuncalpe, O.; et al. Applying GRADE-CERQual to qualitative evidence synthesis findings-paper 2: How to make an overall CERQual assessment of confidence and create a Summary of Qualitative Findings table. *Implement Sci.* **2018**, *13*, 10. [CrossRef] [PubMed]

18. Guasp, A. *Lesbian Gay and Bisexual People in Later Life*; Stonewall: London, UK, 2011.

19. Humphreys, S.; Worthington, V. *Best Practice in Providing Healthcare to Lesbian, Bisexual and Other Women Who Have Sex with Women*; National LGB&T Partnership: Manchester, UK, 2016.

20. Light, B.; Ormandy, P.; Bottomley, R.; Emery, A. *Lesbian, Gay & Bisexual Women in the North West: A Multi-Method Study of Cervical Screening Attitudes, Experiences and Uptake*; University of Salford: Manchester, UK, 2011.

21. Macredie, S. *The Challenge for Change. Health needs of Lesbian, Gay and Bisexual People in Bradford and District*; Equity Partnership: Bradford UK, 2010.

22. River, L. *Appropriate Treatment Older Lesbian, Gay and Bisexual People's Experience of General Practice*; Age of Diversity and Polari: London, UK, 2011.

23. Balding, A. *Young People in Cambridgeshire Schools, the Health-Related Behaviour Survey 2014, a Report for LGBT*; The Schools Health Education Unit: Exeter, UK, 2014.

24. Government Equalities Office (GEO). *National LGBT Survey Research Report*; UK Government Department for Education: Manchester, UK, 2018.

25. Elliott, M.N.; Kanouse, D.E.; Burkhart, Q.; Abel, G.A.; Lyratzopoulos, G.; Beckett, M.K.; Schuster, M.A.; Roland, M. Sexual minorities in England have poorer health and worse health care experiences: A national survey. *J. Gen. Intern. Med.* **2014**, *30*, 9–16. [CrossRef] [PubMed]

26. Lee, E.; Taylor, J.; Raitt, F. 'It's not me, it's them': How lesbian women make sense of negative experiences of maternity care: A hermeneutic study. *J. Adv. Nurs.* **2010**, *67*, 982–990. [CrossRef] [PubMed]

27. Fish, J. *Coming Out about Breast Cancer: Lesbian and Bisexual Women. Policy and Practice Implications for Cancer Services and Social Care Organisations*; National Cancer Action Team and De Montfort University: Leicester, UK, 2010.

28. Formby, E. Sex and relationships education, sexual health, and lesbian, gay and bisexual sexual cultures: Views from young people. *Sex Educ.* **2011**, *11*, 255–266. [CrossRef]

29. Cherguit, J.; Burns, J.; Pettle, S.; Tasker, F. Lesbian co-mothers' experiences of maternity healthcare services. *J. Adv. Nurs.* **2013**, *69*, 1269–1278. [CrossRef]

30. Fenge, L.-A. Developing understanding of same-sex partner bereavement for older lesbian and gay people: Implications for social work practice. *J. Gerontol. Soc. Work* **2014**, *57*, 288–304. [CrossRef]

31. Westwood, S. 'We see it as being heterosexualised, being put into a care home': Gender, sexuality and housing/care preferences among older LGB individuals in the UK. *Health Soc. Care Community* **2016**, *24*, e155–e163. [CrossRef] [PubMed]

32. Carter, L.; Hedges, L.; Congdon, S. Using diversity interventions to increase cervical screening of lesbian and bisexual women. *J. Psychol. Issues Organ. Cult.* **2013**, *3*, 133–145. [CrossRef]

33. Fish, J.; Williamson, I. Exploring lesbian, gay and bisexual patients' accounts of their experiences of cancer care in the UK. *Eur. J. Cancer Care* **2018**, *27*. [CrossRef]

34. Evans, M.; Barker, M. How do you see me? Coming out in counselling. *Br. J. Guid. Counc.* **2010**, *38*, 375–391. [CrossRef]

35. Price, E. Coming out to care: Gay and lesbian carers' experiences of dementia services. *Health Soc. Care Community* **2010**, *18*, 160–168. [CrossRef] [PubMed]

36. Somerville, C. *Unhealthy Attitudes: The Treatment of LGBT People within Health and Social Care Services*; Stonewall: London, UK, 2015.

37. Willis, P.; Ward, N.; Fish, J. Searching for LGBT carers: Mapping a research agenda in social work and social care. *Br. J. Soc. Work* **2011**, *41*, 1304–1320. [CrossRef]

38. Bristowe, K.; Hodson, M.; Wee, B.; Almack, K.; Johnson, K.; Daveson, B.A.; Koffman, J.; McEnhill, L.; Harding, R. Recommendations to reduce inequalities for LGBT people facing advanced illness: ACCESSCare national qualitative interview study. *Palliat. Med.* **2018**, *32*, 23–35. [CrossRef]

39. McDermott, E.; Hughes, E.; Rawlins, V. *Queer futures final report. Understanding Lesbian, Gay, Bisexual and Trans (LGBT) Adolescents' Suicide, Self-Harm and Help-Seeking Behaviour*; Department of Health Policy Research Programme: London, UK, 2016.

40. Urwin, S.; Whittaker, W. Inequalities in family practitioner use by sexual orientation: Evidence from the English General Practice Patient Survey. *BMJ Open* **2016**, *6*, e011633. [CrossRef] [PubMed]

41. Williams, H. *Beyond Babies and Breast Cancer. Health Care Needs of Lesbian and Bisexual Women: An Overview of Available Evidence*; The Lesbian & Gay Foundation: Manchester, UK, December 2013.

42. McNair, R.; Hegarty, K. Guidelines for the Primary Care of Lesbian, Gay, and Bisexual People: A Systematic Review. *Ann. Fam. Med.* **2010**, *8*, 533–541. [CrossRef]

43. Fish, J.; Evans, D.T. Promoting cultural competency in the nursing care of LGBT patients (Editorial). *J. Res. Nurs.* **2016**, *21*, 159–162. [CrossRef]

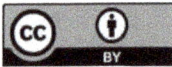

© 2019 by the authors. Licensee MDPI, Basel, Switzerland. This article is an open access article distributed under the terms and conditions of the Creative Commons Attribution (CC BY) license (http://creativecommons.org/licenses/by/4.0/).

International Journal of
*Environmental Research
and Public Health*

MDPI

*Article*

# LGBT+ Health Teaching within the Undergraduate Medical Curriculum

**Jessica Salkind [1,*], Faye Gishen [1,2], Ginger Drage [3], Jayne Kavanagh [1,2] and Henry W. W. Potts [4]**

1   Department, University College London Medical School, London WC1E 6JL, UK
2   Royal Free London NHS Foundation Trust, London NW3 2QG, UK
3   Groundwork London, London SE1 7QZ, UK
4   UCL Institute of Health Informatics, London NW1 2DA, UK
*   Correspondence: jessica.salkind@nhs.net

Received: 13 June 2019; Accepted: 27 June 2019; Published: 28 June 2019

**Abstract:** Introduction: The lesbian, gay, bisexual, and transgender (LGBT+) population experience health and social inequalities, including discrimination within healthcare services. There is a growing international awareness of the importance of providing healthcare professionals and students with dedicated training on LGBT+ health. Methods: We introduced a compulsory teaching programme in a large London-based medical school, including a visit from a transgender patient. Feedback was collected across four years, before (n = 433) and after (n = 541) the session. Student confidence in using appropriate terminology and performing a clinical assessment on LGBT+ people was assessed with five-point Likert scales. Fisher exact tests were used to compare the proportion responding "agree" or "strongly agree". Results: Of the students, 95% (CI 93–97%) found the teaching useful with 97% (96–99%) finding the visitor's input helpful. Confidence using appropriate terminology to describe sexual orientation increased from 62% (58–67%) to 93% (91–95%) (Fisher $p < 0.001$) and gender identity from 41% (36–46%) to 91% (88–93%) ($p < 0.001$). Confidence in the clinical assessment of a lesbian, gay or bisexual patient increased from 75% (71–79%) to 93% (90–95%) ($p < 0.001$), and of a transgender patient from 35% (31–40%) to 84% (80–87%) ($p < 0.001$). Discussion: This teaching programme, written and delivered in collaboration with the LGBT+ community, increases students' confidence in using appropriate language related to sexual orientation and gender identity, and in the clinical assessment of LGBT+ patients.

**Keywords:** LGBT; gay; lesbian; transgender; undergraduate medical education; decolonizing the curriculum; medical education; curriculum development

## 1. Introduction

In many parts of the world, the political and social progress of recent decades has significantly improved the lives of people who are lesbian, gay, bisexual, and transgender (LGBT+, with the "+" indicating inclusion of all sexual and gender minority identities). Despite this progress, even in countries with the most robust legal equality for the LGBT+ population, there remain significant health and social inequalities. Multiple international studies have consistently found higher rates of depression, anxiety, alcohol and drug use, self-harm and suicide, alongside worse physical health outcomes in the LGBT+ community [1–4]. These have been linked to social inequalities stemming from homophobia, biphobia, and transphobia [5]. There is evidence that these inequalities extend to those being treated and working within healthcare systems. For example, in a survey of over 5000 staff within the UK National Health Service (NHS), 25% of staff had heard homophobic language at work and 20% had heard transphobic language at work [6]. Transgender patients have reported being addressed by the wrong names and pronouns, and feeling that they have to educate healthcare professionals [7].

In order to address these inequalities, international organisations including the World Health Organisation [8] and the Association of American Medical Colleges [9] have called for dedicated teaching on LGBT+ health for healthcare students and professionals. Consequently, some healthcare programmes have introduced teaching on LGBT+ health. An example of a comprehensive teaching programme is that offered by the University of Louisville School of Medicine, who have introduced a 50.5 hour integrated programme including a patient panel, with encouraging initial outcomes in terms of reduced implicit bias based on sexuality [10]. A recent systematic review of 15 LGBT+ teaching programmes (seven of which were medical schools) found improvements in knowledge, attitudes and/or practice towards LGBT+ people, however they did not evaluate whether these translated into improvements in the care of LGBT+ patients. The authors reported that the content of the teaching varied between programmes, but in general there was less focus on the specific issues faced by those who are transgender/non-binary and programmes often had no or minimal involvement of LGBT+ people themselves [11].

With this in mind, we introduced a half-day programme for all fifth year medical students (in their penultimate year of the undergraduate course) in a large London medical school. The year before, a pilot programme had been introduced that covered sexual orientation only and was led by senior medical students with no input from LGBT+ patient visitors. The positive feedback to this initial session led to the expansion of the programme. The expanded programme was strongly based on the input of LGBT+ people with an equal focus on sexual orientation and gender identity. The teaching programme aimed to enable students to understand and explore the impact of prejudice and discrimination on LGBT+ people and to consider how medical students and doctors can promote their health and wellbeing.

## 2. Methods

### 2.1. Setting and Context

This half-day teaching programme was embedded within a compulsory fifth year summative teaching week, bringing together key themes from the year's teaching, including obstetrics and gynaecology, paediatrics, general practice, care of the older patient, psychiatry, and palliative care. International guidance recommends embedding LGBT+ teaching throughout the curriculum [12], and this fifth year teaching complements a lecture for first year students on gender identity and sexual orientation, and further teaching on transgender medicine within the 'Child Health' module.

### 2.2. Development of Materials

The teaching materials were developed over several months by Jessica Salkind a junior doctor, using an iterative technique, with input and feedback from self-identifying LGBT+ people. They have subsequently been updated each year in response to student and teacher feedback. As discussed above, many teaching programmes of this kind have placed more onus on sexual orientation, therefore significant effort was made to gain input from transgender and non-binary people who generously shared their stories and helped construct the clinical scenarios to make them as realistic as possible.

### 2.3. Teaching Session Structure

The programme was structured as follows: (1) A 45 minute lecture incorporating key background knowledge, terminology, LGBT+ inequality, legal protection for LGBT+ people and professional guidance; (2) a 45 minute session with a patient visitor who identifies as transgender with the opportunity for students to ask questions about their experiences of accessing healthcare services as well as more general questions; (3) a 1.5 hour seminar to work through four clinical scenarios and generate best practice advice for making services LGBT+ inclusive.

## 2.4. Facilitators

While other models have used senior medical students to facilitate this type of teaching [13,14], within this programme, self-identifying LGBT+ junior doctor facilitators were selected for a number of reasons. Junior doctors have more clinical experience, allowing them to integrate clinical learning into the sessions and answer questions confidently, while still being relatable to students. In addition, there are fewer issues around confidentiality if they choose to share stories about their own experiences, and it has proven easier to ensure the sustainability of the programme. As the majority of the facilitators are cisgender (and identify as lesbian, gay or bisexual), they received additional training on transgender/non-binary issues which may be outside their personal experience. All facilitators had the opportunity to spend time with and learn from the patient visitors. They received a literature pack prior to the teaching with guidance on group facilitation, including what to do if problems occurred, such as disagreement between students or how to handle potentially offensive and/or upsetting comments. They also received guidance from senior university staff with experience of hosting patient visitors in medical student teaching.

## 2.5. Patient Visitors

The patient visitors, who all identify as transgender/non-binary, were recruited through personal networks, LGBT+ national conferences and via social media. The visitors were provided with written guidance, asking them to share their stories of using healthcare services, to explain to students both positive and negative aspects of care they have had and identify times when things were done particularly well or could have been done better. Prior to the teaching, teaching staff discussed the possible impact of sharing potentially distressing personal stories with an unknown group with each visitor. Each group facilitator met their visitor on the day, prior to the teaching, and senior staff were on hand to offer support to visitors if they wished to debrief afterwards, as well as signposting to external sources of support if needed. Three visitors were invited per session to enable smaller discussion groups (maximum 30 students per group). Students were encouraged to think about potential questions for the visitor in advance. Each visitor was asked about their preferred name, pronouns and whether there were any topics that they did not want to be asked about before the session.

## 2.6. Ethical Approval

The UCL Research Ethics Committee approved the anonymised pre and post-session questionnaires. Project ID: 4415/002.

## 2.7. Funding

The programme was awarded a £1470 "Liberating The Curriculum" grant by the University, designed to increase teaching related to equality, diversity and inclusion themes. This money was used to pay for facilitator travel costs, and to pay the visiting speakers for their time and travel costs. Following the positive feedback for programme, these costs are now met by the Medical School.

## 2.8. Questionnaire Design

An anonymous paper-based questionnaire was given to students before and after the session, using a series of statements with a five-point Likert scale from "strongly disagree" to "strongly agree". This assessed their views on the importance of the teaching, their confidence in using appropriate language related to sexual orientation and gender identity, and their confidence in taking a history and examining a lesbian, gay or bisexual patient, and a transgender patient. Other models have used similar scales to evaluate self-perceived confidence in clinical assessment of LGBT+ patients [14]. In addition, the post-session questionnaire, completed directly after the session, explored whether the session was useful and whether the visitor had enhanced students' understanding, with a free-text option for further comments.

Further face-to-face feedback was gathered informally after each session with all visitors and facilitators. Utilising Quality Improvement methodology, a plan-do-study-act cycle approach was taken, using feedback to make rapid changes to content and structure between consecutive sessions and/or days, and asking visitors and facilitators to evaluate those changes, for example, a role play scenario was introduced in response to a number of free text comments.

## 3. Results

Across 2016–2019, 92, 81, 125, and 135 people respectively (433 total) completed the pre-session questionnaire, and 119, 84, 162, and 176 people respectively (541 total) completed the post-session questionnaire (Table 1). To ensure anonymity, responses were not linked to individuals and therefore paired analyses are not possible. Data were combined across the four years, using Fisher exact tests to compare the proportion responding 'agree' or 'strongly agree' before and after the session.

Prior to the session, a small proportion of the group, 9% (CI 6–12%) did not agree with the idea that LGBT+ people face health and social inequalities which are relevant to clinical practice. After the session, this proportion decreased to 1% (1–3%) ($p < 0.001$). There were significant improvements in confidence using appropriate terminology to describe sexual orientation from 62% (58–67%) pre-session to 93% (91–95%) post-session ($p < 0.001$). There was a larger improvement for confidence in using appropriate terminology to describe gender identity, where there was a lower starting confidence pre-session: from 41% (36–46%) to 91% (88–93%) post-session ($p < 0.001$).

Pre-session, 75% (71–79%) of students were confident in the clinical assessment of a lesbian, gay or bisexual patient (including using appropriate language), which increased to 93% (90–95%) post-session ($p < 0.001$). As with terminology, a bigger change was seen with regards to the clinical assessment of a transgender patient, where there was a low initial confidence of 35% (31–40%) pre-session, increasing to 84% (80–87%) post-session ($p < 0.01$).

Overall, nearly all students (95%; CI 93–97%) found the teaching session useful and felt that the visitor had enhanced their understanding of the topics covered in the session (97%; CI 96–99%). In the most recent year, only one student out of 176 did not report the session as useful.

The free text comments were generally positive, with the session described as "a really informative session (which) highlighted the complexity of these issues which I hadn't previously considered" and "something that isn't taught anywhere else in our curriculum, but highly relevant & important to be educated on". Many comments referred directly to the visitors, "I found having a chance to speak with the transgender visitor extremely helpful & insightful", but described wanting more time to ask questions: "could spend even longer discussing issues with them". The feedback from the patient visitors was similarly positive, with one person describing it as "a very empowering experience and more importantly, one that will hopefully help shaping their future attitude towards transgender people, when it comes to it".

**Table 1.** Pre and post-session questionnaire results (2016–2019 data pooled).

| Question | Pre | | Post | | Fisher Exact Test $p$ |
|---|---|---|---|---|---|
| | % Agree/Strongly Agree | 95% CI | % Agree/Strongly Agree | 95% CI | |
| LGBT+ people face health and social inequalities which are relevant to clinical practice | 395/433 (91%) | 88%–94% | 533/540 (99%) | 97%–99% | <0.001 |
| I feel confident using appropriate terminology to describe sexual orientation. | 270/433 (62%) | 58%–67% | 504/540 (93%) | 91%–95% | <0.001 |
| I feel confident using appropriate terminology to describe gender identity. | 176/432 (41%) | 36%–46% | 490/541 (91%) | 88%–93% | <0.001 |
| I would feel confident taking a history from and examining a lesbian, gay or bisexual patient, including using appropriate language. | 326/433 (75%) | 71%–79% | 501/541 (93%) | 90%–95% | <0.001 |
| I would feel confident taking a history from and examining a transgender patient, including using appropriate language. | 153/433 (35%) | 31%–40% | 453/541 (84%) | 80%–87% | <0.001 |
| I found the session useful. | | | 516/541 (95%) | 93%–97% | |
| The visitor enhanced my understanding of topics covered in the session. | | | 527/541 (97%) | 96%–99% | |

grey lines: These questions evaluating the teaching were asked in the post-session questionnaire only, therefore a Fisher test could not be applied.

## 4. Discussion

The results showed marked improvements across all five questions and very positive assessments of the session's usefulness and the value of having the visitor.

There was a significant improvement in confidence in using appropriate terminology to describe people who are LGBT+. This is important, as uncertainty regarding appropriate terminology may underlie the reports of inappropriate and potentially offensive language being used by healthcare professionals to describe those who are LGBT+ [6]. Within the clinical scenarios, students were encouraged to describe ways in which they could challenge inappropriate or offensive language if they overheard it during their clinical placements, for example via the medical school's raising concerns system. The reported increase in confidence in taking a history and examining patients who are LGBT+ is key to ensuring equitable access to healthcare regardless of sexual orientation and gender identity, in line with the Equality Act [15] in the UK. Transgender people have reported being asked inappropriate questions, for example, about their plans for genital surgery when presenting with an unrelated medical problem, and of their gender identity overshadowing an underlying, unrelated problem [7]; this may be mitigated against by a full and appropriate clinical assessment.

The biggest improvements subsequent to the teaching related to describing gender identity and interacting with transgender people, due to initial lower confidence compared with describing sexual orientation and interacting with lesbian, gay and bisexual people. These findings reflect published data that students are more comfortable discussing issues related to sexual orientation than gender identity [16]. The authors propose that the increase in confidence around gender identity may be, in part, due to the time spent with the transgender visitor, with nearly all (97%; CI 95–98%) reporting that the visitor enhanced their understanding of the topics covered, a feeling echoed in the free text comments. Confidence in taking a history and examining a transgender patient, although greatly improved, was the only question that received less than 9 out of 10 positive responses after the session, with 84% agreeing they would feel confident, suggesting this area remains challenging for some students.

To the best of our knowledge, this programme is unique in offering all students within a medical school year cohort the opportunity to hear the stories and ask questions of a visitor who is transgender. The benefit of inviting visitors seems to be two-fold. Intergroup contact theory predicts that exposure to LGBT+ people can reduce prejudice, and there is growing evidence for this in similar settings to this one [17–19]. For all students, it is likely that having the opportunity to ask questions about a group they have potentially had little contact with could reduce discomfort. Evidence from Louisville showed that after an event involving interaction between healthcare professionals and transgender community members, the healthcare professionals felt more confident to work with transgender patients [20]. Furthermore, the real-life expertise provided by the visitors, is likely to provide the most valuable and valid best practice advice for students. This best practice advice is also incorporated into the four clinical scenarios, created from the amalgamation of real life stories shared by LGBT+ patients, as it has been suggested that hypothetical cases can lack the complexity of real clinical cases [21]. In this way, the whole teaching programme directly reflects the lived experiences of LGBT+ people who have been treated recently within the UK NHS. By delivering this teaching in the fifth year, the students have already had sufficient clinical experience and generic history-taking and examination skills to engage meaningfully with the clinical scenarios, consider best practice and contribute their own stories from their clinical placements. By incorporating this training within the core curriculum, its sustainability has been ensured. The model could be easily transferred to other healthcare training settings. While in a large teaching hospital in London, there is a baseline of acceptance towards LGBT+ people and robust legal equality, training of this kind could have even more impact in settings where this is not the case.

A limitation of this work is that, as with other teaching delivered within the same summative teaching week, the teaching session had a relatively low attendance rate of about one third of the year cohort despite it being a mandatory session. It is not currently possible to assess whether this represents selection bias, for example, with those students who are LGBT+ themselves, or those who have friends or family who are, being more likely to attend [22] or if this simply represents a diligent cohort of students who attend all teaching sessions. Efforts are being made by the university to increase attendance through a sign-in sheet. As acknowledged in other work of this kind [11], it is not possible to determine if students' immediate feedback will translate into longer-term change in attitude towards LGBT+ people or a change in clinical practice and improvement in clinical care. The next step is to incorporate LGBT+ scenarios into medical student examinations. There is the potential to use a validated tool to assess students after the teaching—evidence has recently been provided for the lesbian, gay, bisexual, and transgender development of clinical skills scale (LGBT-DOCSS) [23].

## 5. Conclusions

This programme has been positively evaluated by medical students and greatly increases their confidence in using appropriate language related to sexual orientation and gender identity, and in performing clinical assessments on patients who are LGBT+. Further research is required to measure whether improved student confidence translates into improved patient care for the LGBT+ community. This is key for a group with proven healthcare disparities who may disengage from healthcare services if not treated with understanding and respect.

**Author Contributions:** J.S. has recently finished foundation training and is applying for pediatric residency in the USA. She is teaching lead for the LGBT+ health programme at UCL medical school. F.G. is a consultant physician in palliative medicine and the academic lead for Clinical & Professional Practice at UCL Medical School. G.D. is a transgender patient and advocate who has experience working with medical students to improve LGBT+ healthcare and in the third sector. J.K. is a principal clinical teaching fellow at UCL Medical School and a sexual health clinician. She sits on the UCL LGBTQ+ Equality Advisory Group. H.W.W.P. is an associate professor in health informatics at UCL.

**Conflicts of Interest:** The authors declare no conflict of interest.

## Glossary Terms

| | |
|---|---|
| Sexual orientation | describes who a person is sexually attracted to. |
| Homosexual/gay/lesbian | a person who is sexually attracted to people of the same gender. |
| Bisexual | a person who is sexually attracted to people of the same gender and another gender/other genders. |
| Gender identity | how a person identifies in terms of being a man, a woman, both, neither or another identity altogether. |
| Cisgender /cis | a person whose gender identity is consistently congruent with the sex they were assigned at birth. |
| Transgender/trans | a person whose gender identity is not consistently congruent with the sex they were assigned at birth. |
| Non-binary | any gender identity outside of exclusively 'man' or 'woman'; a non-binary person may or may not identify as transgender. |
| Homophobia/biphobia/transphobia | hatred and/or intolerance of people who are homosexual/bisexual/transgender. |

## References

1. Hafeez, H.; Zeshan, M.; Tahir, M.A.; Jahan, N.; Naveed, S. Health Care Disparities Among Lesbian, Gay, Bisexual, and Transgender Youth: A Literature Review. *Cureus* **2017**, *9*, e1184. [CrossRef] [PubMed]
2. Gonzales, G.; Henning-Smith, C. Health Disparities by Sexual Orientation: Results and Implications from the Behavioral Risk Factor Surveillance System. *J. Community Health* **2017**, *42*, 1163–1172. [CrossRef] [PubMed]
3. McKay, B. Lesbian, gay, bisexual, and transgender health issues, disparities, and information resources. *Med. Ref. Serv. Q.* **2011**, *30*, 393–401. [CrossRef] [PubMed]
4. Bonvicini, K.A. LGBT healthcare disparities: What progress have we made? *Patient Educ. Couns.* **2017**, *100*, 2357–2361. [CrossRef] [PubMed]

5.    McDermott, E.; Hughes, E.; Rawlings, V. The social determinants of lesbian, gay, bisexual and transgender youth suicidality in England: A mixed methods study. *J. Public Health (Oxf. Engl.)* **2017**, *40*, e244–e251. [CrossRef] [PubMed]

6.    Somerville, C. *Unhealthy Attitudes: The Treatment of LGBT People Within Health and Social Care Serv*; Stonewall: London, UK, 2015.

7.    McNeill, J.; Bailey, L.; Ellis, S.; Morton, J.; Regan, M. Trans Mental Health Study. Available online: http://www.scottishtrans.org/wp-content/uploads/2013/03/trans_mh_study.pdf (accessed on 28 June 2019).

8.    World Health Organization. *Improving the Health and Well-Being of Lesbian, Gay, Bisexual and Transgender Persons: Report by the Secretariat*; World Health Organization: Geneva, Switzerland, 2013; Available online: http://www.ghwatch.org/sites/www.ghwatch.org/files/B133-6_LGBT.pdf (accessed on 28 June 2019).

9.    AAMC Advisory Committee on Sexual Orientation GI, and Sex Development. *Implementing Curricular and Institutional Climate Changes to Improve Health Care for Individuals Who are LGBT, Gender Nonconforming, or Born with DSD*; AAMC: Washington, DC, USA, 2014.

10.   Leslie, K.F.; Sawning, S.; Shaw, M.A.; Martin, L.J.; Simpson, R.C.; Stephens, J.E.; Jones, V.F. Changes in medical student implicit attitudes following a health equity curricular intervention. *Med. Teach.* **2018**, *40*, 372–378. [CrossRef] [PubMed]

11.   Sekoni, A.O.; Gale, N.K.; Manga-Atangana, B.; Bhadhuri, A.; Jolly, K. The effects of educational curricula and training on LGBT-specific health issues for healthcare students and professionals: A mixed-method systematic review. *J. Int. Aids Soc.* **2017**, *20*, 21624. [CrossRef] [PubMed]

12.   Solotke, M.; Sitkin, N.A.; Schwartz, M.L.; Encandela, J.A. Twelve tips for incorporating and teaching sexual and gender minority health in medical school curricula. *Med. Teach.* **2019**, *41*, 141–146. [CrossRef] [PubMed]

13.   Grosz, A.M.; Gutierrez, D.; Lui, A.A.; Chang, J.J.; Cole-Kelly, K.; Ng, H. A Student-Led Introduction to Lesbian, Gay, Bisexual, and Transgender Health for First-Year Medical Students. *Fam. Med.* **2017**, *49*, 52–56. [PubMed]

14.   Taylor, A.K.; Condry, H.; Cahill, D. Implementation of teaching on LGBT health care. *Clin. Teach.* **2018**, *15*, 141–144. [CrossRef] [PubMed]

15.   Equality Act 2010: Guidance. Available online: https://www.gov.uk/guidance/equality-act-2010-guidance (accessed on 28 June 2019).

16.   Liang, J.J.; Gardner, I.H.; Walker, J.A.; Safer, J.D. Observed Deficiencies in Medical Student Knowledge of Transgender and Intersex Health. *Endocr. Pract.* **2017**, *23*, 897–906. [CrossRef] [PubMed]

17.   Burke, S.E.; Dovidio, J.F.; Przedworski, J.M.; Hardeman, R.R.; Perry, S.P.; Phelan, S.M.; Nelson, D.B.; Burgess, D.J.; Yeazel, M.W.; Van Ryn, M. Do Contact and Empathy Mitigate Bias Against Gay and Lesbian People Among Heterosexual First-Year Medical Students? A Report from the Medical Student CHANGE Study. *Acad. Med. J. Assoc. Am. Med. Coll.* **2015**, *90*, 645–651. [CrossRef] [PubMed]

18.   Phelan, S.M.; Burke, S.E.; Hardeman, R.R.; White, R.O.; Przedworski, J.; Dovidio, J.F.; Perry, S.P.; Plankey, M.; Cunningham, B.A.; Finstad, D.; et al. Medical School Factors Associated with Changes in Implicit and Explicit Bias Against Gay and Lesbian People among 3492 Graduating Medical Students. *J. Gen. Intern. Med.* **2017**, *32*, 1193–1201. [CrossRef] [PubMed]

19.   Walch, S.E.; Sinkkanen, K.A.; Swain, E.M.; Francisco, J.; Breaux, C.A.; Sjoberg, M.D. Using Intergroup Contact Theory to Reduce Stigma Against Transgender Individuals: Impact of a Transgender Speaker Panel Presentation. *J. Appl. Soc. Psychol.* **2012**, *42*, 2583–2605. [CrossRef]

20.   Noonan, E.J.; Sawning, S.; Combs, R.; Weingartner, L.A.; Martin, L.J.; Jones, V.F.; Holthouser, A. Engaging the Transgender Community to Improve Medical Education and Prioritize Healthcare Initiatives. *Teach. Learn. Med.* **2018**, *30*, 119–132. [CrossRef] [PubMed]

21.   Dong, H.; Sherer, R.; Lio, J.; Jiang, I.; Cooper, B. Twelve tips for using clinical cases to teach medical ethics. *Med. Teach.* **2018**, *40*, 633–638. [CrossRef] [PubMed]

22. Nama, N.; MacPherson, P.; Sampson, M.; McMillan, H.J. Medical students' perception of lesbian, gay, bisexual, and transgender (LGBT) discrimination in their learning environment and their self-reported comfort level for caring for LGBT patients: A survey study. *Med. Educ. Online* **2017**, *22*, 1368850. [CrossRef] [PubMed]

23. Bidell, M.P. The Lesbian, Gay, Bisexual, and Transgender Development of Clinical Skills Scale (LGBT-DOCSS): Establishing a New Interdisciplinary Self-Assessment for Health Providers. *J. Homosex.* **2017**, *64*, 1432–1460. [CrossRef] [PubMed]

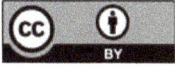

© 2019 by the authors. Licensee MDPI, Basel, Switzerland. This article is an open access article distributed under the terms and conditions of the Creative Commons Attribution (CC BY) license (http://creativecommons.org/licenses/by/4.0/).

International Journal of
*Environmental Research and Public Health*

MDPI

*Article*

# Victimization of Traditional and Cyber Bullying During Childhood and Their Correlates Among Adult Gay and Bisexual Men in Taiwan: A Retrospective Study

Chien-Chuan Wang [1,2], Ray C. Hsiao [3,4] and Cheng-Fang Yen [2,5,*]

1    Zuoying Branch of Kaohsiung Armed Forces General Hospital, Kaohsiung 81342, Taiwan;
     jcwang93@gmail.com
2    Graduate Institute of Medicine and Department of Psychiatry, School of Medicine, College of Medicine,
     Kaohsiung Medical University, Kaohsiung 80708, Taiwan
3    Department of Psychiatry and Behavioral Sciences, School of Medicine, University of Washington,
     Seattle, WA 98195, USA; rhsiao@u.washington.edu
4    Department of Psychiatry, Children's Hospital and Regional Medical Center, Seattle, WA 98105, USA
5    Department of Psychiatry, Kaohsiung Medical University Hospital, Kaohsiung 80708, Taiwan
*    Correspondence: chfaye@cc.kmu.edu.tw

Received: 6 October 2019; Accepted: 19 November 2019; Published: 21 November 2019

**Abstract:** This study examined the associations of timing of sexual orientation developmental milestones, gender role nonconformity, and family-related factors with victimization of traditional and cyber sexuality-related bullying during childhood among gay and bisexual men in Taiwan, in addition to the moderating effects of family-related factors on these associations. A total of 500 homosexual or bisexual men aged between 20 and 25 years were recruited into this study. The associations of early identification of sexual orientation, early coming out, level of masculinity, parental education levels, and perceived family support with victimization of traditional and cyber sexuality-related bullying were evaluated. Early identification of sexual orientation, low self-rated masculinity, and low family support were significantly associated with victimization of traditional bullying. Moreover, low family support, early coming out, and traditional bullying victimization were significantly associated with victimization of cyber bullying. Family support did not moderate the associations of early identification of sexual orientation and low masculinity with victimization of traditional bullying or cyberbullying. The factors associated with victimization of traditional and cyber sexuality-related bullying should be considered when mental health and educational professionals develop prevention and intervention strategies to reduce sexuality-related bullying.

**Keywords:** bullying; sexual minority; sexual orientation; gender role nonconformity; family support

---

## 1. Introduction

Victimization of bullying is one of the most miserable experiences children and adolescents can have and may result in long-term adverse psychological and physical consequences [1]. A meta-analysis study revealed that sexual minority youths, including lesbian, gay, bisexual, transgender, and questioning (LGBTQ) youths, reported higher victimization of bullying rates than heterosexual peers [2]. A review study revealed that victimization of bullying is one of the major factors contributing to mental disorders, suicide, and deliberate self-harm in sexual minority people [3]. Longitudinal studies have similarly demonstrated that victimization of bullying predicts subsequent psychological distress in sexual minority adolescents [4,5]. The aforementioned study findings thus support the implementation of public policy initiatives that reduce bullying and prevent victimization-related effects on the health and well-being of sexual minority youths [6]. Identifying factors that increase the risk of being bullied may provide fundamental knowledge for use in the design, implementation, and evaluation of interventions aiming to reduce bullying of sexual minority youths [4]. Cyber bullying, a new form of bullying, and its associated factors in sexual minority youths have not yet been surveyed thoroughly.

The minority stress hypothesis provides a perspective for understanding the factors related to victimization of bullying in sexual minority individuals. The hypothesis contends that the stigma, prejudice, and discrimination experienced by sexual minority individuals create a hostile social environment that can lead to chronic stress and mental health problems [7]. Being in a sexual minority is itself a minority stressor for LGBTQ youths. One longitudinal study discovered that sexual-minority-specific victimization not only was more prevalent among sexual minority youths compared with heterosexual counterparts but also significantly mediated the effect of sexual minority status on depressive symptoms and suicidality [5]. However, not every sexual minority individual experiences sexuality-related bullying; thus, there may be unique sexual minority stressors that increase the risk of experiencing sexuality-related bullying.

The first aim of the present study was to determine whether the early timing of sexual orientation developmental milestones and gender role nonconformity are sexual minority stressors for sexual minority youths. The major developmental milestones for sexual minorities include first experiencing same-gender attractions, first engaging in sexual behavior with same-gender individuals, first identifying as a sexual minority, first disclosing a sexual minority identity to others, and first same-gender relationship [8,9]. Research has found that the early timing of sexual orientation developmental milestones was associated with negative mental health outcomes such as depression and anxiety among adult lesbians and gay men [10,11], in addition to being associated with homelessness in sexual minority adolescents [12]. The process of sexual minority development differs in that sexual minority individuals face stigma related to sexual minority orientation, which may not only negatively affect the process of forming a minority sexual orientation but also increase the risk of being discriminated by peers. The development of neurocognitive function [13] and social skills [14] is ongoing during early adolescence and is associated with the relatively ineffective coping strategies of individuals in this developmental phase; therefore, early timing of sexual orientation developmental milestones may increase the risk of difficulties in peer interaction in childhood and adolescence. Further study is necessary to determine whether early identification of homosexual or bisexual orientation and early come out are associated with the risk of sexuality-related victimization of bullying among sexual minority individuals. Moreover, a literature review reported that gender role nonconformity significantly increases the risk of experiencing sexuality-related bullying in both heterosexual and sexual minority populations [15]. Individuals are expected to assume the roles and characteristics associated with their respective biological sex [16]. Those who do not assume the expected roles and characteristics of the gender associated with their biological sex are considered to be gender-nonconforming [17]. Gender-nonconforming boys who are more feminine than other boys can be described as those who transgress social gender norms [17].

However, the role played by gender role nonconformity regarding cyber sexuality-related bullying of sexual minority youths has not been examined. Further study is required to determine whether gender role nonconformity plays different roles within traditional face-to-face bullying and cyber bullying.

The socioecological framework developed by Bronfenbrenner [18] provides a perspective for understanding the role of family characteristics in sexuality-related bullying and the buffering effect that family characteristics have between the association of sexuality and gender role characteristics with bullying of sexual minority youths. Homophobic bullying is an ecological phenomenon according to the ecological systems perspective, and such bullying has been established and perpetuated over time as a result of the complex interactions between inter- and intraindividual factors [19]. Family characteristics may have a role for sexuality-related bullying in sexual minority individuals. For example, a study on the United States found that family-level microaggressions increases the risk of polyvictimization for sexual and gender minority adolescents [20].

Research has found that victimization of bullying in young people can be affected by family environment interactions such as domestic violence [21], low parental monitoring [22], and low parental warmth and family cohesion [23]. Given that a low parental educational level is associated with domestic violence and low family monitoring [24], one might hypothesize that young people with a low parental education level would have a higher risk of involvement in bullying than those with a high parental education level. Research found that a higher parental educational status is a protective factor for victimization of bullying in children but not in adolescents [25]. Therefore, the roles of family support and parental education level for victimization of sex-related traditional and cyber bullying warrant further study. Moreover, further study is necessary to determine the moderating effect of family support on the association of early timing of sexual orientation developmental milestones and gender role nonconformity with sexuality-related bullying of sexual minority youths.

People in East Asia are less tolerant of homosexuality than people in the Middle East and Africa; compared with European and North American countries, however, Asian countries generally exhibit much less tolerance of sexual minorities [26]. Due to the Confucian emphasis on family and kinship, homosexuality is regarded by East Asians as a challenge to the family obligations mandated in Confucianism, particularly to the requirement to continue the family bloodline, which explains the low tolerance to homosexuality in East Asian societies [26]. A study on sexual minority men in Japan revealed that 83% and 60% of the men experienced sexuality-related bullying, which increases the risk of attempted suicide [27]. Analysis of a national cross-sectional survey in Chinese adolescents found that victimization of bullying mediated the associations of sexual minority status with suicidality [28] and poor sleep quality [29]. Analysis of the Korea Youth Risk Behavior Web-based Survey found that same- and both-sexes intercourse related suicidality is strongly linked to victimization of bullying among youths [30]. Therefore, factors associated with sexuality-related victimization of bullying during childhood and adolescence in Asian countries warrant further investigation to offer a basis for developing prevention and intervention programs aimed at reducing bullying of sexual minority youths.

The aims of the present study were to examine whether there were differences in the timing of sexual orientation developmental milestones, gender role nonconformity, and family-related factors between gay and bisexual victims and non-victims of traditional and cyber sexuality-related bullying during childhood in Taiwan, in addition to the moderating effects that family factors have on the association of early timing of sexual orientation developmental milestones and gender role nonconformity with being victims of sexuality-related bullying. We had two research hypotheses. First, gay and bisexual victims of traditional and cyber sexuality-related bullying were more likely to identify their homosexual or bisexual orientation earlier, come out earlier, self-rate a lower level of masculinity, perceive lower family support, and have a lower parental education level than non-victims. Second, family support and parental education level moderated the relationships of early timing of sexual orientation developmental milestones and gender role nonconformity with being victims of sexuality-related bullying (Figure 1).

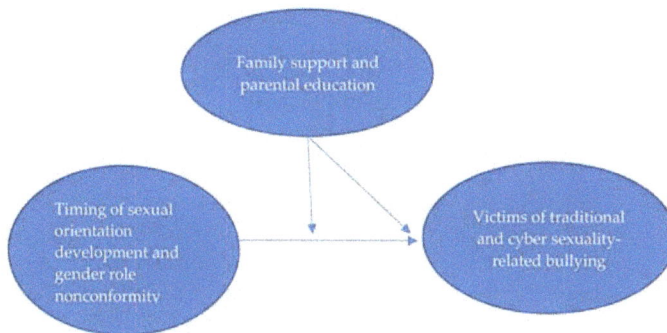

**Figure 1.** Hypothesized model of the associations among timing of sexual orientation development, gender role nonconformity, family-related factors, and victimization of traditional and cyber sexuality-related bullying.

## 2. Methods

### 2.1. Participants

Participants were recruited using an online advertisement posted on Facebook, a bulletin board system, and the home pages of five health promotion and counseling centers for gay, lesbian, bisexual, and transgender (LGBT) individuals from August 2015 to July 2017. Print versions of the advertisement were also mailed to the LGBT student clubs of 25 colleges. A master-degree research assistant explained the study aims and procedures to potential participants who were interested in this study face-to-face and excluded two potential participants (one with impaired intellect and one with the smell of alcohol) who had difficulties in understanding the study's purpose or and method to complete the questionnaire. In total, 500 participants (371 homosexual and 129 bisexual men) were recruited into this study. The mean age of the participants was 22.9 years (standard deviation (SD): 1.6 years). The sample size was calculated based on a previous study in Taiwan with the prevalence of traditional bullying 8.4% [31]. The estimated sample size was 426 with 80% power, 95% confidence interval (CI), and statistically significant level ($\alpha$) at 5% [32]. The sample of 500 participants was thus determined as adequate. Informed consent was obtained from all participants prior to the assessment. The study was approved by the Institutional Review Board of Kaohsiung Medical University Hospital.

### 2.2. Measures

#### 2.2.1. Chinese Version of the School Bullying Experience Questionnaire

We used six items from the Chinese version of the self-report School Bullying Experience Questionnaire (C-SBEQ) to evaluate the participants' experience of traditional sexuality-related victimization of bullying due to gender nonconformity and sexual orientation at school, in afterschool classes, at tutoring schools, and at part-time workplaces while they were a primary school and junior and senior high school student [33]. Two types of traditional bullying were surveyed, namely verbal ridicule and relational exclusion (three items: Social exclusion, being called a mean nickname, and being spoken ill of; for example, "How often have others spoken ill of you because they thought of you as a sissy [they found you homosexual or bisexual] in childhood or adolescence?") and physical aggression and theft of belongings (three items: Being beaten up, being forced to do work, and having money, school supplies, or snacks taken away; for example, "How often have others beaten you up because they thought of you as a sissy [they found you homosexual or bisexual] in childhood or adolescence?") These six items were rated on a 4-point Likert scale with 0 indicating *never*, 1 indicating *just a little*, 2 indicating *often*, and 3 indicating *all the time*. The psychometrics of the C-SBEQ have been examined elsewhere, and the results show that the C-SBEQ has good reliability and validity [33]. The total McDonald's $\omega$ values of the scales for measuring the two types of victimization of traditional bullying due to gender nonconformity and sexual orientation were 0.85 and 0.92, respectively. According to the original study, participants who answered 2 or 3 to any item were identified as self-reported victims of traditional bullying [16].

#### 2.2.2. Cyberbullying Experiences Questionnaire

We employed three items from the Cyberbullying Experiences Questionnaire to assess the participants' experience of cyber sexuality-related bullying victimization due to gender nonconformity and sexual orientation while a primary school and junior and senior high school student [34]. The three items addressed experience of mean or hurtful comments being posted about the participant; pictures, photos, or videos being posted that upset someone; and the spreading of rumors online through e-mails, blogs, social media (Facebook/Twitter/Plurk), pictures, or videos; for example, "How often have other students posted mean or hurtful comments on you through emails, blogs, or social media because they thought of you as a sissy (they found you homosexual or bisexual) in childhood or adolescence?" The items were rated on a 4-point Likert scale with 0 indicating *never*, 1 indicating *just a little*, 2 indicating *often*, and 3 indicating *all the time*. The total McDonald's $\omega$ values of the scales for measuring victimization of cyber bullying due to gender nonconformity and sexual orientation were 0.76 and 0.80, respectively. According to the original study, participants who answered 1 or higher to any item were identified as self-reported victims of cyber bullying [34].

### 2.2.3. Timing of Sexual Orientation Developmental Milestones and Gender Role Nonconformity

We collected the participants' sexual orientation (homosexual or bisexual), age of identification of sexual orientation, and timing of coming out. Those who came out while in junior high school or earlier were classified as having come out early, whereas those who came out while in senior high school or after were classified as having come out late. We also evaluated the participants' self-rated level of masculinity during childhood and adolescence using one item and a 5-point Likert scale ranging from 1 (*very low*) to 5 (*very high*).

We collected the participants' sexual orientation (homosexual or bisexual), age of identification of sexual orientation (*"When did you firstly identify yourself as a gay or bisexual?"*), and timing of coming out (*"When did you firstly disclose your sexual identity to others?"*). Those who came out while in junior high school or earlier were classified as having come out early, whereas those who came out while in senior high school or after were classified as having come out late. We also evaluated the participants' self-rated level of masculinity using one item (*"Compared to other boys who are your same age, do you see yourself during childhood and adolescence as: Much more feminine (1), more feminine (2), about the same (3), more masculine (4), or much more masculine (5)?"*) [17].

### 2.2.4. Family-Related Factors

We examined the participants' parental education levels and perceived family support during childhood and adolescence. In Taiwan, the duration of compulsory fundamental education is nine years. The participants were divided into those who had a high paternal and maternal education level (completing nine years of compulsory fundamental education) and those who had a low paternal and maternal education level (completing less than nine years of compulsory fundamental education). We employed the 5-item Chinese version of the Family Adaptation, Partnership, Growth, Affection, Resolve Index (APGAR) to measure the participants' perceived family support using a 4-point Likert scale ranging from 0 (*never*) to 3 (*always*) [35,36]. High total scores indicate the perception of favorable family support. The total McDonald's ω of APGAR in this study was 0.90.

### 2.3. Procedure and Data Analysis

A master-degree research assistant was responsible for administrating the research questionnaire after completing the training program. The questionnaire was administrated in the interview rooms of the research center that the principal investigator (CFY) worked at. The research assistant explained to the participants that the aims of this questionnaire-surveyed study was to explore the prevalence and risk factors of victimization of homophobic bullying among gay and bisexual men in Taiwan, and the results of this study might provide knowledge for use in the design, implementation, and evaluation of interventions aiming to reduce bullying of sexual minority youths. Then, the research assistant explained to the participants individually how to complete the questionnaires. The participants could ask questions when they encountered problems completing the questionnaires, and the research assistants would resolve their problems. The average time that the data collection process took overall was 30 min. Data analysis was performed using the SPSS 20.0 statistical software (SPSS Inc., Chicago, IL, USA).

The proportions of participants with experience of victimization of traditional and cyber sexuality-related bullying due to gender nonconformity and sexual orientation were calculated. The factors associated with traditional and cyber victimization of bullying were examined using two steps. First, differences in age, family characteristics, timing of sexual orientation developmental milestones, and level of masculinity between victims and nonvictims of traditional and cyber bullying were examined using chi-square and *t*-tests. A *p*-value of 0.05 or lower was used to indicate significance.

The significant factors were then entered into multiple logistic regression analysis. Odds ratios (ORs) and 95% CIs were used to indicate statistical significance.

We also used the standard criteria proposed by Baron and Kenny [37] to examine the moderating effects of family-related factors on the association of early timing of sexual orientation developmental milestones and gender role nonconformity with sexuality-related bullying. According to these criteria, moderation occurred when the term representing interaction between the predictor (early timing of sexual orientation developmental milestones and gender role nonconformity) and the hypothesized moderator (family-related factors) was significantly associated with the dependent variable (sexuality-related bullying) after we controlled for the main effects of both the predictors and hypothesized moderator variables. If early timing of sexual orientation developmental milestones, gender role nonconformity, and family-related factors were significantly associated with sexuality-related bullying, the interactions (early timing of sexual orientation developmental milestones × family-related factors or gender role nonconformity × family-related factors) were incorporated into the regression analysis to examine the moderating effects.

## 3. Results

All 500 participants completed the research questionnaire without omission. The age, family characteristics, timing of sexual orientation developmental milestones, level of masculinity, and rates of victimization of traditional and cyber sexuality-related bullying of the 500 participants are presented in Table 1. In total, 23% and 22.4% of participants had a low paternal maternal education level, respectively. The mean (SD) of perceived family support on the APGAR was 8.5 (3.8). Regarding timing of sexual orientation developmental milestones, the mean (SD) of age to firstly identify sexual orientation was 13.8 (3.6) years old; 27.2% came out early. The mean (SD) level of self-rated masculinity was 2.7 (0.8). Regarding victimization of sexuality-related bullying during their childhood and adolescence, 34.8% and 17% reported to be victims of traditional bullying due to gender non-conformity and sexual orientation, respectively; 27% and 22.4% reported to be victims of cyber bullying due to gender non-conformity and sexual orientation, respectively. In total, 190 (38%) and 163 (32.6) participants reported themselves to be victims of traditional and cyber sexuality-related bullying, respectively.

The differences in age, family characteristics, sexual orientation developmental milestones, and the level of masculinity between the victims and non-victims of traditional and cyber bullying due to gender role nonconformity or sexual orientation during childhood and adolescence, obtained using chi-square and *t*-tests, are displayed in Tables 2 and 3. Victims of traditional bullying had lower paternal and maternal education levels, perceived lower family support, were more likely to be gays, identified their sexual orientation earlier, came out earlier, and self-rated lower masculinity than non-victims of traditional bullying (Table 2).

Moreover, victims of cyber bullying perceived lower family support, came out earlier, and were more likely to be the victims of traditional bullying than non-victims of cyber bullying (Table 3).

The significant correlates of victimization of traditional bullying in chi-square and *t*-tests were entered into Model I of multiple logistic regression (Table 4). The results confirmed that lower family support, earlier identification of sexual orientation, and a lower level of masculinity were significantly associated with victimization of traditional bullying. The moderating effects of family support on the associations of early identification of sexual orientation and low masculinity with victimization of traditional bullying were further examined in Model II. The results of Model II revealed that neither the interaction variable of low family support × early identification of sexual orientation nor the interaction variable of low family support × low masculinity was significantly associated with victimization of traditional bullying, indicating that family support did not moderate the associations of early identification of sexual orientation and low masculinity with victimization of traditional bullying.

**Table 1.** Age, family characteristics, sexual orientation developmental milestones, level of masculinity, and traditional and cyber bullying victimization (*n* = 500).

| Variables | *n* (%) | Mean (SD) | Range |
|---|---|---|---|
| Age (years) | | 22.9 (1.6) | 20–25 |
| Paternal education level | | | |
| High | 385 (77) | | |
| Low | 115 (23) | | |
| Maternal education level | | | |
| High | 388 (77.6) | | |
| Low | 112 (22.4) | | |
| Perceived family support on the APGAR | | 8.5 (3.8) | 0–15 |
| Sexual orientation | | | |
| Bisexuality | 129 (25.8) | | |
| Homosexuality | 371 (74.2) | | |
| Age of identification of sexual orientation (years) | | 13.8 (3.6) | 6–23 |
| Timing of coming out | | | |
| Late (senior high school or after) | 364 (72.8) | | |
| Early (junior high school or before) | 136 (27.2) | | |
| Self-rated level of masculinity | | 2.7 (0.8) | 1–5 |
| Victims of traditional bullying | | | |
| Due to gender non-conformity | 174 (34.8) | | |
| Due to sexual orientation | 85 (17) | | |
| Either | 190 (38) | | |
| Victims of cyber bullying | | | |
| Due to gender non-conformity | 135 (27) | | |
| Due to sexual orientation | 112 (22.4) | | |
| Either | 163 (32.6) | | |

**Table 2.** Correlates of victimization of traditional bullying during childhood and adolescence: Chi-square and *t*-tests (*n* = 500).

| Variables | Traditional Bullying | | | | |
|---|---|---|---|---|---|
| | No (*n* = 310) | Yes (*n* = 190) | $\chi^2$ or *t* | *p* | Cohen's d |
| Paternal education level, *n* (%) | | | | | |
| High (*n* = 385) | 250 (64.9) | 135 (35.1) | 6.121 | 0.013 | |
| Low (*n* = 115) | 60 (52.2) | 55 (47.8) | | | |
| Maternal education level, *n* (%) | | | | | |
| High (*n* = 388) | 250 (64.4) | 138 (35.6) | 4.352 | 0.037 | |
| Low (*n* = 112) | 60 (53.6) | 52 (46.4) | | | |
| Perceived family support, mean (SD) | 9.1 (3.6) | 7.5 (4.0) | 4.809 | <.001 | 0.44 |
| Sexual orientation, *n* (%) | | | | | |
| Bisexuality (*n* = 129) | 95 (73.6) | 34 (26.4) | 10.004 | 0.002 | |
| Homosexuality (*n* = 371) | 215 (58.0) | 156 (42.0) | | | |
| Age of identification of sexual orientation (years), mean (SD) | 14.3 (3.4) | 13.0 (3.7) | 4.099 | <0.001 | 0.37 |
| Timing of coming out, *n* (%) | | | | | |
| Late (senior high school or after) (*n* = 364) | 237 (65.1) | 127 (34.9) | 5.493 | 0.019 | |
| Early (junior high school or before) (*n* = 136) | 73 (53.7) | 63 (46.3) | | | |
| Self-rated level of masculinity, mean (SD) | 2.9 (0.8) | 2.3 (0.8) | 7.882 | <0.001 | 0.72 |
| Victims of traditional bullying, *n* (%) | | | | | |
| No (*n* = 310) | | | | | |
| Yes (*n* = 190) | | | | | |

**Table 3.** Correlates of victimization of cyber bullying during childhood and adolescence: $X^2$ and *t*- tests ($n = 500$).

| Variables | Cyber Bullying | | $X^2$ or $t$ | $p$ | Cohen's d |
|---|---|---|---|---|---|
| | No ($n = 299$) | Yes ($n = 201$) | | | |
| Paternal education level, $n$ (%) | | | | | |
| High ($n = 385$) | 229 (59.5) | 156 (40.5) | 0.071 | 0.790 | |
| Low ($n = 115$) | 70 (60.9) | 45 (39.1) | | | |
| Maternal education level, $n$ (%) | | | | | |
| High ($n = 388$) | 237 (61.1) | 151 (38.9) | 1.185 | 0.276 | |
| Low ($n = 112$) | 62 (55.4) | 50 (44.6) | | | |
| Perceived family support, mean (SD) | 8.9 (3.8) | 7.8 (3.8) | 3.148 | 0.002 | 0.29 |
| Sexual orientation, $n$ (%) | | | | | |
| Bisexuality ($n = 129$) | 75 (58.1) | 54 (41.9) | 0.199 | 0.655 | |
| Homosexuality ($n = 371$) | 224 (60.4) | 147 (39.6) | | | |
| Age of identification of sexual orientation (years), mean (SD) | 14.1 (3.5) | 13.5 (3.7) | 1.779 | 0.076 | |
| Timing of coming out, $n$ (%) | | | | | |
| Late (senior high school or after) ($n = 364$) | 231 (63.5) | 133 (36.5) | 7.463 | 0.006 | |
| Early (junior high school or before) ($n = 136$) | 68 (50) | 68 (50) | | | |
| Self-rated level of masculinity, mean (SD) | 2.7 (0.8) | 2.6 (0.9) | 1.374 | 0.170 | |
| Victims of traditional bullying, $n$ (%) | | | | | |
| No ($n = 310$) | 218 (70.3) | 92 (29.7) | 35.575 | <0.001 | |
| Yes ($n = 190$) | 81 (42.6) | 109 (57.4) | | | |

**Table 4.** Correlates of victimization of traditional bullying during childhood and adolescence: Multiple logistic regression ($n = 500$).

| Variables | Victims of Traditional Bullying | | | |
|---|---|---|---|---|
| | Model I | | Model II | |
| | OR | 95% CI of OR | OR | 95% CI of OR |
| Low paternal education | 1.439 | 0.859–2.411 | 1.444 | 0.861–2.421 |
| Low maternal education | 1.084 | 0.646–1.822 | 1.085 | 0.646–1.823 |
| Perceived family support | 0.894 | 0.847–0.943 | 0.843 | 0.647–1.098 |
| Homosexuality (bisexuality as reference) | 1.262 | 0.768–2.074 | 1.270 | 0.772–2.091 |
| Age of identification of sexual orientation | 0.939 | 0.884–0.998 | 0.912 | 0.794–1.046 |
| Early coming out | 1.122 | 0.704–1.788 | 1.122 | 0.703–1.791 |
| Self-rated level of masculinity | 0.401 | 0.302–0.532 | 0.388 | 0.206–0.734 |
| Perceived family support × Age of identification of sexual orientation | | | 1.004 | 0.989–1.019 |
| Perceived family support × Level of masculinity | | | 1.004 | 0.932–1.082 |
| −2 log likelihood | 570.916 | | 570.672 | |
| Nagelkerke $R^2$ | 0.231 | | 0.232 | |
| Walds $\chi^2$ | 28.232 | | 28.232 | |
| $p$ | <0.001 | | <0.001 | |

The significant correlates of victimization of cyber bullying in chi-square and *t*-tests were entered into multiple logistic regression models in two steps (Table 5). In the first step perceived family support and timing of coming out were selected into Model III. The results of Model III confirmed that low family support and early coming out were significantly associated with victimization of cyber bullying. In the second step, victimization of traditional bullying was further selected into Model IV. The results of Model IV revealed that victims of traditional bullying were more likely to also be victims of cyber bullying. The moderating effects of family support on the associations of early coming and victimization of traditional bullying with victimization of cyber bullying were further examined in Model V.

**Table 5.** Correlates of victimization of cyber bullying during childhood and adolescence: Multiple logistic regression ($n$ = 500).

| Variables | Victims of Cyber Bullying | | | | | |
| --- | --- | --- | --- | --- | --- | --- |
| | Model III | | Model IV | | Model V | |
| | OR | 95% CI of OR | OR | 95% CI of OR | OR | 95% CI of OR |
| Perceived family support | 0.928 | 0.885–0.974 | 0.952 | 0.906–1.001 | 0.865–1.002 | 0.865–1.002 |
| Early coming out | 1.729 | 1.156–2.584 | 1.585 | 1.045–2.403 | 0.391–2.875 | 0.391–2.875 |
| Victims of traditional bullying | | | 2.868 | 1.949–4.221 | 1.012–6.199 | 1.012–6.199 |
| Perceived family support × Early coming out | | | | | 0.921–1.126 | 0.921–1.126 |
| Perceived family support × Victims of traditional bullying | | | | | 0.942–1.170 | 0.942–1.170 |
| −2 log likelihood | | 656.919 | | 627.830 | | 626.891 |
| Nagelkerke $R^2$ | | 0.045 | | 0.119 | | 0.121 |
| Walds $\chi^2$ | | 18.958 | | 18.958 | | 18.958 |
| $p$ | | <0.001 | | <0.001 | | <.001 |

## 4. Discussion

The present study discovered that early identification of sexual orientation, low self-rated masculinity, and low family support were significantly associated with victimization of traditional bullying. Moreover, low family support, early coming out, and victimization of traditional bullying were significantly associated with victimization of cyber bullying. Family support did not moderate the associations of early identification of sexual orientation and low masculinity with victimization of traditional or cyber bullying.

The results of the present study supported the hypothesis that early identification of sexual orientation and early coming out are sexual minority stressors that may increase the risk of victimization of sexuality-related bullying. The developmental perspective may partially explain these results [11,38]. First, because of immature neurocognitive function and social skills, those who identify their sexual orientation or come out in early adolescence may be less able to cope effectively with stressors related to the stigma of sexual minority identification or to deal with bullying incidents compared with those who reach sexual orientation milestones in late adolescence or young adulthood. Research has found that early timing of sexual orientation developmental milestones was associated with negative mental health outcomes such as depression and anxiety among adult lesbians and gay men [10,11]. Second, individuals reaching sexual orientation developmental milestones earlier might have less access to supportive resources [11], which may increase their risk of being bullied. One study discovered that early timing of sexual orientation developmental milestones was significantly associated with homelessness among sexual minority adolescents [12]. The finding of the present study highlights the importance of developing strategies for the prevention and early detection of sexuality-related bullying of sexual minority youths who identify their sexual orientation or come out in early adolescence. Mental-health services providers and education professionals should provide sexual minority individuals who come out early the critical resources, including gay-straight alliances, inclusive curricular resources, supportive educators, and comprehensive bullying/harassment policies [39].

Low self-rated masculinity was significantly associated with victimization of traditional but not cyber bullying among sexual minority youths. Gender role conformity is a major component of heteronormativity, which prescribes gender norms and determines peer interactions [40]. One previous study found that endorsement of heteronormative culture or behavior contributes to the extent of homophobic bullying directed against sexual minority youths [41]. Boys who exhibit nonconformal gender characteristics such as low masculinity may be perceived as "gay" in face-to-face interactions and then be targets of homophobic bullying, whereas such characteristics may be considered less "odd" in cyber environments wherein gender role nonconformity is perceived or judged to a lesser extent. Sexual minority youths who exhibit obvious gender role nonconformity may perceive cyberspace as a safe environment compared with the face-to-face context and thus spend considerable time there. However, sexual minority youths are more likely to experience online peer victimization than heterosexual youths [42]. Moreover, cyber bullying is not easily detected by parents and school employees. Detection and intervention may not be possible until cyber bullying has severe consequences, especially in sexual minority youths without substantial gender role nonconformity.

The present study discovered that low family support was significantly associated with both victimization of traditional and cyber sexuality-related bullying of gay and bisexual youths. A similar result was obtained by a previous study; specifically, family acceptance reduced the effect of sexuality-based discrimination in gay and bisexual men [43]. There are several possible explanations for these results. First, low family support may make sexual minority youths feel uncomfortable about discussing with their families how to cope with the homophobic harassment they face. Repeated and prolonged harassment may then progress to homophobic bullying. Second, low family support may prevent youths from learning a mature and effective strategy from their parents that enables them to cope with the maltreatment from their peers. Third, sexual minority youths perceiving low family support may rely more heavily on peers than family members [44], and consequently, the risk of victimization of bullying increases. Fourth, low family support may co-occur with mental health problems, which may further increase the risk of being bullied. Contrary to our hypothesis, family support did not moderate the associations of early identification of sexual orientation and low masculinity with victimization of traditional or cyber bullying. Many sexual minority youths fear family rejection because of their sexual identity [45]. Thus, family buffering effects may be slight. The results of the present study indicate that interventions that help families become more accepting of young sexual minority family members may have beneficial mental health effects and reduce sexuality-related bullying.

Contrary to the hypothesis, this study did not find a significant association between low family support and victimization of sex-related traditional and cyber bullying in gay and bisexual men. Although research found that a higher parental educational status was a protective factor for victimization of bullying in children [25], the effect of parental education levels on adolescent victimization of bullying may abate as individuals grow up. Research found that most of people identify their sexual orientation during adolescence [46]. Therefore, the influence of parental educational level on victimization of sex-related bullying may be attenuated.

The present study found that victimization of traditional sexuality-related bullying increased the risk of victimization of cyber sexuality-related bullying among sexual minority youths. Previous studies have reported that cyberbullying perpetration is an extension of traditional bullying perpetration, particularly psychological, relational, and indirect forms of bullying in cyberspace [47,48]. Compared with traditional bullying perpetrators, cyberbullying perpetrators can remain virtually anonymous [49]. Being cruel and malicious using digital harassment is also easier because of the physical distance separating the offender and the victim [47]. All of these cyber activity characteristics may extend bullying perpetration from face-to-face interactional situations to cyberspace. The results of this study are a reminder to mental health and education professionals of the necessity of evaluating whether an individual is being bullied in the face-to-face context when addressing victimization of cyber bullying among sexual minority youths. Furthermore, because cyber bullying is less detectable by adults than traditional bullying is [50] and because most cyber bullying victims do not report such bullying to an adult or use digital tools to prevent online incidents [51], experiencing traditional bullying may be used as an indicator for detecting the occurrence of cyber bullying among sexual minority youths.

The present study is one of the first to examine the roles played by early timing of sexual orientation developmental milestones, gender role nonconformity, and family support regarding victimization of cyber sexuality-related bullying in sexual minority youths. The results of the present study also provided knowledges to the factors associated with sexuality-related victimization of bullying among sexual minority youths in Asian countries. However, the present study had several limitations. First, this study retrospectively obtained data on participants' victimization of sexuality-related bullying, timing of sexual orientation developmental milestones, and family support; therefore, recall bias may have been introduced. Moreover, whether victimization of homophobic bullying in childhood and adolescence has adverse effects on victims' memory in emerging adulthood warrants further study. Second, the study data were exclusively self-reported. The use of only a single data source may have influenced our findings and resulted in shared-method variances. Third, we did not examine the perpetrators of sexuality-related bullying. Fourth, the participants were gay or bisexual men who responded to the advertisements and participated in this study. Whether the results of this study can be generalized to those who did not respond to the advertisements warrants further study. Fifth, the cut-offs for identifying victims of traditional bullying (two or higher on the C-SBEQ) and cyber bullying (one or higher on the Cyberbullying Experiences Questionnaire) were not the same. Although the present study did not aim to compare the rates of victims between traditional bullying and cyber bullying, further study examining whether the relationship of traditional bullying with cyber bullying may vary if the cut-offs are changed may provide insights to the formation of cyber bullying.

Based on the results of the present study, we recommended further study to examine the mediators of the associations of early identification of sexual orientation, early come out, low masculinity, and low family support with victimization of traditional and cyber sexuality-related bullying. The identification of mediators not only provides knowledge to the occurrence of victimization of homophobic bullying but also serves as the target of prevention and intervention programs. Further prospective study is also needed to establish the temporal relationships among victimization of bullying and related individual and environmental factors, especially the relationship between victimization of traditional bullying and cyber bullying. Moreover, what kinds of cyberspace and cyber activities in which cyber homophobic bullying may occur also warrants further study. Sexual minority may experience not only homophobic bullying but also bullying related to other identity minority, for example, ethnicity, gender, and religion. Further study is needed to examine the experiences of victimization in double or multiple identity minority in Taiwan. Although parental educational levels were not significantly associated in the victimization of homophobic bullying in the present study, we were concerned that there may be other family factors, for example, parent-child bonding and parental knowledge and attitude toward sexual minority that relate to victimization of homophobic bullying in LGB individuals. We suggest further study to examine.

## 5. Conclusions

Based on the results of the present study, we suggest that factors associated with victimization of traditional and cyber sexuality-related bullying be considered when mental health and educational professionals develop a comprehensive approach to providing a positive school and community climate and reducing sexuality-related bullying [52]. Sexual minority youths who identify their sexual orientation and come out early could receive additional peer support from gay–straight alliances to reduce prejudice, discrimination, and bullying within schools [53]. Interventions that enhance family support for sexual minority youths may have beneficial mental health effects and reduce sexuality-related bullying. Whether sexual minority victims of cyber bullying also experience traditional bullying warrants routine surveying.

**Author Contributions:** C.-C.W., R.C.H., and C.-F.Y. wrote the paper; C.-F.Y. conceived of and performed the study; C.-F.Y. analyzed the data.

**Funding:** This study was supported by the grant MOST 104-2314-B-037-024-MY3 awarded by the Ministry of Science and Technology, Taiwan, R.O.C., and the grants KMUH104-4R60 and KMUH105-5R59 awarded by Kaohsiung Medical University Hospital.

**Conflicts of Interest:** The authors declare no conflict of interest. The founding sponsors had no role in the design of the study; in the collection, analyses, or interpretation of the data; in the writing of the manuscript; nor in the decision to publish the results.

# References

1. Olweus, D. *Bullying at School: What We Know and What We Can. Do*; Blackwell Publishers: Hoboken, NJ, USA, 1993.
2. Katz-Wise, S.L.; Hyde, J.S. Victimization experiences of lesbian, gay, and bisexual individuals: A meta-analysis. *J. Sex Res.* **2012**, *49*, 142–167. [CrossRef] [PubMed]
3. King, M.; Semlyen, J.; Tai, S.S.; Killaspy, H.; Osborn, D.; Popelyuk, D.; Nazareth, I. A systematic review of mental disorder, suicide, and deliberate self harm in lesbian, gay and bisexual people. *BMC Psychiatry* **2008**, *8*, 70. [CrossRef] [PubMed]
4. Birkett, M.; Newcomb, M.E.; Mustanski, B. Does it get better? A longitudinal analysis of psychological distress and victimization in lesbian, gay, bisexual, transgender, and questioning youth. *J. Adolesc. Health* **2015**, *56*, 280–285. [CrossRef] [PubMed]
5. Burton, C.M.; Marshal, M.P.; Chisolm, D.J.; Sucato, G.S.; Friedman, M.S. Sexual minority-related victimization as a mediator of mental health disparities in sexual minority youth: A longitudinal analysis. *J. Youth Adolesc.* **2013**, *42*, 394–402. [CrossRef]
6. Coulter, R.W.; Herrick, A.L.; Friedman, M.R.; Stall, R.D. Sexual-orientation differences in positive youth development: The mediational role of bullying victimization. *Am. J. Public Health* **2016**, *106*, 691–697. [CrossRef]
7. Meyer, I.H. Prejudice, social stress, and mental health in lesbian, gay, and bisexual populations: Conceptual issues and research evidence. *Psychol. Bull.* **2003**, *129*, 674. [CrossRef]
8. D'Augelli, A.R. Developmental and contextual factors and mental health among lesbian, gay, and bisexual youths. In *Sexual Orientation and Mental Health: Examining Identity and Development in Lesbian, Gay, and Bisexual People*; Omoto, A.M., Kurtzman, H.S., Eds.; American Psychological Association: Washington, DC, USA, 2006; pp. 37–53.
9. Garnets, L.D.; Kimmel, D.C. Lesbian and gay male dimensions in the psychological study of human diversity. In *Psychological Perspectives on Lesbian and Gay Male Experience*; Garnets, L.D., Kimmel, D.C., Eds.; Columbia University Press: New York, NY, USA, 1993; pp. 1–51.
10. Friedman, M.S.; Marshal, M.P.; Stall, R.; Cheong, J.; Wright, E.R. Gay-related development, early abuse and adult health outcomes among gay males. *AIDS Behav.* **2008**, *12*, 891–902. [CrossRef]
11. Katz-Wise, S.L.; Rosario, M.; Calzo, J.P.; Scherer, E.A.; Sarda, V.; Austin, S.B. Associations of timing of sexual orientation developmental milestones and other sexual minority stressors with internalizing mental health symptoms among sexual minority young adults. *Arch. Sex. Behav.* **2017**, *46*, 1441–1452. [CrossRef]
12. Rosario, M.; Schrimshaw, E.W.; Hunter, J. Risk factors for homelessness among lesbian, gay, and bisexual youths: A developmental milestone approach. *Child. Youth Serv. Rev.* **2012**, *34*, 186–193. [CrossRef]
13. Alikasifoglu, M.; Erginoz, E.; Ercan, O.; Uysal, O.; Albayrak-Kaymak, D. Bullying behaviours and psychosocial health: Results from a cross-sectional survey among high school students in Istanbul, Turkey. *Eur. J. Pediatr.* **2007**, *166*, 1253–1260. [CrossRef]
14. Casey, B.J.; Jones, R.M.; Hare, T.A. The adolescent brain. *Ann. N. Y. Acad. Sci.* **2008**, *1124*, 111–126. [CrossRef] [PubMed]
15. Hong, J.S.; Garbarino, J. Risk and protective factors for homophobic bullying in schools: An application of the social–ecological framework. *Educ. Psychol. Rev.* **2012**, *24*, 271–285. [CrossRef]
16. Grossman, A.H.; D'Augelli, A.R. Transgender youth: Invisible and vulnerable. *J. Homosex.* **2006**, *51*, 111–128. [CrossRef] [PubMed]
17. Toomey, R.B.; Ryan, C.; Diaz, R.M.; Card, N.A.; Russell, S.T. Gender-nonconforming lesbian, gay, bisexual, and transgender youth: School victimization and young adult psychosocial adjustment. *Dev. Psychol.* **2010**, *46*, 1580–1589. [CrossRef]
18. Bronfenbrenner, U. Ecological systems theory. In *Six Theories of Child. Development: Revisited Formulations and Current Issues*; Vasta, R., Ed.; Jessica Kingsley Press: London, UK, 2002; pp. 221–288.
19. Espelage, D.L.; Swearer, S.M. *Bullying in North. American Schools: A Social-Ecological Perspective on Prevention and Intervention*, 2nd ed.; Routledge Press: New York, NY, USA, 2010.
20. Sterzing, P.R.; Ratliff, G.A.; Gartner, R.E.; McGeough, B.L.; Johnson, K.C. Social ecological correlates of polyvictimization among a national sample of transgender, genderqueer, and cisgender sexual minority adolescents. *Child Abuse Negl.* **2017**, *67*, 1–12. [CrossRef]

21. Bowes, L.; Arseneault, L.; Maughan, B.; Taylor, A.; Caspi, A.; Moffitt, T.E. School, neighborhood, and family factors are associated with children's bullying involvement: A nationally representative longitudinal study. *J. Am. Acad. Child Adolesc. Psychiatry* **2009**, *48*, 545–553. [CrossRef]

22. Gage, J.C.; Overpeck, M.D.; Nansel, T.R.; Kogan, M.D. Peer activity in the evenings and participation in aggressive and problem behaviors. *J. Adolesc. Health* **2005**, *37*, 517. [CrossRef]

23. Bowers, L.; Smith, P.K.; Binney, V. Perceived family relationships of bullies, victims and bully/victims in middle childhood. *J. Soc. Pers. Relatsh.* **1994**, *11*, 215–232. [CrossRef]

24. Garcia-Moreno, C.; Jansen, H.; Ellsberg, M.; Heise, L.; Watts, C.H. WHO Multi-country Study on Women's Health and Domestic Violence against Women Study Team. Prevalence of intimate partner violence: Findings from the WHO multi-country study on women's health and domestic violence. *Lancet* **2006**, *368*, 1260–1269. [CrossRef]

25. Von Rueden, U.; Gosch, A.; Rajmil, L.; Bisegger, C.; Ravens-Sieberer, U. Socioeconomic determinants of health related quality of life in childhood and adolescence: Results from a European study. *J. Epidemiol. Community Health* **2006**, *60*, 130–135. [CrossRef]

26. World Value Survey Association (WVSA). World Value Survey Wave 6: 2010–2014. Available online: http://www.worldvaluessurvey.org/WVSOnline.jsp (accessed on 6 October 2019).

27. Hidaka, Y.; Operario, D. Attempted suicide, psychological health and exposure to harassment among Japanese homosexual, bisexual or other men questioning their sexual orientation recruited via the internet. *J. Epidemiol. Community Health* **2006**, *60*, 962–967. [CrossRef] [PubMed]

28. Huang, Y.; Li, P.; Lai, Z.; Jia, X.; Xiao, D.; Wang, T.; Guo, L.; Lu, C. Association between sexual minority status and suicidal behavior among Chinese adolescents: A moderated mediation model. *J. Affect. Disord.* **2018**, *239*, 85–92. [CrossRef] [PubMed]

29. Li, P.; Huang, Y.; Guo, L.; Wang, W.; Xi, C.; Lei, Y.; Luo, M.; Pan, S.; Deng, X.; Zhang, W.H.; et al. Is sexual minority status associated with poor sleep quality among adolescents? Analysis of a national cross-sectional survey in Chinese adolescents. *BMJ Open* **2017**, *7*, e017067. [CrossRef]

30. Kim, G.H.; Ahn, H.S.; Kim, H.J. Type of sexual intercourse experience and suicidal ideation, plans, and attempts among youths: A cross-sectional study in South Korea. *BMC Public Health* **2016**, *16*, 1229. [CrossRef] [PubMed]

31. Yen, C.F.; Kim, Y.S.; Wang, P.W.; Lin, H.C.; Tang, T.C.; Wu, Y.Y. Socio-demographic correlates of involvement in school bullying among adolescents in southern Taiwan. *Taiwan. J. Psychiatry* **2012**, *26*, 197–206.

32. Hsieh, F.Y. Sample size tables for logistic regression. *Stat. Med.* **1989**, *8*, 795–802. [CrossRef] [PubMed]

33. Yen, C.F.; Kim, Y.S.; Tang, T.C.; Wu, Y.Y.; Cheng, C.P. Factor structure, reliability, and validity of the Chinese version of the School Bullying Experience Questionnaire. *Kaohsiung J. Med. Sci.* **2012**, *28*, 500–505. [CrossRef]

34. Yen, C.F.; Chou, W.J.; Liu, T.L.; Ko, C.H.; Yang, P.; Hu, H.F. Cyberbullying among male adolescents with attention-deficit/hyperactivity disorder: Prevalence, correlates, and association with poor mental health status. *Res. Dev. Disabil.* **2014**, *35*, 3543–3553. [CrossRef]

35. Chen, Y.C.; Hsu, C.C.; Hsu, S.H.; Lin, C.C. A preliminary study of family Apgar index. *Acta. Paediatr. Sin.* **1980**, *21*, 210–217.

36. Smilkstein, G. The family APGAR: A proposal for a family function test and its use by physicians. *J. Fam. Pract.* **1978**, *6*, 1231–1239.

37. Baron, R.M.; Kenny, D.A. The moderator-mediator variable distinction in social psychological research: Conceptual, strategic, and statistical considerations. *J. Personal. Soc. Psychol.* **1986**, *51*, 1173–1182. [CrossRef]

38. Smith, P.K.; Madsen, K.C.; Moody, J.C. What causes the age decline in reports of being bullied at school? Towards a developmental analysis of risks of being bullied. *Educ. Res.* **1999**, *41*, 267–285. [CrossRef]

39. Kosciw, J.G.; Greytak, E.A.; Giga, N.M.; Villenas, C.; Danischewski, D.J. *The 2015 National School Climate Survey: The Experiences of Lesbian, Gay, Bisexual, Transgender, and Queer Youth in Our Nation's Schools*; GLSEN: New York, NY, USA, 2016.

40. Toomey, R.B.; McGuire, J.K.; Russell, S.T. Heteronormativity, school climates, and perceived safety for gender nonconforming peers. *J. Adolesc.* **2011**, *35*, 187–196. [CrossRef] [PubMed]

41. Nadal, K.L.; Issa, M.A.; Leon, J.; Meterko, V.; Wideman, M.; Wong, Y. Sexual orientation microaggressions: "Death by a thousand cuts" for lesbian, gay, and bisexual youth. *J. LGBT Youth* **2011**, *8*, 234–259. [CrossRef]

42. Ybarra, M.L.; Mitchell, K.J.; Palmer, N.A.; Reisner, S.L. Online social support as a buffer against online and offline peer and sexual victimization among US LGBT and non-LGBT youth. *Child Abuse Negl.* **2015**, *39*, 123–136. [CrossRef] [PubMed]

43. Diaz, R.M.; Ayala, G.; Bein, E.; Henne, J.; Marin, B.V. The impact of homophobia, poverty, and racism on the mental health of gay and bisexual Latino men: Findings from 3 US cities. *Am. J. Public Health* **2001**, *91*, 927–932.

44. Munõz-Plaza, C.; Quinn, S.C.; Rounds, K.A. Lesbian, gay, bisexual and transgender students: Perceived social support in the high school environment. *High Sch. J.* **2002**, *85*, 52–63. [CrossRef]

45. Savin-Williams, R.C.; Ream, G.L. Sex variations in the disclosure to parents of same-sex attractions. *J. Fam. Psychol.* **2003**, *17*, 429–438. [CrossRef]

46. Katz-Wise, S.L.; Rosario, M.; Calzo, J.P.; Scherer, E.A.; Sarda, V.; Austin, S.B. Endorsement and timing of sexual orientation developmental milestones among sexual minority young adults in the growing up today study. *J. Sex. Res.* **2017**, *54*, 172–185. [CrossRef]

47. Patchin, J.W.; Hinduja, S. Bullies move beyond the schoolyard: A preliminary look at cyberbullying. *Youth Violence Juv. Justice* **2006**, *4*, 148–169. [CrossRef]

48. Patchin, J.W.; Hinduja, S. Traditional and nontraditional bullying among youth: A test of general strain theory. *Youth Soc.* **2011**, *43*, 727–751. [CrossRef]

49. Kowalski, R.M.; Limber, S.P. Electronic bullying among middle school students. *J. Adolesc. Health* **2007**, *41*, S22–S30. [CrossRef] [PubMed]

50. Williams, K.R.; Guerra, N.G. Prevalence and predictors of Internet bullying. *J. Adolesc. Health* **2007**, *41*, S14–S21. [CrossRef] [PubMed]

51. Juvonen, J.; Gross, E.F. Extending the school grounds? bullying experiences in cyberspace. *J. Sch. Health* **2008**, *78*, 496–505. [CrossRef] [PubMed]

52. Wilson, S.J.; Lipsey, M.W. School-based interventions for aggressive and disruptive behavior: Update of a meta-analysis. *Am. J. Prev. Med.* **2007**, *33*, S130–S343. [CrossRef] [PubMed]

53. Goodenow, C.; Szalacha, L.; Westheimer, K. School support groups, other school factors, and the safety of sexual minority adolescents. *Psychol. Sch.* **2006**, *43*, 573–589. [CrossRef]

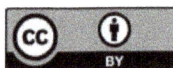

© 2019 by the authors. Licensee MDPI, Basel, Switzerland. This article is an open access article distributed under the terms and conditions of the Creative Commons Attribution (CC BY) license (http://creativecommons.org/licenses/by/4.0/).

International Journal of
*Environmental Research*
*and Public Health*

MDPI

*Article*

# Education First: Promoting LGBT+ Friendly Healthcare with a Competency-Based Course and Game-Based Teaching

Hsing-Chen Yang

Graduate Institute of Gender Studies, Kaohsiung Medical University, Kaohsiung 80708, Taiwan;
yhckmu@gmail.com

Received: 30 October 2019; Accepted: 20 December 2019; Published: 22 December 2019

**Abstract:** How, apart from by conveying professional knowledge, can university medical education nurture and improve the gender competency of medical students and thereby create an LGBT+ friendly healthcare environment? This study explored the use of game-based teaching activities in competency-based teaching from the perspective of competency-based medical education (CBME) and employed a qualitative case-study methodology. We designed an LGBT+ Health and Medical Care course in a medical school. Feedback was collected from two teachers and 19 medical students using in-depth interviews and thematic analysis was used to analyze the collected data. The findings of this study were as follows: (1) Games encouraged student participation and benefited gender knowledge transmission and transformation through competency learning, and (2) games embodied the idea of assessment as learning. The enjoyable feeling of pressure from playing games motivated students to learn. Using games as both a teaching activity and an assessment tool provided the assessment and instant feedback required in the CBME learning process. Game-based teaching successfully guided medical students to learn about gender and achieve the learning goals of integrating knowledge, attitudes, and skills. To fully implement CBME using games as teaching methods, teaching activities, learning tasks, and assessment tools, teachers must improve their teaching competency. This study revealed that leading discussions and designing curricula are key in the implementation of gender competency-based education; in particular, the ability to lead discussions is the core factor. Game-based gender competency education for medical students can be facilitated with discussions that reinforce learning outcomes to achieve the objectives of gender equality education and LGBT+ friendly healthcare. The results of this study indicated that game-based CBME with specific teaching strategies was an effective method of nurturing the gender competency of medical students. The consequent integration of gender competency into medical education could achieve the goal of LGBT+ friendly healthcare.

**Keywords:** assessment as learning; medical student; game-based teaching; gender competency; LGBT+ friendly healthcare

---

## 1. Introduction

Gender is a major source of concern in healthcare environments. A psychiatrist with 10 years of practical experience, including with numerous LGBT+ patients, contended that doctors are able to more easily help patients who are willing to fully reveal their true selves and share their feelings [1]. However, the extent to which LGBT+ patients feel comfortable revealing themselves and the additional help that doctors can provide depend on numerous conditions and factors; of these, doctors' gender competency is a key factor.

In many places, good health is considered to be a basic human right to which everyone is entitled. From the perspective of gender equality and medical human rights, gender-competent doctors with adequate knowledge and understanding of gender and sexual orientation can, in the core spirit of holistic medicine, care for patients as if they were family members. Thus, creating an LGBT+ friendly healthcare environment demonstrates a commitment to equality and social justice. An LGBT+ friendly healthcare environment must start with medical education reform. As Verdonk, Mans, and Lagro-Janssen [2] indicated, gender equality must be incorporated into policies and education. Medical professionals must understand the relationship between gender and health, and the ideas concerning gender must be addressed through gender courses in medical education. The promotion and implementation of gender equality and LGBT+ friendly healthcare can be achieved only incrementally through education, thereby necessitating the reform of courses.

In addition, because of rapid changes in society and living environments, various educational and learning method reforms have been proposed worldwide. Newly emerged competency-based medical education (CBME) demands the innovation of education and curricula [3–5]. Competency has become a prominent education concept in the field. CBME emphasizes the integration of knowledge, attitudes, and skills and the application of these to real life and medical practices [4–7]. Integrating gender education with CBME requires more research and practical teaching experience. Moreover, the key component of successful education reform is truly the determination of how to inspire medical students to willingly participate in gender-related education and courses.

In particular, we face the following challenges present in contemporary educational environments: (1) Learning has become complex because of diversified learning environments, spaces, and resources, and (2) learning must be immediate, interactive, and fun. In such an environment, medical education professionals must establish effective teaching methods with which to inspire students to learn about gender and to nurture their gender competency. Yang [8] indicated that students who grew up in the digital era only responded to learning methods that were delivered in real time, required participation, and were fun. This requires game-based learning. Students do not want to be inculcated with certain ideologies or values, but rather prefer to be consulted, entertained, and inspired.

Overall, the expertise of teachers in competency-based education and gender education is critical for medical students to understand the importance of gender equality, to enhance gender competency, and to promote the health and well-being of the LGBT+ community in particular.

### 1.1. Competency-Based Medical Education and Gender Competency

Competency refers to the knowledge, attitudes, and skills that learners acquire from education and that enable the handling of complex personal or social scenarios, demands, or endeavors [9–12]. Mulder et al. [10] proposed characteristics of competency according to an integral perspective and indicated the following points: (1) Competency refers to the collective integration of knowledge, skills, and attitudes; (2) when exhibited in certain professional fields, organizations, tasks, roles, scenarios, and endeavors, competency enables a person to effectively solve problems; (3) competency is embedded in certain situations, and its meaning and accomplishment criteria are given by the specific task context; and (4) competency is demonstrated through behaviors or task orientations.

To effectively care for the health needs of the general public, education reform on the basis of CBME emerged. CBME emphasizes a learner-centered teaching method and entails changing education methods with respect to course development, instructional design, and frequent and formative evaluations that focus on the application of knowledge to practicing skills [3,9]. Teaching and evaluations in CBME focus on the development of integrated abilities in students. The establishment of evaluation and feedback mechanisms during the process of learning teaches students to apply their competencies to real medical scenarios. CBME endeavors to transform knowledge-centered learning methods in conventional school education into integral learning that focuses on cultivating students' knowledge, attitudes, and problem-solving abilities to accommodate future changes in society and medical practices [3,6].

In 2004, Taiwan implemented the Gender Equity Education Act, which clearly established that gender equity education must include sexuality education, gay and lesbian education, and relationship education. Taiwanese scholars and practitioners of gender equity education include gay and lesbian education in their use of the terms gender education and gender competency. In other words, gender equity education is a general term and includes gay and lesbian education. Therefore, the connotations of the term "gender competency" used in this study include basic gender-related concepts and education regarding sexual orientation and gender identify.

To integrate gender into medical education, Yang and Yen [13] adopted the theory of CBME and gender competency to develop medical education and gender competency indicators (MEGCIs) as a tool for curriculum guidance and instructional design. The MEGCIs framework was divided into three educational phases containing 8 domains, 20 themes, and 79 competence indicators. The domains included "sex and gender", "gender, health, and medicine", "diagnosis and treatment", and "psychiatry and gender." The themes included "gender and society", "sexual and gender minorities", "gender-friendly medical care", "equality, differences, and power", and "common sex and gender issues in clinical services" [13]. Yang and Yen argued that the gender competency of medical students comes from the integration of learning regarding gender knowledge, attitude, and skills and the development of abilities relating to appropriate actions. Yang and Yen replaced skills with actions to highlight the connotations of skills and to emphasize that the goal of gender equality education is for students to apply their learned skills to practice and actions.

Many scholars also require medical education to instill correct knowledge of and positive attitudes toward LGBT+ into medical students or healthcare professionals [14–20]. Many studies revealed the importance of teaching medical students to understand basic LGBT+ concepts and terminology and focused on guiding students toward establishing friendly attitudes toward LBGT+ in their courses [18,19], including inviting LGBT+ community members to participate in curriculum development, lesson planning, or teaching assistance [18]. Some studies demonstrated multiple approaches to providing students with teaching on LGBT+ health in medical education curricula, such as didactic lectures, student-led presentations, patient panels, and small-group sessions [17,20].

Keuroghlian, Ard, and Makadon proposed sexual health education and provided LGBT affirming healthcare environments to advance LGBT health equity. They addressed the mastering of basic LGBT concepts and terminology and the demonstration of openness toward LGBT people as core components of LGBT health education in clinical training programs [19]. Salkind, Gishen, Drage, Kavanagh, and Potts introduced a compulsory curriculum in a medical school to provide undergraduate students with LGBT+ health-related education, including talks from transgender patients as guest speakers. The respective research results showed that students learned to use appropriate language to explain and discuss sexual orientation and gender identity [18].

This study confirms that the teaching of basic LGBT+ concepts and terminology is the first step toward developing medical students and healthcare professionals' LGBT+ competency and LGBT+ friendly healthcare. This study also asserts that in the process of learning basic LGBT+ concepts, students also learn positive attitudes and skills relevant to LGBT+ healthcare in medical curricula. It adopts the doctrines of CBME and the reasoning that neither curricula and teaching nor teaching and learning are separate in education; competency-based gender curricula and teaching involve a teaching implementation process in which curriculum design and teaching plans are considered simultaneously.

*1.2. Game-Based Teaching*

Game-based teaching and learning is a participatory educational approach in which students brainstorm together to solve problems. Studies indicated that teaching activities involving games stimulate active learning and enhance learning motivation and outcomes [5,21–24].

Gee [25,26] stated that a successful game-based teaching approach features the following characteristics: (1) Identification, wherein participants establish a sense of identification in the game; (2) interaction; (3) risk-taking, that is, compared with real life, failing in a game does not incur serious consequences, thereby giving participants the freedom to take risks; (4) autonomy, that is participants have control over the game; (5) well-ordered problems, that is, the game is properly designed to include problems that are related and that enable participants to gradually grow and develop; (6) challenging, whereby the game is designed to have problems that challenge the existing professional knowledge of students; (7) instant feedback, whereby students instantaneously obtain necessary information to improve their ability of critical thinking; (8) situated and meaningful learning, that is, students can learn new concepts through game scenarios; (9) pleasantly frustrating; (10) exploration, in-depth understanding, and rethinking, whereby the game forces players to expand contextual knowledge to conduct comprehensive and in-depth thinking; (11) opportunities and environment for team-work; and (12) problem-based learning, where game-based teaching is also a type of problem-based learning which develops the problem-solving abilities of students. The instant feedback from the game helps students to improve and apply their problem-solving skills.

The present study contends that teaching and learning are two sides of the same coin, as learning involves the interaction between learners and teaching content, including teaching activities and media, and this interaction determines what the students learn or experience. Therefore, adopting appropriate teaching methods is crucial.

In summary, in today's educational environment, medical education professionals must develop an appropriate teaching method to facilitate the development of student gender competency. If CBME is an education approach involving ability-integration learning and if game-based teaching is a powerful method for active learning, then the integration of these methods to teach CBME gender courses could yield novel insights based on the disclosure and review of practical knowledge at the teaching site.

Using the CBME perspective and gender courses in psychiatric clinical education, this study explores whether the application of game-based teaching activities promotes gender learning and improves the gender competency of students. Moreover, on this basis, suggestions are offered regarding competency-based teaching methods. The results of this study could enable teachers to understand which teaching methods and strategies nurture the gender competency of medical students and may help teachers to develop professional skills and competency-based teaching through which to further promote LBGT-friendly healthcare environments.

## 2. Materials and Methods

This study adopted a qualitative case-study methodology, with Kaohsiung Medical University (KMU) as the research setting. KMU is a long-established medical university with affiliated medical centers and institutions. Taiwan has three gender institutes across the country, one of which is KMU. KMU has also committed itself to promoting gender mainstreaming in higher education, including reforms in gender and medical education. The characteristics of case studies are that the cases themselves are empirically or theoretically representative. By analyzing situations, events, or exceptions of general significance, a case study can grasp and present insights at the grand or macro level [27]. Favorable case studies have universal and general requirements and have the effect of echoing and improving theory or practice.

### 2.1. Teaching Design and Implementation

Taiwan's clinical education is a part of undergraduate medical education and is taught in the fifth or sixth year of college. Medical students in the fifth or sixth year are both students and interns. KMU arranges for a fifth-year or sixth-year medical student to go to psychiatry for one month of clinical education and practice in psychiatry.

Psychiatric clinical education training includes six courses on clinical topics in psychiatry. The six course topics and content include: (1) Communication skills, including mental examination, suicide, and violence assessment; (2) psychopharmacology; (3) cognitive dysfunction, including dementia, delirium, and Mini-Mental State Examination testing; (4) anxiety disorder; (5) substance abuse; and (6) depression. These six courses are taught by different teachers, each for one hour at a time. With the consent of the administrative department of clinical education in psychiatry, the research course, LGBT+ Health and Medical Care (LGBT+ HMC), was added to the psychiatric clinical education training for one academic year. During this year, students entering psychiatric clinical education training were required to take seven courses. Of these seven courses, LGBT+ HMC was the only two-hour course.

This study adopted the CBME perspective and MEGCIs [13] to design the LGBT+ HMC, with an aim of cultivating and enhancing gender competency in medical students through game-based teaching. The teaching objectives of LGBT+ HMC were as follows: (1) To understand how social structures, culture, and other relevant influences affect the lives of LGBT+ individuals, and (2) to perceive the influences of sexual orientation, gender expression, and sexual discrimination on the physical and mental health of LGBT+ patients.

LGBT+ HMC content included basic concepts of gender, such as sexual orientation, LGBT+ issues, sexual and gender identity, the history and social medical background of homosexuality being removed from DSM-5, and related psychopathological theories. The LGBT+ HMC also included content based on the aforementioned teaching goals, such as discussions around how stigma affects LGBT+ mental health, medical assistance to promote LGBT+ health, and more. After the course content was planned, effective design and transformation was still required to promote student learning effectiveness. Therefore, the typical teaching procedure of the course was as follows: Warm up, concept explanation (e.g., what is LGBT+), storytelling (LGBT+ individuals were invited to share their life and healthcare experiences), teaching activities, and course conclusion. This course was conducted by two teachers in rotation, and both teachers were also psychiatrists and attending doctors.

According to the competency-based course and teaching design ideas, a 3 × 3-grid game was designed as the warm-up game for LGBT+ HMC. Apart from stimulating learning motivation, this game served as an evaluative tool, functioning as a pretest and a formative evaluation. The aim of this game was to prompt learning motivation. It was designed to assess students' prior LGBT+ knowledge, which provided feedback that served to inform the adjustment of the course and the improvement of learning conditions.

The 3 × 3-grid game contained nine questions. Based on the concepts in CBME, these questions were designed to elicit responses regarding students' understanding of LGBT+ healthcare and mental health issues and could be answered from the perspectives of knowledge, attitudes, and skills. This game was played in teams. The teacher first divided students into two teams that would compete against each other. After the starting order was decided (using the game "rock–paper–scissors"), one member from each team took a turn selecting and answering questions. After an item number was selected, the teacher revealed the question by clicking on the number. The student was required to answer the question within a limited amount of time. The team that gave the correct answer could continue selecting questions, and the team that connected a line of correct answers won. In some instances, the game was adapted into an individual competition with the same rules and procedures. In addition, teachers could ask students to elaborate on certain answers or to answer other relevant questions, introducing real LGBT+ healthcare scenarios and prompting students to consider whether different responsive measures were required for different scenarios and cases. The teacher could also consider the answers from the students to discern their knowledge, attitudes, and skills regarding LGBT+ medical and healthcare.

*2.2. Participants, Data Collection, and Data Analysis*

A total of 230 students entered psychiatric clinical education training and were taught in stages during one academic year. The number of students per stage was 8–12. The LGBT+ HMC was conducted from September 2017 to May 2018, and two teachers were responsible for teaching the course.

Because of concerns regarding research ethics, such as the disclosure of students' grades, the participants were invited to be interviewed only after the end of the academic year. Invitations to participate in this study were issued only after May 2018. However, some students received invitations to interview almost one year after the end of the course, at which time some had left the school, were undertaking internships at other hospitals, or were preparing for exams and unable to participate in this study. Finally, 19 medical students and two teachers participated in this study (Table 1). In addition to being medical teachers and psychiatrists, the two instructors were also lecturers on gender education courses, often giving speeches on LGBT+ related topics and medical education.

**Table 1.** The basic sociodemographic data of the participants.

| Participants | Sex | | Years of Study | | Age Range | In Total |
|---|---|---|---|---|---|---|
| | Male | Female | Fifth year | Sixth year | 23–30 | |
| Students | 11 | 8 | 11 | 8 | 19 | 19 |
| Teachers | 2 | 0 | | | | 2 |

Through semi-structured, in-depth interviews, this study interviewed 19 medical students and two teachers from LGBT+ HMC to obtain feedback and reflections regarding learning and teaching for this topic. Teachers and students were interviewed individually. For each interviewee, one or two interviews were conducted; each interview lasted between 1 and 2 hours. The interviewers used voice recordings and took notes during the interview process, allowing participants to talk freely. The interview data were transcribed by research assistants and translated verbatim.

The researcher participated in each course and took down field notes. The field notes were used to check the interviewees' feedback on teaching and learning for the course. Field notes were also used as a reference for data analysis. In addition, although few students participated in this study, saturation of information was achieved from qualitative interviews when similar content was repeatedly collected and new information was no longer obtained from respondents.

Data analysis used the perspectives of CBME, gender competency, and game-teaching methods. Thematic analysis was used to analyze the data and themes were identified from the interview data.

*2.3. Ethical Considerations*

To enable students to comment freely on the course, the researcher invited students to participate in interviews only after the course completely ended. Therefore, some students received interview invitations almost one year after the end of the course, some received invitations six months later, and some received invitations one month later. However, at the time when they participated in this research interview, students had completed clinical education and internships at KMU. In addition, all student interviews were conducted by research assistants. The students knew that the researcher was a KMU teacher, that the course was designed by the researcher, and that the researcher participated in each class. Considering these factors, as well as the possibility that students' responses or opinions were influenced by the need to give socially desirable answers, student participants were interviewed by research assistants. The first interview between the two teachers was also conducted by research assistants. Based on the results of the first interview, the researcher conducted a second interview with the teachers to complete the data collection.

With respect to the disclosure of informed consent, the researchers informed the participants of the place and manner in which the interview would be conducted, that the interview would be recorded and a transcript produced, and that the participants could withdraw from the research at any time. To ensure the research ethics and anonymity, all of the cited interview data were presented as codes. In addition, some quotes were moderately edited, without alteration of the original meaning, for readability.

**3. Results**

*3.1. Games Gave Students a Sense of Participation and Benefited Knowledge Transmission and Transformation*

This study determined that the 3 × 3-grid game successfully provoked learning motivation by arousing curiosity and drawing attention to LGBT+ healthcare issues.

Playing the 3 × 3-grid game at the beginning of the course drew our attention. We could roughly understand what this course was about. (Student C)

With the 3 × 3-grid game, we were more concentrated in class because the game had our attention at the beginning. Normally in a block course we are always playing with our phones.

So yes, I think that game was quite important ... Because the way this game proceeded was with competition. We like competitive games; these games draw our attention. (Student A)

The slides following the game explain the questions in the 3 × 3-grid game ... I remember the teacher talked about the process of removing homosexuality from being listed as a mental disease ... Although I know that homosexuality is not a disease, I did not know this revolution process and historical development, etc. When the teacher explained the process, I was like, oh ... oh ... , it was like this! One of the questions mentioned that homosexual and bisexual individuals experience higher [rates of] mental troubles compared with heterosexual individuals. I found this information quite informative ... I think these questions should be considered for people to assess why are they like that. (Student D)

The learning behaviors and learning outcomes of students were easily affected by the teaching method [28]. Students repeatedly mentioned that "playing games caught our attention from the beginning," that games "drew our attention," and that "the 3 × 3-grid game made us concentrate." The research thus determined that game-based teaching effectively reduced students' resistance to learning about LGBT+ subjects.

The students stated that, in courses conveying knowledge in conventional lecture form, they often played with their phones. Moreover, the competitiveness and participation involved in games attracted students to participate in learning and motivate them to acquire previously unknown knowledge. As already described, students who grew up in the digital era only react to learning methods that are delivered in real time, are interactive, and are fun [8]; game-based learning satisfies these criteria. These students desire guidance, entertainment, and inspiration. The 3 × 3-grid game, which enabled students to participate, interact, challenge, and take risks, represents such a teaching and learning context.

In addition, using this game as a teaching activity aimed to achieve two objectives: To trigger the learning motivation of students and encourage them to proceed to concept learning, and to prevent lecturing on LGBT+ concepts from becoming an instance of the "banking education" [29]. Student responses also revealed that game-based teaching helped teachers convey and integrate knowledge or concepts into a game; students connected with the course content and experienced knowledge transformation to achieve positive learning outcomes [30]. Game-based teaching not only helped the transmission of knowledge but also provoked thinking and exploration for students. Students were able to learn about LGBT+ related topics in a game that expanded their existing cognition, attitudes, and skills.

With respect to LGBT+ medical and healthcare issues, within the context of a game, students were able to express and discuss their correct, incorrect, or even biased understandings regarding LGBT+ communities without being overly concerned with providing politically correct answers. These interactions and dialogues led to meaningful learning. Moreover, students expressed their desire to conduct further dialogue and learning.

There was one question where the teacher just gave out the answer. I think the teacher should let us discuss it before telling us the answer or the teacher's point of view; we can listen to why some people think it is bad. However, doing so may have one disadvantage, which is the lack of time; also the discussion might lead to some intense arguments, hehe, just like that ... I think the time reserved for the 3 × 3-grid game was too short. I wish the discussion time could be longer ... The teacher should not talk all the time and appear to be superior ... I wish for more discussion time because I would like to hear from people holding different opinions; I would like to know why they insist on their own point of view regarding LGBT+ communities. (Student X)

Weinert [12] indicated that competency was only formed through learning processes rather than through direct inculcation. This study revealed that not only LGBT+ concepts, but also attitudes such as respect for the healthcare rights of LGBT+ individuals, awareness of sexism, and respect for gender equality, must be taught through enlightenment. Moreover, the mere transmission of knowledge without encouraging the learning process provoked no transformation in attitudes, because such teaching methods constituted mere preaching or inculcation of students with unquestioned ideologies.

This study revealed that competency requires a learning process. Teaching and learning were situated in an intensely and dynamically uncertain interactive scenario, and teachers were required to respond to dynamic tensions and challenges according to students' performance. This topic is discussed in the following section.

*3.2. Games Embodied the Idea of Assessment as Learning; the Pleasant Frustration from the Game Motivated Students to Learn*

The most critical step in a competency-based curriculum project is the identification of students' abilities [9]. Therefore, the 3 × 3-grid game constituted a teaching activity as well as a learning task. The concepts of assessment as learning (AaL) were employed, and the assessment was designed to be part of the game. The purpose of AaL is to help teachers obtain feedback on their teaching on the basis of adjusting their teaching methods to help students learn [31]. Therefore, AaL emphasizes the integration of assessment into the process of teaching and learning and transforms the assessment into part of the teaching activity and learning process.

In fact, students were clearly aware of the assessment purpose of the 3 × 3 grid game after taking this course.

> Actually, the 3 × 3-grid game is kind of like a pretest to test everyone's understanding of this issue. (Student A)

> I prefer the 3 × 3-grid game ... because it is unlike other classes. Most of the other classes only involve the teacher explaining slides to us and this kind of interaction is rare ... Lectures are for us to absorb information, or rather, teachers throw us information without us having to think about it. The game involves more interactions and gives us a chance to weigh our knowing with LBGT medical care. (Student W)

Assessments can be performed in numerous forms, including exams, pencil and paper tests, or presentations. Block curricula, which medical departments often employ, usually adopt exams as the formative or conclusive evaluation. The response from students indicated that the integration of competitive games into the interactive process of teaching and learning and games as an assessment tool was popular. Games provided an indication of learning objectives to students. As stated by one student: "We could roughly understand what this course was about." This statement revealed that AaL is a two-way street: Teachers could determine the abilities of students, and students could also evaluate their own understanding of course topics.

The game served as a warm-up activity to stimulate learning motivation and to enhance students' concentration. It also enabled teachers to obtain instant feedback. The assessment was therefore helpful for both teaching and learning, engendering positive interactions and a reflection circle. The game serving as AaL was helpful for the teacher to determine students' abilities, prior knowledge, and relevant understandings regarding LGBT+ healthcare.

For example, when the researcher and the teachers were designing the questions for the 3 × 3-grid game, the answers to some of the questions were considered basic knowledge that students must know and be capable of understanding. Surprisingly, none of these students, who had already commenced their internships in a hospital, could state the year in which homosexuality was removed from the classification of mental diseases. Numerous students did not know what "transgender" meant, and a few students were unfamiliar with the meaning of LGBT+.

> I think the 3 × 3-grid game was quite fun, compared with lectures. On one hand, the game made us think and was interactive ... Because in the medical department, regular classes are carried out by the teacher lecturing without knowing whether the students are listening.

However, I think starting a course with this game was very intriguing. For example, one of the questions asked in which year homosexuality was removed from the classification of mental diseases and we really did not know that ... Then, you become curious about what the other questions are ... I feel like it drew my attention. I think it was quite interesting. (Student D)

As previously stated, successful game-based learning is adequately challenging and pleasantly frustrating [26]. In games, students are frustrated by not being able to answer a question. Experiencing challenges is also positively stimulating in a game and provokes motivation to learn among students; for example, one student stated that "You become curious about what the other questions are, and that draws my attention." The students were more focused and invested in the following section of the course, which explained the concepts of LGBT+ health issues and psychiatry. The game achieved the exploratory function of game-based learning and provoked active thinking in students.

Learning outcomes refer to quality experiences/knowledge/practices that students accumulate through meaningful learning in a situation; they emphasize the true abilities of students rather than scores or grades [32]. This study revealed that the 3 × 3-grid game, which served as the teaching activity and assessment tool, also supported learning and teaching. The game helped with learning by identifying difficulties and misconceptions experienced by students, which enabled the timely provision of instructional scaffolding to enhance efficacy. For example, the course was designed to conduct concept teaching after the game, and the concepts included the history of the removal of homosexuality from the classification of mental diseases (including the modification of DSM-5) and an introduction to LGBT+ communities. The teachers also invited LGBT+ individuals to the class to share their own medical experiences. These real-life experiences gave the answers to the questions in the game and helped the students with the integration of knowledge, attitudes, and skills.

In addition, the game facilitated teaching because the design of the game allowed for the integration of assessment into teaching, which made the assessment part of the teaching method and teaching activity rather than a supplementary evaluative tool. In fact, both aspects of the game enhanced assessment for teaching and exhibited value in terms of instant feedback obtained in the CBME and game-based learning.

*3.3. Discussion is the Key to Deepen Competency Learning and Improve Teaching and Learning Effectiveness*

I felt like we had more time to think this time, like the 3 × 3-grid game at the beginning gave us some questions to think about. Before, classes were infinite lectures without giving us any time to think about why we think like this or act like this ... Now that we could truly think about LGBT+ issues through discussions, learning will not be just listening to what the teacher has to say and forgetting about it immediately. (Student B)

Conventional learning models require students to learn first instead of undertaking any practical activities and testing their abilities. By contrast, in game-based teaching, learning and skills are acquired actively through games [25,26].

I think the 3 × 3-grid game can be mixed with group discussions. The teacher should hold on to the answer and even withdraw from nodding or showing any emotions. The teacher should simply ask: "Why do you think like this?" So, everyone knows we can express our opinions. Otherwise, if the person answering the question happens to know the answer, the teacher will not be able to listen to opinions or answers from other people. So, the teacher can obtain feedback that there are other ideas. Besides, I like and want to have open discussions. Some questions have no correct answers. Sometimes, even if there is a correct answer, you can still listen to the other opinions or thoughts. In certain moments, these other opinions or thoughts are maybe what we really need to pay attention to. (Student K)

Student feedback revealed that the process of teaching is extremely complex and unpredictable. Any planned teaching activities could be altered at the teacher's discretion, and decisions regarding follow-up teaching plans or actions were influenced by the engagement levels of students during implementation at the education site. Student feedback also revealed that they wanted further discussion of LGBT+ healthcare issues after the game. As such, the teachers were asked how they thought this desire for discussion was inspired by the game.

> Time management is essential. Whenever I had to sacrifice something in class, it was usually the discussion part. (Teacher A)

> Arranging such interactive activities are great, but I think it is not easy. It is not easy because course design, choosing teaching materials, and designing an activity take a lot of time. The preparation alone demands the investment of a huge amount of time. Then, the process of teaching also consumes time and energy. Giving a lecture or simply talking is easy. However, activities involve a lot of uncertainty at the site, such as lack of response from students or a great variety of responses. The teacher must be able to handle the responses and respond to them cleverly. Whenever I failed to handle a response or give a proper response, I would feel so frustrated afterwards. Therefore, having an activity is more energy-consuming than simply giving a lecture. (Teacher B)

According to Rovegno [33], determining the teaching knowledge of teachers requires an understanding of events in the classroom. Because CBME focuses on the learner and the process of learning, teaching activities must be modified accordingly [6]. The feedback from the teachers and students revealed that a well-designed teaching activity, such as the 3 × 3-grid game, could indeed inspire students to think and provoke student participation and teacher–student interactions, potentially prompting interrelated questions and more discussions. The student feedback revealed that the discussions offered room for reflection in competency-based learning and improved the effectiveness of game-based learning. However, teachers may not always be available to conduct discussion promptly in the classroom.

Reasons for unavailability to conduct discussions included a lack of confidence by teachers with respect to conducting discussions or the anxiety of being unable to handle situations following discussions. The 3 × 3-grid game was a teaching activity and a teaching method. Whether to conduct discussions or increase discussion time depends on the scope and depth of a teacher's teaching knowledge, such as being familiar with numerous methods by which to conduct a discussion or being able to lead and respond during discussions.

CBME emphasizes the integral learning of knowledge, attitudes, and skills. The present study revealed that, for gender competency learning, although these three aspects can be separated, they coexist and interact. This was explained in student feedback: "Sometimes, even if there is an answer, you can still listen to other opinions. At certain moments, these other opinions may be what we really need to pay attention to." This statement revealed that discussions not only clarify education on aspects of LGBT+ healthcare, but also change attitudes toward LGBT+ communication and LGBT+ friendly healthcare provision.

Discussions are a teaching method involving cognition, attitudes, and skills. Moreover, leading discussions is a learning process that transforms attitudes and changes opinions. One aspect of competency-based teaching is for students to participate in or conduct discussions [34]. Therefore, teachers must focus on discussions in competency-based teaching and use discussion and dialogue as a basis for all education, reflection, and action. Integrating games into gender competency courses and teaching requires follow-up discussions to clarify the gender competency abilities of students during the interactive aspects of the game.

## 4. Discussion

In 2004, Taiwan implemented the Gender Equity Education Act, which clearly established that gender equity education must include sexuality education, gay and lesbian education, and relationship education. Gender equity education began to encounter huge obstacles in 2014 (i.e., 10 years after the Gender Equity Education Act was created and came into force). Numerous religious groups and parents used "traditional family values" as an excuse to oppose gay and lesbian education. They claimed that only two genders exist, men and women, and that gay and lesbian education could transform children into gays or lesbians. In Taiwan, people who disapproved of gays or lesbians severely opposed gay or lesbian allies. In 2018, Taiwan held a referendum. The voting results constituted an overwhelming victory for opponents of gay and lesbian education. In addition, a referendum proposition that gender equity education be enhanced failed to pass, accompanying the requests to revise the Gender Equity Education Act and to prohibit the use of the words "gay and lesbian education". Extremely varied understandings of and attitudes toward the LGBT+ communities exist in Taiwan.

The question is whether students are mature enough to understand LGBT+ issues. Students' feedback cited in the article indicated that they did not fully understand LGBT+ issues. Using students' responses on page 8 as an example, this study found that some medical students did not even understand what the acronym LGBT+ represents or what the term transgender means. The course in question was provided for clinical education in psychiatry. The researcher participated in observing the course for an entire academic year. When questioned regarding which year homosexuality ceased to be considered a disease, almost no students could answer. According to Student D, students who participated in this study indicated that they did not understand the history of how homosexuality ceased to be considered a disease, and they had no knowledge in this area. By interviewing students, it was observed that numerous medical students had prejudices against LGBT+ people or exhibit hostile attitudes toward these communities.

It is for this reason that the purpose of this study was to emphasize the importance of education first. Medical doctors have a high level of social prestige and status in Taiwanese society and are highly influential. This study aimed to explore effective courses and teaching designs and methods to integrate gender equity education into medical education, thereby cultivating students' gender competency and achieving the ultimate purpose of LGBT+ friendly medical care.

Undoubtedly, games motivate students to learn. A well-designed game, especially one that corresponds to the learning characteristics of complements students' learning styles such as competitiveness, achieves the learning objective regarding the integration of multiple abilities in CBME. The 3 × 3-grid game used competitions and contests to guide students' thinking, exploration, and development of relevant concepts and enhanced students' participation and active learning. In addition, the game inspired students' desire to learn and opened up opportunities and spaces for discussion between teachers and students.

Nevertheless, using games as a teaching method and a teaching activity requires relevant knowledge of teaching design. A factor that limits opportunities for discussion is a lack of time. In fact, this problem is related to course planning and decision-making in classes, and these aspects are part of teaching design. Each teaching activity is designed to help students achieve certain learning objectives and learning outcomes. However, these objectives and students' accomplishments do not always align in reality, which is a challenge of competency-based teaching. The 3 × 3-grid game featured the AaL attribute. Therefore, in addition to providing positive feedback and encouragement to students regarding their responses in class, teachers were required to pay attention to ideas, misconceptions, or values that the students presented and provide further guidance in terms of thinking and conducting discussions.

In game-based teaching, teachers play a crucial role. Teaching has been conceptualized as a design science [35], where teachers are designers of learning [25]. Gee emphasized that games are a useful tool, but the way in which positive learning outcomes are facilitated using such tools and methods must be determined [22,25]. In fact, all teaching design models generally include the five steps of analysis, design, development, execution, and evaluation. Thinking, exploration, interactions, and discussions all require time for implementation, organization, and reflection. Adequate time to learn and assimilate are indispensable learning moments, even when a game is fast-paced, and must be incorporated into the teaching design, planning, and execution.

Gee indicated that students must experience all types of situations to benefit from learning activities [22]. A well-designed game provides numerous educational experiences. In particular, a successful learning activity requires participation in social groups. Games offer the experience of sharing and interaction with others through discussions, conversations, interactions, and modeling between peers and teachers. With specific experiences, learning brings in-depth understandings and improved problem-solving abilities. A well-designed game-based learning activity provokes reflection as well as the reconsideration and reconstruction of specific values, and benefits the learning of cognition, attitudes, and skills. This was demonstrated, for example, in the above-mentioned quote from a student who expressed a desire for further exploration of the ideas relating to the questions they had already answered.

Overall, a successful game-based teaching approach must be designed by the teacher and integrated into appropriate courses for students to receive meaningful learning outcomes. In this manner, playing a game can be an effective learning approach rather than just a form of entertainment. In particular, teachers must analyze, design, develop, and evaluate students' learning performances and allocate adequate learning time for them to experience all learning moments to optimize the effectiveness of CBME and game-based teaching.

A limitation of this study was that, although 19 student participants allowed for "saturation," the quality of the research results could have been enhanced by using more participating students to achieve "sufficiency". Also, whether the study's voluntary student participants exhibited a degree of selection bias was unable to be evaluated; for example, whether these participating students had friendlier attitudes toward LGBT+ communities or were interested in LGBT+ related subjects. As discussed previously, teaching is a methodology [35]. Effective teaching effectively transfers course content to students through effective teaching methods and the design of teaching activities to achieve predetermined learning results. If a teaching method fails to attract the attention of and motivate students that are interested in a topic, the teaching method and strategy are deemed invalid.

LGBT+ education is a highly controversial education issue in Taiwan. Students who were willing to participate in this study half a year or one year after the end of their courses, while also graduating or preparing for national examinations, were potentially more likely than most people to care about LGBT+ related subjects and LGBT+ healthcare. If game-based teaching promoting LGBT+-friendly healthcare gained the academic interest of these students and motivated them to participate in this study, their opinions are likely meaningful and valuable. This reinforces the spirit and benefit of case studies.

Comparatively, the small number of students participating may have reflected the shortage of students concerned regarding LGBT+ friendly healthcare. This was the purpose of the CBME education reform. In response to criticism that medical education overlooked social responsibility in the past, CBME emphasizes social accountability and effective care for the health needs of the general public [3,4]. The results of this study indicated that game-based teaching and CBME could be used to effectively provide students with teaching regarding gender and LGBT+ competency. Students interested in LGBT+ issues can act as seeds. For young people, the influence of peer education sometimes exceeds that of formal education and curricula. If students' attitudes regarding LGBT+ issues can be understood in the process of data collection, a more complete reference might be available for analysis and interpretation of this study, thereby preventing bias.

Finally, the teacher's feedback indicated that, although game-based teaching is an effective method to engage students in gender and medical competency education courses, investing in such teaching methods poses quite a challenge for teachers. Teachers' professional development must rely on institutional support systems and the resources provided by schools.

## 5. Conclusions

In the current education environment, effective gender competency learning for medical students requires strategic teaching methods that integrate gender into courses and create integral learning of knowledge, attitudes, and skills through interactive teaching activities. The present study revealed that designing gender competency courses by incorporating games enhanced the concentration and interest of students. Moreover, the instant assessment and feedback enabled students to understand their achievements and directions in learning. The challenge and pleasant frustration experienced during the game were stimulating and encouraged learning. At the same time, students were willing to actively think and explore, thereby taking initiative in the learning process and providing a multifaceted learning and reflection process that established cognition, attitudes, and skills. In this competency-based course and teaching approach, the game served as the teaching method, teaching activity, and assessment tool.

Moreover, this study revealed that game-based teaching was helpful to convey and integrate knowledge. One objective of the gender education course was the elimination of bias and discrimination against LGBT+ communities and in LGBT+ healthcare. Game-based teaching activities and learning tasks familiarized students with LGBT+ related knowledge and concepts. Also, these knowledge and concepts could be immediately transformed into attitudes and skills.

However, this study also revealed that applying game-based teaching in a competency-based curriculum challenged the teacher's ability to design courses and steer discussions. In the course of teaching, where the environment changes but the learning content remains, teachers must be flexible enough to handle the essentials of teaching design and improve their knowledge and practical abilities regarding discussion-leading. This ability is a core proficiency for teachers in the practice of CBME. The teacher's ability to lead a discussion is a key factor to deepen and affect the gender competency learning of students. If a teacher cannot truly master the challenges of leading classroom discussions and facilitating the acquisition of practical knowledge and experiences, the teacher's professional knowledge on education remains suspended in the meaningless realm of abstraction.

This study revealed that, for teachers to improve their ability to lead a discussion and design a teaching activity, they must strengthen their pedagogical knowledge of theories and professional proficiency; more critically, they must reflect on, react to, and exploit their teaching practice experiences, thereby modifying their teaching strategies and transforming their teaching knowledge to improve teaching effectiveness and achieve change.

For gender and medical education professionals, social changes refer to the goals of eliminating sexism and ushering in a gender-equal society through relevant courses and classroom teaching. In light of the trends and developments in CBME, the results of this study provide a reference for teachers on the basis of how to learn or improve their abilities to teach gender competency so that the spirit of equality can be encouraged in medical students.

This study addressed the application of games in regard to the development of teaching activities, the design of learning assessments, the reform of teaching methods, the improvement of teacher knowledge, and the enhancement of pedagogical proficiency. The actual improvements in gender competency exhibited by medical students who participated in this research demonstrate the design of gender competency CBME courses with game-based teaching. Moreover, this study provides a reference for medical teachers and professionals seeking a novel means by which to integrate gender competency into clinical education and improve teaching knowledge.

**Funding:** The present study was based on research conducted as part of a project titled "Gender mainstreaming and medical education: Developing gender competence indicators and integrating gender into the psychiatric clerkship teaching program", which was funded by the Ministry of Science and Technology of Taiwan.

**Acknowledgments:** Thanks to Y. Y. Chen for assisting with data collection. Thanks to all participants for sharing their thoughts and insights. Special thanks to the reviewers for all of the comments to enhance the quality of this paper.

**Conflicts of Interest:** The authors declare no conflict of interest.

## References

1. Wang, T.H.; Cheng, L.F. Friendly healthcare for lesbians, gays, bisexual, transgender and other sexual minorities. *Formos. J. Med.* **2012**, *16*, 295–301.

2. Verdonk, P.; Mans, L.J.L.; Lagro-Janssen, T.L.M. How is gender integrated in the curricula of Dutch medical schools? A quick-scan on gender issues as an instrument for change. *Gend. Educ.* **2006**, *18*, 399–412. [CrossRef]

3. Bansal, P.; Supe, A.; Sahoo, S.; Vyas, R. Faculty development for competency based medical education: Global, national and regional perspectives. *Natl. J. Integr. Res. Med.* **2017**, *8*, 89–95.

4. Frank, J.R.; Snell, L.S.; Cate, O.T.; Holmboe, E.S.; Carraccio, C.; Swing, S.R.; Harris, P.; Glasgow, N.J.; Campbell, C.; Dath, D.; et al. Competency-based medical education: Theory to practice. *Med. Teach.* **2010**, *32*, 638–645. [CrossRef] [PubMed]

5. Walsh, A.; Koppula, S.; Antao, V.; Bethune, C.; Cameron, S.; Cavett, T.; Clavet, D.; Dove, M. Preparing teachers for competency-based medical education: Fundamental teaching activities. *Med. Teach.* **2018**, *40*, 80–85. [CrossRef]

6. Shah, N.; Desai, C.; Jorwekar, G.; Badyal, D.; Singh, T. Competency-based medical education: An overview and application in pharmacology. *Indian J. Pharm.* **2016**, *48*, 5–9.

7. Swing, S.R. Perspectives on competency-based medical education from the learning sciences. *Med. Teach.* **2010**, *32*, 663–668. [CrossRef]

8. Yang, H.C. Teaching sexual matters in Taiwan: The analytical framework for popular culture and youth sexuality education. *Asia Pac. J. Educ.* **2014**, *34*, 49–64. [CrossRef]

9. Modi, J.N.; Gupta, P.; Singh, T. Competency-based medical education, entrustment and assessment. *Indian Pediatrics* **2015**, *52*, 413–420. [CrossRef]

10. Mulder, M.; Gulikers, J.; Biemans, H.; Wesselink, R. The new competence concept in higher education: Error or enrichment? *J. Eur. Ind. Train.* **2009**, *33*, 755–770. [CrossRef]

11. Trilling, B.; Fadel, C. *21st Century Skills: Learning for Life in Our Times*; Wiley: San Francisco, CA, USA, 2009.

12. Weinert, F.E. Concept of competence: A conceptual clarification. In *Defining and Selecting Key Competencies*; Rychen, D.S., Salganik, L.H., Eds.; Hogrefe & Huber: Göttingen, Germany, 2001; pp. 93–120.

13. Yang, H.C.; Yen, C.F. Integrating gender into medicine: Research on the construction of gender competence indicators in medical education. *Taiwan J. Soc. Educ.* **2018**, *18*, 91–145.

14. Chapman, R.; Watkins, R.; Zappia, T.; Nicol, P.; Shields, L. Nursing and medical students' attitude, knowledge and beliefs regarding lesbian, gay, bisexual and transgender parents seeking health care for their children. *J. Clin. Nurs.* **2012**, *21*, 938–945. [CrossRef] [PubMed]

15. Sanchez, N.F.; Rabatin, J.; Sanchez, J.P.; Hubbard, S.; Kalet, A. Medical students' ability to care for lesbian, gay, bisexual, and transgendered patients. *Fam. Med.* **2006**, *38*, 21–27. [PubMed]

16. Sawning, S.; Steinbock, S.; Croley, R.; Combs, R.; Shaw, A.; Ganzel, T. A first step in addressing medical education curriculum gaps in lesbian-, gay-, bisexual-, and transgender-related content: The university of louisville lesbian, gay, bisexual, and transgender health certificate program. *Educ. Health* **2017**, *30*, 108–114. [CrossRef]

17. Cooper, M.B.; Chacko, M.; Christner, J. Incorporating LGBT health in an undergraduate medical education curriculum through the construct of social determinants of health. *MedEdPORTAL* **2018**, *14*, 10781. [CrossRef]

18. Salkind, J.; Gishen, F.; Drage, G.; Kavanagh, J.; Potts, H. LGBT+ health teaching within the undergraduate medical curriculum. *Int. J. Environ. Res. Public Health* **2019**, *16*, 2305. [CrossRef]

19. Keuroghlian, A.S.; Ard, K.L.; Makadon, H.L. Advancing health equity for lesbian, gay, bisexual and transgender (LGBT) people through sexual health education and LGBT-affirming health care environments. *Sex. Health* **2017**, *14*, 119–122. [CrossRef]

20. Grosz, A.M.; Gutierrez, D.; Lui, A.A.; Chang, J.J.; Cole-Kelly, K.; Ng, H. A student-led introduction to lesbian, gay, bisexual, and transgender health for first-year medical students. *Fam. Med.* **2017**, *49*, 52–56.

21. Admiraal, W.; Huizenga, J.; Akkerman, S.; Dam, G. The concept of flow in collaborative game-based learning. *Comput. Hum. Behav.* **2011**, *27*, 1185–1194. [CrossRef]

22. Gee, J. Learning and games. In *The Ecology of Games: Connecting Youth, Games, and Learning*; Salen, K., John, D., Catherine, T., Eds.; The MIT Press: Cambridge, MA, USA, 2008; pp. 21–40.

23. Horsley, T.L. Education theory and classroom games: Increasing knowledge and fun in the classroom. *J. Nurs. Educ.* **2010**, *49*, 363–364. [CrossRef]

24. Virvou, M.; Katsionis, G.; Manos, K. Combining software games with education: Evaluation of its educational effectiveness. *Educ. Tech. Soc.* **2005**, *8*, 54–65.

25. Gee, J. *What Video Games Have to Teach Us about Learning and Literacy*; St. Martin's Griffin: New York, NY, USA, 2007.

26. Legends of Learning. James Paul Gee's 16 Principles for Good Game Based Learning. Available online: https://www.legendsoflearning.com/blog/james-paul-gees-16-principles-for-good-game-based-learning/ (accessed on 15 November 2018).

27. Stake, R. Case studies. In *Handbook of Qualitative Research*; Norman, K.D., Yvonna, S.L., Eds.; Sage: Thousand Oaks, CA, USA, 2000; pp. 435–454.

28. Lin, C.T. Active teaching strategies and practice: A perspective of pedagogical content and learning content knowledge. *Curric. Instr. Quart.* **2019**, *22*, 1–16.

29. Freire, P. *Pedagogy of the Oppressed*; Continuum: New York, NY, USA, 1970.

30. Day-Black, C.; Merrill, E.B.; Konzelman, L.; Williams, T.T.; Hart, N. Gamification: An innovative teaching-learning strategy for the digital nursing students in a community health nursing course. *ABNF J.* **2015**, *26*, 90–94. [PubMed]

31. Dann, R. Assessment as learning: Blurring the boundaries of assessment and learning for theory, policy and practice. *Assess. Educ. Princip. Policy Pract.* **2014**, *21*, 149–166.

32. Spady, W. *Outcome-Based Education: Critical Issues and Answers*; American Association of School Administrators: Arlington, VA, USA, 1994.

33. Rovegno, I. Teachers' knowledge construction. In *Student Learning in Physical Education*, 2nd ed.; Silverman, S.J., Ennis, C.D., Eds.; Human Kinetics: Champaign, IL, USA, 2003; pp. 295–310.

34. Wu, P.C.; Chan, J.C. Reflecting on the perspective transformation of competency-based education. *J. Educ. Res. Dev.* **2018**, *14*, 35–64.

35. Laurillard, D. *Teaching as a Design Science*; Routledge: New York, NY, USA, 2012.

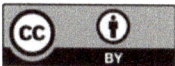

© 2019 by the author. Licensee MDPI, Basel, Switzerland. This article is an open access article distributed under the terms and conditions of the Creative Commons Attribution (CC BY) license (http://creativecommons.org/licenses/by/4.0/).

MDPI

St. Alban-Anlage 66

4052 Basel

Switzerland

Tel. +41 61 683 77 34

Fax +41 61 302 89 18

www.mdpi.com

*International Journal of Environmental Research and Public Health* Editorial Office

E-mail: ijerph@mdpi.com

www.mdpi.com/journal/ijerph

www.ingramcontent.com/pod-product-compliance
Lightning Source LLC
Chambersburg PA
CBHW051840210326

41597CB00033B/5716